A. Lippa

# MOLECULAR PHARMACOLOGY
# OF NEUROTRANSMITTER RECEPTORS

*Advances in Biochemical Psychopharmacology*
*Volume 36*

*Advances in Biochemical Psychopharmacology*

Series Editors

E. Costa, M.D.
*Chief, Laboratory of Preclinical Pharmacology*
*National Institute of Mental Health*
*Washington, D.C.*

Paul Greengard, Ph.D.
*Professor of Pharmacology*
*Yale University School of Medicine*
*New Haven, Connecticut*

# Molecular Pharmacology of Neurotransmitter Receptors

*Advances in Biochemical Psychopharmacology Volume 36*

Volume Editors

Tomio Segawa, Ph.D.
*Professor of Pharmacology
Department of Pharmacology
Institute of Pharmaceutical Sciences
Hiroshima University School
  of Medicine
Hiroshima, Japan*

Henry I. Yamamura, Ph.D.
*Professor of Pharmacology
Departments of Pharmacology,
Biochemistry, Psychiatry, and
The Arizona Research Laboratories
The University of Arizona
Health Sciences Center
Tucson, Arizona*

Kinya Kuriyama, M.D.
*Professor of Pharmacology
Department of Pharmacology
Kyoto Prefectural University
School of Medicine
Kyoto, Japan*

Raven Press ■ New York

Raven Press, 1140 Avenue of the Americas, New York, New York 10036

© 1983 by Raven Press Books, Ltd. All rights reserved. This book is protected by copyright. No part of it may be reproduced, stored in a retrieval system, or transmitted, in any form or by any means, electronic, mechanical, photocopying, recording, or otherwise, without the prior written permission of the publisher.

Made in the United States of America

**Library of Congress Cataloging in Publication Data**
Main entry under title:

Molecular pharmacology of neurotransmitter receptors.

(Advances in biochemical psychopharmacology; v. 36)
Includes bibliographical references and index.
1. Neurotransmitter receptors—Addresses, essays, lectures.  2. Neuropharmacology—Addresses, essays, lectures.  I. Segawa, Tomio, 1927–  . II. Yamamura, Henry I.  III. Kuriyama, Kinya, 1932–  . IV. Series.
[DNLM: 1. Neuroregulators.  2. Synaptic receptors. W1 AD437 v.36 /WL 102.8 M718]
RM315.A4   vol. 36       615'.78s       [615'.78]       83-3084
[QP364.7]
ISBN 0-89004-736-7

Great care has been taken to maintain the accuracy of the information contained in the volume. However, Raven Press cannot be held responsible for errors or for any consequences arising from the use of the information contained herein.

Materials appearing in this book prepared by individuals as part of their official duties as U.S. Government employees are not covered by the above-mentioned copyright.

# Preface

The concept of drug receptors was postulated in the early twentieth century. In the last decade, by use of the radio-ligand binding assays, great advances have been made in the understanding of neurotransmitter and drug receptors. Initial radio-ligand binding studies provided their identification and characterization; recent studies show an increasing receptor heterogeneity and complexity of receptor mechanisms.

For example, it has been shown that guanine nucleotides, ions, and sulfhydryl reagents modulate ligand binding to the receptor. These modulation studies have yielded new insights into receptor heterogeneity. In some tissues, guanine nucleotides and sodium ions selectively reduce the binding of some agonists to their specific receptors. The binding is characterized by the conversion of a heterogeneous population of antagonist binding sites into a predominantly lower affinity homogeneous population of receptors. On the other hand, sulfhydryl reagents and magnesium ions can have the effect of increasing the binding of some agonists.

An unexpected result of new radio-ligand binding sites is the apparent heterogeneity of agonist binding sites. In this case, guanine nucleotides appear to cause an increase in antagonist binding by an apparent conversion of low- to high-affinity antagonist site.

A very recent area of intense receptor research has to do with receptor interactions. In the heart, for example, the β-adrenergic and muscarinic cholinergic receptors apparently interact through a guanine nucleotide protein that regulates adenylate cyclase activity.

It was our intent that this book clarify some of these recently discovered receptor complexities. It provides a detailed and comprehensive study of the molecular pharmacology of the receptors for a range of neurotransmitters. Subject sections include acetylcholinesterase and acetylcholine receptors, subtypes and regulation of adrenergic receptors, serotonin release and receptor mechanisms, heterogeneity and regulation of dopamine receptors, benzodiazepine receptors, and amino acid receptors and their involvement in disease, and the localization and functional aspects of receptor binding.

This volume will be of interest to neuroscientists, pharmacologists, and other researchers working in the broad-based field of receptor research.

*Tomio Segawa, Ph.D.*
*Henry I. Yamamura, Ph.D.*
*Kinya Kuriyama, M.D.*

# Acknowledgments

We acknowledge generous support from the following: American Cyanamid Company, Hoffman-LaRoche Laboratories, Merrell-Dow Research Laboratories, New England Nuclear Corporation, Sandoz, Basle, and Taisho Pharmaceutical Company, Japan.

We are indebted to the many assistants in the laboratory of Dr. Segawa and Dr. Kuriyama for their help.

# Contents

1 Introduction
*J.J.C. Jacob*

## Acetylcholinesterase and Acetylcholine Receptors

7 Recent Advances in Identification and Isolation of Acetylcholinesterase and a Cholinergic Receptor Protein
*P.G. Waser, W.H. Hopff, M.C. Schaub, and A. Hofmann*

15 Recent Advances in Muscarinic Receptor Heterogeneity and Regulation
*William R. Roeske, Frederick J. Ehlert, Diana S. Barritt, Kyozo Yamanaka, Lois B. Rosenberger, Shizuo Yamada, Susan Yamamura, and Henry I. Yamamura*

31 Muscarinic Acetylcholine Receptors in Smooth Muscles: Regulation of Contraction and Molecular Nature
*Shuji Uchida, Kunio Takeyasu, Hiroshi Higuchi, Kazuo Matsumoto, and Hiroshi Yoshida*

43 Presynaptic Muscarinic Cholinergic and Postsynaptic β-Adrenergic Receptors in Splenic Tissue
*Shizuo Yamada, Eiichi Hayashi, Henry I. Yamamura, and William R. Roeske*

## Adrenergic Receptors: Subtypes and Regulation

53 $\alpha_2$-Adrenergic Receptor: Multiple Affinity States and Regulation of a Receptor Inversely Coupled to Adenylate Cyclase
*David C. U'Prichard, Joan C. Mitrius, Deborah J. Kahn, and Bruce D. Perry*

73 β-Adrenergic Receptor Subtypes in Rat Brain
*Kenneth P. Minneman, Barry B. Wolfe, Randall N. Pittman, and Perry B. Molinoff*

83 Possible Influence of Noradrenaline on β-Adrenergic and Muscarinic Cholinergic Receptors in Rat Heart: Effects of 6-Hydroxydopa, Isoproterenol, and Desmethylimipramine
*Yasuyuki Nomura, Hiroko Kajiyama, and Tomio Segawa*

## CONTENTS

### Serotonin Release and Receptor Mechanisms

91 Modulation of *In Vivo* Nigral 5HT Release in the Cat
   *T.D. Reisine, P. Soubrie, S. Bourgoin, F. Artaud, and J. Glowinski*

103 $^3$H-Serotonin Binding Sites: Pharmacological and Species Differences
   *David L. Nelson, Rick Schnellmann, and Mark Smit*

115 Central Serotonin Receptors: Regulation Mechanism at the Molecular Level
   *Gilles Fillion*

### Dopamine Receptors: Heterogeneity and Regulation

125 Dopamine Receptors in the Central Nervous System
   *Ian Creese, David R. Sibley, Mark W. Hamblin, and Stuart E. Leff*

135 Identification and Localization of the Recognition Binding Subunit of the $D_1$ Dopamine Receptor
   *C. Tanaka, T. Kuno, T. Mita, and T. Ishibe*

147 Demonstration of a Complex Subunit Composition of a Unitary Dopamine Receptor: Effects of Lesions and Proteolytic Enzymes on Stereospecific Binding
   *J.E. Leysen, W. Gommeren, and P. Van Gompel*

163 Two Distinct Classes of Dopamine Receptor Mediating Actions of Antipsychotics: Binding and Behavioral Studies
   *P. Sokoloff, M.P. Martres, P. Protais, J. Costentin, and J.C. Schwartz*

175 Dopamine Receptor System Involving Adenylate Cyclase in Canine Caudate Nucleus
   *Hiroo Maeno, Kenji Sano, Koji Nishikori, Osamu Noshiro, Akiro Sato, Takashi Yoneda, Shinjii Usuda, and Sumio Iwanami*

185 Modification of Dopaminergic Transmission by Thyrotropin-Releasing Hormone
   *Shigehiko Narumi and Yuji Nagawa*

199 Inhibition of VIP-Sensitive Adenylate Cyclase by Dopamine in Rat Anterior Pituitary
   *Pierluigi Onali, Joan P. Schwartz, and E. Costa*

## Benzodiazepine Receptors: Heterogeneity and Regulation

209 The Benzodiazepine Receptor: Complex Binding Properties and the Influence of GABA
*Frederick J. Ehlert, William R. Roeske, Susan H. Yamamura, and Henry I. Yamamura*

221 Endogenous Modulating Mechanism of Cerebral Benzodiazepine Receptor: Roles of Membrane Phospholipids
*Eiko Ueno and Kinya Kuriyama*

## Amino Acid Receptors

233 Glycine Receptors in the Human Brain: Characterization of ³H-Strychnine Binding and Status in Pathological Conditions
*K.G. Lloyd, G. De Montis, F. Javoy-Agid, K. Beaumont, A. Lowenthal, J. Constantinidis, and Y. Agid*

239 Specific Binding of Cysteine Sulfinic Acid to Synaptic Membrane Fractions
*Heitaroh Iwata and Akemichi Baba*

## Localization and Functional Aspects of Receptor Binding

245 Morphological Studies of Neurotransmitter Receptors in Rat Brain
*Shozo Kito, Eiko Itoga, Takenobu Kishida, and Masanori Togo*

259 Involvement of Sulfyhydryl Groups in the Functional Integrity of Opiate Receptors of Neuroblastoma × Glioma Hybrid NG108-15.
*Arthur J. Blume, D. Mullikin-Kilpatrick, and N.E. Larsen*

269 Structural Modifications of the Ergopeptine Molecule and Their Differential Influence on the Affinities to Different Receptor Binding Sites—A Structure Affinity Analysis
*A. Closse, G. Bolliger, A. Dravid, W. Frick, D. Hauser, P. Pfäffli, A. Sauter, and H.J. Tobler*

281 Labeling of a GTP-Binding Regulatory Protein of Rat Brain Adenylate Cyclase System by Cholera Toxin-Catalyzed ADP-Ribosylation
*Keiichi Enomoto and Takeo Asakawa*

295 Subject Index

# Contributors

**Y. Agid**
Hôpital Pitié-Salpétrière
75013 Paris, France

**F. Artaud**
INSERM U. 114, Group NB
College de France
75231 Paris Cedex 5, France

**Takeo Asakawa**
Department of Pharmacology
Saga Medical School
Saga 840-01, Japan

**Akemichi Baba**
Department of Pharmacology
Faculty of Pharmaceutical Sciences
Osaka University
Osaka 565, Japan

**Diana Barritt**
Departments of Pharmacology, Internal
 Medicine, and Psychiatry
The University of Arizona Health
 Sciences Center
Tucson, Arizona 85724

**K. Beaumont**
Department of Pharmacology
University of North Carolina
Raleigh, North Carolina 27607

**Arthur J. Blume**
Department of Physiological Chemistry
 and Pharmacology
Roche Institute of Molecular Biology
Nutley, New Jersey 07110

**G. Bolliger**
Preclinical Research
SANDOZ Ltd.
CH-4002 Basle, Switzerland

**S. Bourgoin**
INSERM U. 114, Groupe NB
College de France
75231 Paris Cedex 5, France

**A. Closse**
Preclinical Research
SANDOZ Ltd.
CH-4002 Basle, Switzerland

**J. Constantinidis**
Clinique Psychiatrique Bel-Air
Geneva, Switzerland

**E. Costa**
Laboratory of Preclinical Pharmacology
National Institute of Mental Health
Saint Elizabeths Hospital
Washington, D.C. 20032

**J. Costentin**
UER de Médecine et de Pharmacie
76800 St. Etienne du Rouvray, France

**Ian Creese**
Department of Neurosciences
University of California, San Diego
School of Medicine
La Jolla, California 92093

**G. De Montis**
2nd Institute of Pharmacology
University of Cagliari
Cagliari, Italy

**A. Dravid**
Preclinical Research
SANDOZ Ltd.
CH-4002 Basle, Switzerland

**Frederick J. Ehlert**
Departments of Pharmacology, Internal
 Medicine, and Psychiatry
The University of Arizona Health
 Sciences Center
Tucson, Arizona 85724

**Keiichi Enomoto**
Department of Pharmacology
Saga Medical School
Saga 840-01, Japan

# CONTRIBUTORS

**Gilles Fillion**
Laboratory of Pharmacology
Pasteur Institute
75724 Paris Cedex 15, France

**W. Frick**
Preclinical Research
SANDOZ Ltd.
CH-4002 Basle, Switzerland

**J. Glowinski**
INSERM U. 114, Groupe NB
College de France
75231 Paris Cedex 5, France

**W. Gommeren**
Department of Biochemical
 Pharmacology
Janssen Pharmaceutica Research
 Laboratories
B-2340 Beerse, Belgium

**Mark W. Hamblin**
Department of Neurosciences
University of California, San Diego
School of Medicine
La Jolla, California 92092

**D. Hauser**
Preclinical Research
SANDOZ Ltd.
CH-4002 Basle, Switzerland

**Eiichi Hayashi**
Department of Pharmacology
Shizuoka College of Pharmaceutical
 Sciences
Shizuoka 422, Japan

**Hiroshi Higuchi**
Department of Pharmacology I
Osaka University School of Medicine
Osaka 530, Japan

**A. Hofmann**
Institute of Pharmacology
University of Zurich
Gloriastrasse 32A
CH-8006 Zurich, Switzerland

**W. H. Hopff**
Institute of Pharmacology
University of Zurich
Gloriastrasse 32A
CH-8006 Zurich, Switzerland

**T. Ishibe**
Department of Pharmacology
Kobe University School of Medicine
Osaka 530, Japan

**Eiko Itoga**
Third Department of Internal Medicine
Hiroshima University School of Medicine
Hiroshima 732, Japan

**Sumio Iwanami**
Department of Pharmacology and
 Biochemistry
Central Research Laboratories
Yamanouchi Pharmaceutical
 Company, Ltd.
Tokyo 174, Japan

**Heitaroh Iwata**
Department of Pharmacology
Faculty of Pharmaceutical Sciences
Osaka University
Osaka 565, Japan

**J. J. C. Jacob**
Laboratory of Pharmacology and
 Toxicology
Pasteur Institute
F75724 Paris Cedex 15, France

**F. Javoy-Agid**
Hôpital Pitié-Salpétrière
75013 Paris, France

**Deborah J. Kahn**
Department of Pharmacology
Northwestern University School of
 Medicine
Chicago, Illinois 60611

**Hiroko Kajiyama**
Department of Pharmacology
Institute of Pharmaceutical Sciences
Hiroshima University School of Medicine
Hiroshima 734, Japan

**Takenobu Kishida**
Third Department of Internal Medicine
Hiroshima University School of Medicine
Hiroshima 734, Japan

**Shozo Kito**
Third Department of Internal Medicine
Hiroshima University School of Medicine
Hiroshima 734, Japan

# CONTRIBUTORS

**T. Kuno**
Department of Pharmacology
Kobe University School of Medicine
Kobe 650, Japan

**Kinya Kuriyama**
Department of Pharmacology
Kyoto Prefectural University of Medicine
Kyoto 602, Japan

**N. E. Larsen**
Hematology Research
Boston, Massachusetts 02118

**Stuart E. Leff**
Department of Neurosciences
University of California, San Diego
School of Medicine
La Jolla, California 92093

**J. E. Leysen**
Department of Biochemical
    Pharmacology
Janssen Pharmaceutica Research
    Laboratories
B-2340 Beerse, Belgium

**K. G. Lloyd**
Neuropharmacology Unit
Synthelabo LERS
Bagneu 92220, France

**A. Lowenthal**
University of Antwerp
Antwerp, Belgium

**Hiroo Maeno**
Department of Pharmacology and
    Biochemistry
Central Research Laboratories
Yamanouchi Pharmaceutical
    Company, Ltd.
Tokyo 174, Japan

**M. P. Martres**
Centre Paul Broca de l' INSERM
Unité 109 de Neurobiologie
75014 Paris, France

**Kazuo Matsumoto**
Department of Pharmacology I
Osaka University School of Medicine
Osaka 530, Japan

**Kenneth P. Minneman**
Department of Pharmacology
Emory University Medical School
Atlanta, Georgia 30322

**T. Mita**
Department of Pharmacology
Kobe University School of Medicine
Kobe 650, Japan

**Joan C. Mitrius**
Department of Pharmacology
Northwestern University School of
    Medicine
Chicago, Illinois 60611

**Perry B. Molinoff**
Department of Pharmacology
University of Pennsylvania School of
    Medicine
Philadelphia, Pennsylvania 19104

**D. Mullikin-Kilpatrick**
Department of Physiological Chemistry
    and Pharmacology
Roche Institute of Molecular Biology
Nutley, New Jersey 07110

**Yuji Nagawa**
Central Research Division
Takeda Chemical Industries, Ltd.
Osada 532, Japan

**Shigehiko Narumi**
Central Research Division
Takeda Chemical Industries, Ltd.
Osada 532, Japan

**David L. Nelsen**
Department of Pharmacology and
    Toxicology
College of Pharmacy
University of Arizona
Tucson, Arizona 85721

**Koji Nishikori**
Department of Pharmacology and
    Biochemistry
Central Research Laboratories
Yamanouchi Pharmaceutical
    Company, Ltd.
Tokyo 174, Japan

**Yasuyuki Nomura**
Department of Pharmacology
Institute of Pharmaceutical Sciences
Hiroshima University School of Medicine
Hiroshima 734, Japan

**Osamu Noshiro**
Department of Pharmacology and
 Biochemistry
Central Research Laboratories
Yamanouchi Pharmaceutical
 Company, Ltd.
Tokyo 174, Japan

**Pierluigi Onali**
Laboratory of Preclinical Pharmacology
National Institute of Mental Health
Saint Elizabeths Hospital
Washington, D.C. 20032

**Bruce D. Perry**
Department of Pharmacology
Northwestern University School of
 Medicine
Chicago, Illinois 60611

**P. Pfäffli**
Preclinical Research
SANDOZ Ltd.
CH-4002 Basle, Switzerland

**Randall N. Pittman**
Department of Pharmacology
University of Colorado Medical Center
Denver, Colorado 80262

**P. Protais**
UER de Médecine et de Pharmacie
76800 St. Etienne du Rouvray, France

**T. D. Reisine**
INSERM U. 114, Groupe NB
College de France
75231 Paris Cedex 5, France

**William R. Roeske**
Departments of Internal Medicine and
 Pharmacology
The University of Arizona Health
 Sciences Center
Tucson, Arizona 85724

**Lois B. Rosenberger**
Mead Johnson Corporation
Evansville, Indiana 47721

**Kenji Sano**
Department of Pharmacology and
 Biochemistry
Central Research Laboratories
Yamanouchi Pharmaceutical
 Company, Ltd.
Tokyo 174, Japan

**Akiko Sato**
Department of Pharmacology and
 Biochemistry
Central Research Laboratories
Yamanouchi Pharmaceutical
 Company, Ltd.
Tokyo 174, Japan

**A. Sauter**
Preclinical Research
SANDOZ Ltd.
CH-4002 Basle, Switzerland

**M. C. Schaub**
Institute of Pharmacology
University of Zurich
Gloriastrasse 32A
CH-8006 Zurich, Switzerland

**Rick Schnellmann**
Department of Pharmacology and
 Toxicology
College of Pharmacy and Department of
 Pharmacology
College of Medicine
University of Arizona
Tucson, Arizona 85721

**J. C. Schwartz**
Centre Paul Broca de l'INSERM
Unité 109 de Neurobiologie
75014 Paris, France

**Joan P. Schwartz**
Laboratory of Preclinical Pharmacology
National Institute of Mental Health
Saint Elizabeths Hospital
Washington, D.C. 20032

**Tomio Segawa**
Department of Pharmacology
Institute of Pharmaceutical Sciences
Hiroshima University School of Medicine
Hiroshima 734, Japan

# CONTRIBUTORS

**David R. Sibley**
Department of Neurosciences
University of California, San Diego
School of Medicine
La Jolla, California 92093

**Mark Smit**
Department of Pharmacology and
 Toxicology
College of Pharmacy and Department of
 Pharmacology
College of Medicine
University of Arizona
Tucson, Arizona 85721

**P. Sokoloff**
Centre Paul Broca de l'INSERM
Unité 109 de Neurobiologie
75014 Paris, France

**P. Soubrie**
INSERM U. 114, Groupe NB
Collège de France
75231 Paris Cedex 5, France

**Kunia Takeyasu**
Department of Pharmacology I
Osaka University School of Medicine
Osaka 530, Japan

**C. Tanaka**
Department of Pharmacology
Kobe University School of Medicine
Kobe 650, Japan

**H. J. Tobler**
Preclinical Research
SANDOZ Ltd.
CH-4002 Basle, Switzerland

**Masanori Togo**
Third Department of Internal Medicine
Hiroshima University School of Medicine
Hiroshima 734, Japan

**Shuji Uchida**
Department of Pharmacology I
Osaka University School of Medicine
Osaka 530, Japan

**Eiko Ueno**
Department of Pharmacology
Kyoto Prefectural University of Medicine
Kyoto 602, Japan

**David C. U'Prichard**
Department of Pharmacology
Northwestern University
Chicago, Illinois 60611

**Shinji Usuda**
Department of Pharmacology and
 Biochemistry
Central Research Laboratories
Yamanouchi Pharmaceutical
 Company, Ltd.
Tokyo 174, Japan

**P. Van Gompel**
Department of Biochemical
 Pharmacology
Janssen Pharmaceutica Research
 Laboratories
B-2340 Beerse, Belgium

**P. G. Waser**
Institute of Pharmacology
University of Zurich
Gloriastrasse 32A
CH-8006 Zurich, Switzerland

**Barry B. Wolfe**
Department of Pharmacology
University of Pennsylvania
School of Medicine
Philadelphia, Pennsylvania 19104

**Shizuo Yamada**
Department of Pharmacology
Shizuoka College of Pharmaceutical
 Sciences
Shizuoka 422, Japan

**Henry I. Yamamura**
Departments of Pharmacology,
 Biochemistry, Psychiatry, and the
 Arizona Research Laboratories
The University of Arizona Health
 Sciences Center
Tucson, Arizona 85724

**Susan H. Yamamura**
Departments of Pharmacology, Internal Medicine, and Psychiatry
The University of Arizona Health Sciences Center
Tucson, Arizona 85724

**Kyozo Yamanaka**
Department of Pharmacology
Fukui Medical School
Matsuoka, Japan

**Takashi Yoneda**
Department of Pharmacology and Biochemistry
Central Research Laboratories
Yamanouchi Pharmaceutical Company, Ltd.
Tokyo 174, Japan

**Hiroshi Yoshida**
Department of Pharmacology I
Osaka University School of Medicine
Osaka 530, Japan

*Molecular Pharmacology of Neurotransmitter Receptors*, edited by T. Segawa et al.
Raven Press, New York © 1983.

# Introduction

## J. J. C. Jacob

*Laboratory of Pharmacology and Toxicology, Pasteur Institute, F75724 Paris Cedex 15, France*

The existence of specific receptors was postulated as early as 1905 by Langley (14) and 1906 by Ehrlich (7), and an equation describing the rate of formation of a drug–receptor complex in terms of the law of mass action was formulated in 1909 by Hill (11) before Michaelis and Menten published their model of enzyme kinetics. It is remarkable—but not fortuitous—that the publications of Langley and of Hill concerned nicotine and curare, i.e., drugs acting on neurotransmitter receptor systems which are the topic of this volume.

The concept rapidly gained a wide acceptance because it satisfied the opinion that when a chemical is exerting effects with low amounts or concentrations, it does so through a chemical reaction with some discrete endogenous structure. This point was quantified later; in particular, the first approximation was made by Clark (4) who calculated that $5.10^{-6}$ of the heart cell surface was covered with threshold concentrations of acetylcholine. Since then, many examples have been accumulated, including drugs acting in the picomolar range of doses and substances triggering olfaction with very few molecules.

The notion of competitive antagonists, i.e., compounds inhibiting the effects of other ones at the level of receptors, also developed readily, the first instance being the ergot alkaloids as suggested by Sir Henri Dale (6).

The specificity of the receptors was inherent to the concept and was further supported by innumerable studies of structure–action relationships, which described, in general, rather strict requirements, one of the most impressive being stereospecificity. This proceeds from the steric configuration of the amino acids of the receptors; it can be present even when the natural agonist has no optical activity (e.g., acetylcholine, dopamine) and uncovered by the use of other agonists (e.g., acetyl-β-methylcholine) or antagonists (e.g., butaclamol).

The use of various agonists and antagonists acting on various *in vivo* and *in vitro* preparations disclosed classes of receptors and for each class, different subtypes. This important taxonomic work began early with the distinction between muscarinic and nicotinic cholinergic receptors and is still currently effected: Important and classical steps for the different receptors of opiates and opioids, β-agonists, and serotonin have been the distinction between the α- and β-adrenergic, the $H_1$ and $H_2$ histaminergic, and the pre- and postsynaptic receptors. Problems of specificity often remain difficult. The notion of families of receptors was also proposed and might still be useful.

Quantitative treatment of drug–receptor interactions has also been much developed by Clark (5), Gaddum (9), Schild (15), Ariëns (1), and Jacob (13). It has led to distinguishing various classes of antagonists (competitive, noncompetitive, physiological, uncompetitive, etc.) and many subtypes—possibly too many, however, because the experimental errors do not always allow for choosing among different possible subtypes. Further, the biological responses result from several steps and thus cannot truly reflect the sole reactions with the receptors. Gaddum pointed out clearly that most experimental curves were smoothed integrative ones, which could correspond precisely to integrations more than to particular steps. Ariëns had the merit to distinguish between affinity and "intrinsic activity"; this conception as well as that of "spare receptors" were later embodied and their modalities can still guide biochemical work.

All these studies based on the receptor complex have allowed and still allow for important pharmacological, biological, and therapeutical progress. In particular, they are still in use for biological dosages of various substances. They were and are at the basis of the discovery of various biological substances, from acetylcholine to leucotrienes going through, e.g., substance P, prostaglandins and enkephalins, the purification of which was followed by Hughes (12) with the use of an isolated organ and of a specific antagonist.

This concept has lead also to the successful search for the receptor entities themselves. The initial attempts at this discovery were numerous but unsuccessful due to the use of markers that bound essentially to structures other than the specific receptors. Examples are the attempts to isolate the nicotinic receptors with radiocurare by Chagas et al. (2); the pioneer study of Goldstein et al. (10), who described the process for characterizing the opiates' receptors, but did not have a suitable ligand at their disposal; and the failure of many scientists in the field of catecholamines, which bound mostly to structures reacting with the catechol moiety and not with the amines themselves. This latter problem has recently received some solutions, but in general the study of the binding of several biological neurotransmitters or modulators themselves is still difficult and, in our opinion, this represents one of the major pitfalls of current research.

Characterization and sometimes solubilization, isolation, and analyses of the receptors have been possible with the availability of specific ligands with sufficient specific radioactivity and a higher affinity for the receptor than for other structures, specific (enzymes) or not. Furthermore, a high affinity for the receptors facilitates the separation of bound from free radioactivity in the experimental procedure; "irreversible" ligands have been particularly favorable for isolation purposes.

The criterion for biochemical characterization is saturability, and that criterion, which was postulated for the pharmacological characterization, i.e., structural specificity (most often stereospecificity), drug specificity, uneven distribution and, not least, triggering by agonist of a primary effector system, which is the opening (or closing) of an ion channel or the activation of an adenylate cyclase or some other still unknown step. If an agonist has no effect, it is not an agonist, or the binding site cannot yet be considered as the regulatory site of a pharmacological receptor system.

The high affinity of a specific ligand is also often considered to be an important criterion. This is true in many cases, but interesting exceptions exist for agonists: Carbaminoylcholine binds with the nicotinic cholinergic receptor with a $K_D$ of the order of $10^{-4}$ M. This low affinity is considered by Changeux (3) as a prerequisite for biological activity because the $K_D$ corresponds to the concentration of acetylcholine in the synaptic cleft and higher affinity would imply a dissociation much slower than deduced from the electrical events.

As will be illustrated in this volume, the major lines of research concern (a) attempts to isolate and assess the molecular structure of the receptors, (b) the functional relations between binding sites and primary effectors, and between this complex (or parts of it) and the adjacent molecules of the membranes or of the cells, (c) the characterization of new classes or subtypes, and (d) the regulation of the affinity and/or numbers of receptors.

Although the knowledge of the structure and interactions among the various (sub)units of the receptor systems and the adjacent molecules is the key for a thorough understanding and even—in some cases—for the validation of all other works, I will comment briefly only about the latter.

The characterization of new classes or subtypes of receptors proceeds most often— as in previous pharmacological work—with the use of various ligands (agonists or antagonists) and preparations. It was and remains a truism to assert that no drug has a single effect; this is valid for the affinity of any ligand, an example being the affinity of various dopaminergic ligand for 5-HT receptors. The complexity of the pharmacological responses is paralleled by that of most so-called plasma membrane preparations. Only isolation and structure analysis and studies of molecular mechanism will embody many of the current suggestions and hypotheses. For instance, as outlined in 1975 by Changeux (3), subtypes might correspond to different conformation and not to distinct recognition units. The use of nonnatural ligands always raises the question of the artifactual or biological nature of the corresponding binding site (or conformation).

Meanwhile, just as in classical pharmacology, such works have also led to the discovery of natural ligands (e.g., opioids) and will probably continue to do so. Their provisional conclusions help in understanding the functioning of the nervous system and will guide more fundamental work. The results obtained thus far account, at least in part, for the discovery of some mechanisms of various therapeutic drugs and will facilitate them and aid in finding new ones, as was the case—the classical line of approach—for the antihistamines, the β-blockers, and the anti-$H_2$.

Regulation may be effected through changes in the conformation or in the number of binding sites, in the coupling of the latter with the effector [in particular, by the action of guanosine triphosphate (GTP), and possibly by other substances on the protein regulating the adenylate cyclase], or in the effector system itself. Regulatory loops must also be taken into consideration; transconformations and modifications of the number of sites deserve some comments.

Incubation with agonists increases the affinity for their own binding, as shown first by Changeux (3) for the nicotinic receptor, and later by Fillion (8) for the serotoninergic receptor. Changeux has speculated that such increases of affinity occurred in two steps: The first corresponding to the transition resting state → active state, and the second to the transition active state → desensitized state, the latter being in relation to the loss of tissue responsiveness to the agonist. Antagonists often bind with high affinities on sites that might represent different structural conformations. It has been ascertained that they do not produce the modifications observed with agonists, but this does not exclude other possible changes.

The conformation of binding sites can also be modified noncompetitively, e.g., Fillion and Fillion (8) have shown that antidepressants increase the affinity of serotonin for the serotoninergic postsynaptic receptor (and thus probably desensitize it) with concentrations that do not bind to the serotoninergic-specific binding site. Considering the existence of imipramine receptors, the question arises as to whether a natural ligand exists which would modulate the serotoninergic postsynaptic receptor. Other noncompetitive modulators are ions, which are well known for the opioids and glycine receptors; local anesthetics, which bind to the ionophore, increase the affinity of the nicotinic cholinergic regulatory unit for agonists. Those peptides that are generally considered as modulators might act through similar mechanisms.

The number of binding sites measured *in vivo* has been shown to be decreased by agonists and also decreased when agonists were lacking (denervation), or when their binding was prevented by antagonists. Again, noncompetitive substances can be involved (e.g., hormones). It is well known that hyperthyroidism increases the number of β-adrenergic binding sites, hypothyroidism has the opposite effect.

Opiates and opioids have not yet been shown to modify either the affinity or the number of their own receptors, but do increase the number of binding sites of various neurotransmitters, possibly through a denervationlike process. This effect alone can hardly account for tolerance and abstinence phenomena, and direct or indirect modifications of adenylate cyclases and/or ion channels are, *inter alia*, also to be considered.

Ontogenesis is a particularly interesting aspect of the modifications of the number and structures of receptors; some of the factors involved are suspected, e.g., the innervation might correspond to a diminution of the number of receptors.

These variations in the number of receptors are progressively analyzed with studies concerning their synthesis—which can be very rapid—and their masking or destruction, the first step being internalization.

We have insisted on the crucial value of fundamental biochemical and molecular research in this field; the development and progress of *ex vivo* studies is also urgently needed so as to establish the physiological and pharmacological relevance of *in vitro* experiments.

## REFERENCES

1. Ariëns, E. J., van Rossum, J. M., and Simonis, A. M. (1957): Affinity, intrinsic activity and drug interactions. *Pharmacol. Rev.*, 9:218.
2. Chagas, C., Penna-Franca, E., Nishie, K., and Garcia, E. J. (1958): A study of the specificity of the complex formed by gallamine triethiodide with a macromolecular constituent of the electric organ. *Arch. Biochem. Biophys.*, 75:251.
3. Changeux, J. P. (1979): Some principles of neuronal regulation at the postsynaptic level. In: *Central Regulation of the Endocrine System*, edited by Kjell Juxe, Tomas Hökfelt, and Rolf Luft. Plenum Press, New York.
4. Clark, A. J. (1926): The reaction between acetylcholine and muscle cells. *J. Physiol. (Lond.)*, 61:530–546.
5. Clark, A. J. (1937): General pharmacology. In: *Heffter's Handbuch der experiment pharmakologie*, Vol. IV. Springer, Berlin.
6. Dale, H. H. (1906): On some physiological actions of ergot. *J. Physiol. (Lond.)*, 34:163–206.
7. Ehrlich, P. (1962): Address delivered at the dedication of the George-Speyer-Haus, 1906. In: *Readings in Pharmacology*, edited by L. Schuster, pp. 231–244. Little, Brown, Boston.
8. Fillion, G., and Fillion, M. P. (1982): Modulation of affinity of postsynaptic serotonin receptors by antidepressant drugs. *Nature (in press)*.
9. Gaddum, J. H. (1957): Drug antagonism. *Pharmacol. Rev.*, 9:211.
10. Goldstein, A., Lowney, L. I., and Pal, K. (1971): Stereospecific and nonspecific interactions of the morphine congener levorphanol in subcellular fractions of mouse brain. *Proc. Natl. Acad. Sci. USA*, 68:1742–1747.
11. Hill, A. V. (1909): The mode of action of nicotine and curare determined from the contraction curve and the method of temperature coefficients. *J. Physiol. (Lond.)*, 39:361–373.
12. Hughes, J. (1975): Isolation of an endogenous compound from the brain with pharmacological properties similar to morphine. *Brain Res.*, 88:295–308.
13. Jacob, J. (1963): Quelques problèmes pharmacologiques posés par l'antagonisme médicamenteux. *Thérapie*, 18:1031–1049.
14. Langley, J. N. (1905): On the reaction of cells and nerve-endings to certain poisons, chiefly as regards the reaction of striated muscle to nicotine and to curare. *J. Physiol. (Lond.)*, 33:374–413.
15. Schild, H. O. (1957): Drug antagonism and pAx. *Pharmacol. Rev.*, 9:242.

*Molecular Pharmacology of Neurotransmitter Receptors*, edited by T. Segawa et al.
Raven Press, New York © 1983

# Recent Advances in Identification and Isolation of Acetylcholinesterase and a Cholinergic Receptor Protein

P. G. Waser, W. H. Hopff, M. C. Schaub, and A. Hofmann

*Institute of Pharmacology, University Zurich, CH-8006 Zurich, Switzerland*

The identification of specific proteins in the excitable membrane of synapses is based on different steps of experimental procedure. First, highly specific compounds with strong pharmacodynamic actions have to be found or synthesized. Then the labeled compounds have to be bound by enzymes or receptors following dose-effect relationships and with saturation characteristics. Affinity and uniformity of receptor population must be shown. The agonist will interact with competitive antagonists on this uniform receptor population, always in relation to the pharmacodynamic or biochemical effects. Finally, the isolation of an unchanged reactive protein, in a global form or in parts, can be tried. But only the biological change of this protein under the influence of agonists will prove its receptor specificity.

This is currently—in our view—the missing link and the most difficult part of receptor characterization. It depends mostly on our knowledge of membrane structure and the architecture of the complex membrane components responsible for the different membrane functions, such as ion flux, transport mechanisms, endo- and exocytosis, enzymatic activities, plasticity for learning and memory processes, and regeneration. The binding of agonists or antagonists represents the first step of a complex mechanism of the information process through the membrane and its coupling to the effector sites in the cytoplasm.

Specific labeling of cholinergic receptors or curare binding sites and of acetylcholinesterase was possible years ago (8). Lately, we were able to show in a combined experiment with electrophysiology and autoradiography the localization and number of $^{14}C$-toxiferine molecules on the postsynaptic membrane and, at the same time, its effect on the endplate potential (1). Saturation of the excitable membrane was achieved with $10^{-6}$ M toxiferine; but at a lower concentration ($3 \times 10^{-7}$ molar) the muscle was already paralyzed to nerve stimulation and no action potentials of contracting muscle fibers were recorded. Only endplate potentials were apparent, diminishing in number with increasing toxiferine concentration and disappearing completely with $10^{-6}$ M toxiferine in the bath fluid. This naturally means that the postsynaptic membrane is no longer depolarizable.

As we have seen earlier, a higher concentration of cholinergic compounds is needed for complete block by depolarization, i.e., acetylcholine $5 \times 10^{-3}$ M (with neostigmine), diazoacetylcholine $5 \times 10^{-5}$ M, carbachol $2.5 \times 10^{-5}$ M. Even with the classical depolarizing muscle relaxant decamethonium, a concentration of $10^{-5}$ M is needed for complete block. Furthermore, the number of depolarizing molecules at the excitable membrane of the endplate is much higher ($70 \times 10^6$/endplate) than with different stabilizing curare molecules (toxiferine, tubocurarine, pancuronium; $5 \times 10^6$ molecules/endplate). Additionally, the distribution of radioactive molecules shows a considerable spread of depolarizing molecules around the endplates compared with the narrow concentration of radioactivity of classical curare molecules in the synaptical cleft only.

Acetylcholinesterase, concentrated mainly in the postsynaptic membrane and in its folds, has a definite number of active centers as determined with the irreversible fixation of $^{14}$C-diisopropyl-fluorophospate. As each enzyme unit carries four active centers, the number of enzyme molecules can be determined ($10^7$/endplate) in combination to the curare binding sites, but not in direct relation to the cholinergic receptor sites (Fig. 1).

This morphological-functional model of the cholinoceptive unit in the postjunctional membrane is currently accepted by many scientists. But only the isolation of acetylcholinesterase and its identification as enzyme has been fully successful. The isolation of receptor proteins and ionophores is, in our opinion, still in the early stage of technical and methodological difficulties. We have followed a purely biochemical approach without the use of toxins and will discuss this strategy below.

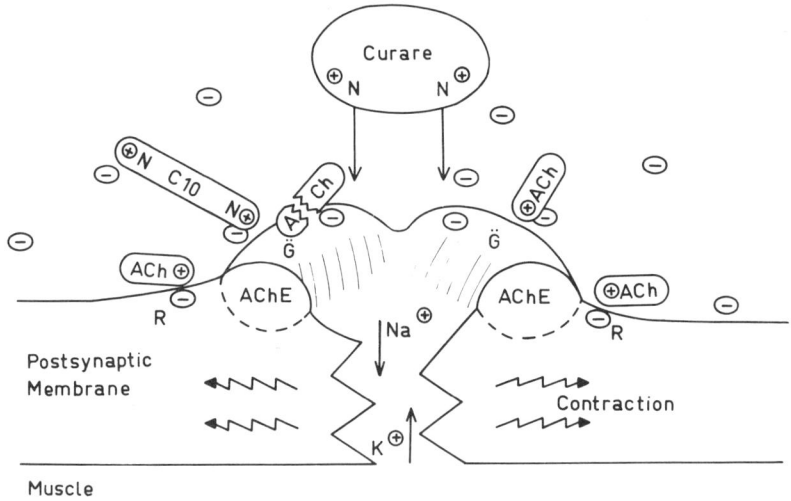

**FIG. 1.** Schematic cross section of receptor area. The pore permitting ion flux in the depolarized state of the postsynaptic membrane is enclosed by molecules of acetylcholinesterase (AchE) with four active centers (—,G̈). It may be blocked by the large curare molecules. Acetylcholine (Ach) or decamethonium (C10) molecules attack the many cholinergic receptors (R), of which 10 are located near the cholinesterase, perhaps in close contact with its protein outside the active center. An allosteric action changes the structure of the membrane (contraction) and opens the pores. The juxta-junctional cholinergic receptor further out might belong to inactive isoenzymes of AchE.

## ACETYLCHOLINESTERASE

The homogenate of the electric organ of *Torpedo marmorata* and electric eel contains the synaptical membranes with the tetrameric enzyme molecules bound to it in 1 to 3 units by some kind of long collagenous chains (6). Toluene extraction brings the enzyme into solution without the tails. Chromatography on Sephadex G-100 and centrifugation of the active fraction at $30'000 \times g$ gives a clear solution. The important step is the following run of this solution through a special affinity chromatography column, with a long (46 Å) spacer and a final quaternary trimethylammonium group (Fig. 2). Elution with tetramethylammonium bromide from this column in one step yielded 93% recovery of enzyme activity. After a second filtration through Sephadex G-200 the specific enzyme activity was $18'650$ μMU. The enzyme crystallized slowly from a 2-M ammonium sulfate solution (3,4).

Amino acid analysis of the purified acetylcholinesterase was performed according to standard procedures. Tryptophan was determined after hydrolysis with *p*-toluenesulfonic acid (Table 1). Carbohydrates were identified as methylglycosides by gas liquid chromatography (Table 2). It is worth noting that the amino acid compositions of acetylcholinesterase from the two species are almost identical. So far, no collagen was found in our enzyme preparations. In preliminary experiments, pure acetylcholinesterase was inhibited by sarin and diisopropylfluorophosphate (DFP). The inactivation rate was 200 times faster for sarin in relation to DFP. Sarin inactivates one active site per one subunit (MW: $70'000$) in a stoichiometric way. Essentially the same result was obtained with a slight surplus of DFP. This confirms the suggestion that each subunit bears one active site. We will use this approach for labeling the active center of acetylcholinesterase.

The total carbohydrate weight was approximately 12% of the protein. Acetylcholinesterase (AchE) clearly is a glycoprotein. The carbohydrates may belong to the associated ionophore, or might simply be part of the basement membrane. In

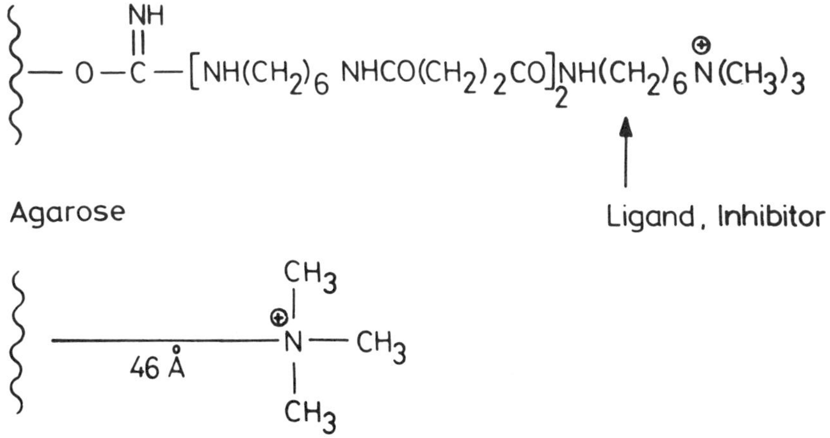

**FIG. 2.** Spacer and inhibtor group for affinity chromatography of AchE.

TABLE 1. Amino acid composition of AchE from
T. marmorata and electric eel

| Amino acid | No. of residues per $10^5$ g/protein | |
|---|---|---|
| | Torpedo | Eel |
| Cys | 26 | 23 |
| Asp | 90 | 97 |
| Thr | 47 | 50 |
| Ser | 69 | 72 |
| Glu | 108 | 110 |
| Pro | 60 | 67 |
| Gly | 83 | 82 |
| Ala | 41 | 43 |
| Val | 56 | 52 |
| Met | 22 | 20 |
| Ile | 47 | 36 |
| Leu | 83 | 73 |
| Tyr | 29 | 28 |
| Phe | 41 | 43 |
| Lys | 41 | 42 |
| His | 19 | 19 |
| Arg | 39 | 40 |
| Trp | 15 | 17 |

the lipid fraction, lecithin, cholesteroltryglyceride, and phosphatidylinositol are predominant (9). They may be important not only for the stability, but also for the functioning of the membrane. At the moment we are trying to investigate the active center of the enzyme with suitable substrates in order to get more information on the amino acids involved in its structure and functioning.

## CHOLINERGIC RECEPTOR PROTEIN

After using diazoacetylcholine as specific affinity label to the cholinergic receptor, we started to isolate receptor proteins from the homogenate of electric organs of T. marmorata after solubilization with the nonionic detergents. Instead of using neurotoxins on an affinity chromatography column, we preferred chemically defined inhibitors for adsorption of the specific protein. We first synthesized several ligands of the depolarizing type, again linked to agarose by a long spacer (Fig. 3). Decamethonium proved to the best suited ligand group (Fig. 4). The protein fraction that was retained on the column and eluted with tetramethylammonium had no cholinesterase activity. In contrast to former experiments with membrane fragments

TABLE 2. Carbohydrate composition
of AchE from T. marmorata

| Carbohydrate | % Values (w/w) |
|---|---|
| Mannose | 2.7 |
| Galactose | 2.4 |
| Glucose | 1.4 |
| Glucosamine | 4.0 |
| N-acetylneuraminic acid | 2.0 |

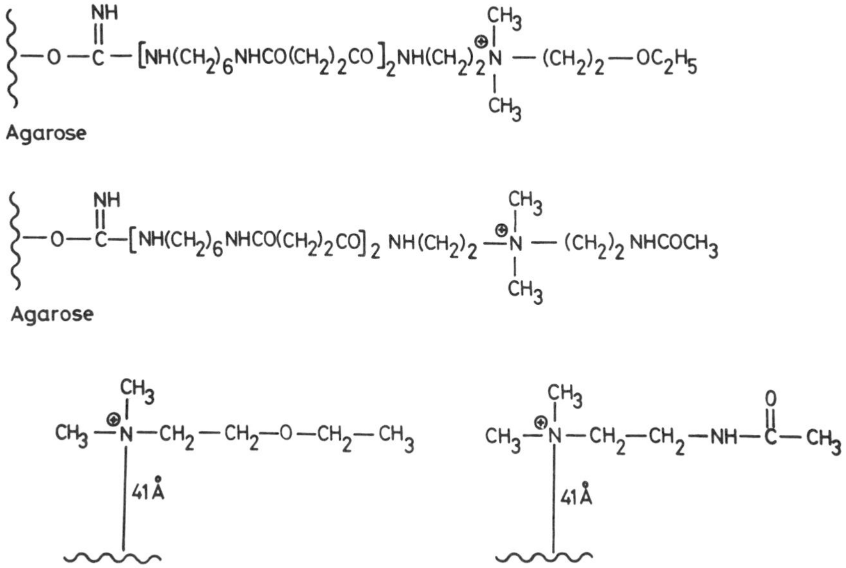

**FIG. 3.** Spacer and ligand groups for affinity chromatography of cholinergic receptor protein.

of electric organs (7), the $^3$H-acetylcholine binding capacity with an affinity of $K = 5,3 \times 10^6$ M$^{-1}$ was practically lost. The high affinity binding state may be obtained with immediate extraction of fresh electric organs, but it is lost, perhaps by conformational changes, within hours. Reactivation by convertion into the active conformational state was not achieved.

## CURARE BINDING PROTEIN

In order to investigate the curare (or nondepolarizing) binding protein, we synthesized a gallamine inhibitor for affinity chromatography which was different from

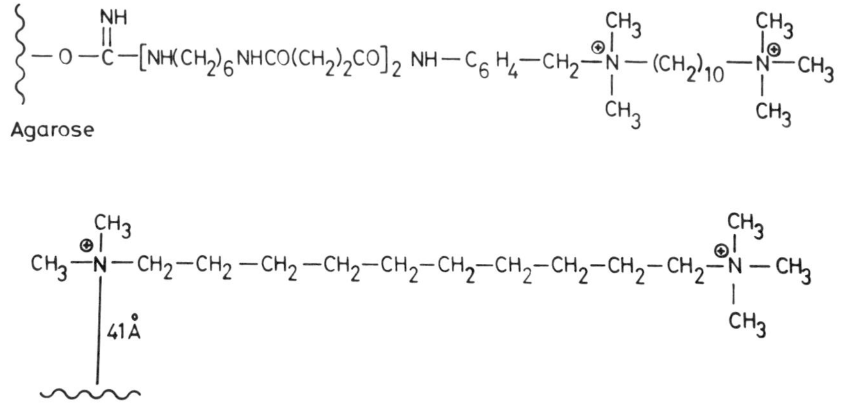

**FIG. 4.** Decamethonium as ligand for affinity chromatography of cholinergic receptor protein.

the one used by Olson (6). In our case, all three side arms of the phenyl group are free (Fig. 5). Careful protective measures had to be taken to prevent changes or degradation of the binding protein (2). Separation of this binding protein from acetylcholinesterase was possible after inactivation of the latter by methylisopropylfluorophosphate (sarin). The crude protein solution was prepurified by a "double reversed" gel filtration and concentrated again by ultrafiltration. Then sarin was added and the solution run over the gallamine column. AchE appeared with the bulk of non-specific proteins at the front of the elution profile. The column was then washed for several days with buffer solution containing 0.5 M NaCl without loss of detectable amounts of protein. Finally, the elution of the specific gallamine-binding protein was achieved with free gallamine which acted as specific desorbant. For preparation of freeze-dried curare binding protein (CBP) the free gallamine was removed by ultrafiltration and by final gel filtration.

The overall yield of this CBP protein calculated on the basis of wet weight of electric organ was 0.02%. Samples showed good binding of α-bungarotoxin with high affinity ($K = 1,3 \times 10^8 \text{ M}^{-1}$). The amino acid composition shows significant differences from that calculated by Lindstrom and co-workers (5) who isolated their binding protein complex from *Torpedo californica* with a najatoxin affinity column (Table 3). At present we are further investigating possible differences between the CBP and the toxin binding protein complex. The carbohydrate content of the CBP was found to be approximately 13% by weight (Table 4).

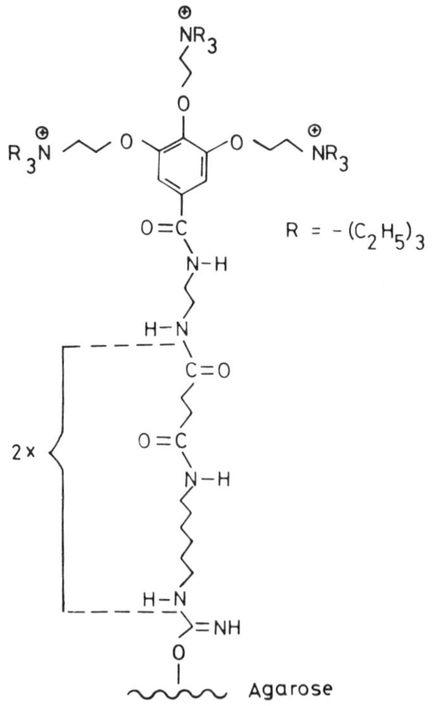

**FIG. 5.** Gallamine as inhibitor for affinity chromatography of CBP.

TABLE 3. *Amino acid composition of cholinergic binding proteins purified by affinity chromatography from T. marmorata and T. californica*

| Amino acid | No. of residues per $10^5$ g protein | |
|---|---|---|
| | Gallamine specific binding, elution, with gallamine[a] | Naja toxin binding, elution with benzoquinonium[b] |
| Asp | 75 | 105 |
| Thr | 80 | 55 |
| Ser | 78 | 49 |
| Glu | 115 | 85 |
| Pro | 51 | 53 |
| Gly | 49 | 41 |
| Ala | 55 | 40 |
| Val | 49 | 63 |
| Met | 30 | 20 |
| Ile | 46 | 66 |
| Leu | 61 | 81 |
| Tyr | 21 | 34 |
| Phe | 34 | 41 |
| Lys | 53 | 51 |
| His | 23 | 21 |
| Arg | 30 | 38 |
| Trp | 9 | 13 |

[a] Data from Hopff et al., ref. 2, with permission.
[b] Values calculated from Lindstrom et al., ref. 5, with permission.

TABLE 4. *Carbohydrate composition of CBP from T. marmorata*

| Carbohydrate | % Values (w/w) |
|---|---|
| Mannose | 0.95 |
| Galactose | 3.37 |
| Glucose | 0.57 |
| Glucosamine | 4.52 |
| N-acetylneuraminic acid | 4.19 |

## ACKNOWLEDGMENTS

We gratefully acknowledge the financial help of the Swiss National Foundation for Scientific Research (Grant 3.086.076) and the technical help of Dr. G. Riggio, Mrs. H. Meier, Mrs. E. Schönberger, and Mr. G. Engler.

## REFERENCES

1. Caratsch, C. G., Waser, P. G., Spiess, C., and Schönenberger, E. (1979): Quantitative correlation between complete block of nicotinic acetylcholine receptors and saturation of the motor endplate with $^{14}$C-toxiferine. *Naunyn Schmiedebergs Arch. Pharmacol.*, 306:17–21.
2. Hopff, W. H., Hofmann, A. A., Riggio, G., and Waser, P. G. (1981): Cholinergic receptor isolation. In: *Cholinergic Mechanisms*, pp. 323–332. Plenum Press, New York.

3. Hopff, W. H., Riggio, G., and Waser, P. G. (1973): Affinity chromatography of acetylcholine acetyl-hydrolase. EC 3.1.1.7. A new straight chain aliphatic inhibitor. *FEBS LETT.*, 35:220–222.
4. Hopff, W. H., Riggio, G., and Waser, P. G. (1975): Progress in isolation of acetylcholinesterase. In: *Cholinergic Mechanisms*, edited by P. G. Waser, pp. 293–298. Raven Press, New York.
5. Lindstrom, J., Merlie, J., and Yogeeswaran, G. (1979): Biochemical properties of acetylcholine receptor subunits from *Torpedo Californica*. *Biochemistry*, 18:4465–4470.
6. Olsen, R., Meunier, J. C., Weber, W., and Changeux, J. P. (1972): Characterization, isolation and purification of the cholinergic receptor protein from electrophorus electric organ. *FEBS Lett.*, 28:96–100.
7. Taylor, P., Lwebuga-Mukasa, J., Lappi, S., and Berman, H. A. (1978): Structure of acetylcholinesterase: Its relationship to the postsynaptic membrane. In: *Cholinergic Mechanisms and Psychopharmacology*, edited by D. J. Jenden, pp. 239–251. Plenum Press, New York.
8. Walser, J. T., Schaub, M. C., and Waser, P. G. (1975): Binding Studies on Membrane Fragments of Electroplax from *Torpedo Marmorata*. In: *Cholinergic Mechanisms*, edited by P. G. Waser, pp. 365–374. Raven Press, New York.
9. Waser, P. G. (1970): On receptors in the post synaptic membrane of the motor endplate. In: *Ciba Foundation Symposium on Molecular Drug Receptors*, pp. 59–75. Churchill, London.
10. Werner, G., Wojnarowski, W., Hopff, W. H., and Waser, P. G. (1978): Constituents of acetylcholinesterase. *Cholinergic Mechanisms and Psychopharmacology*, edited by D. J. Jenden, pp. 231–237. Plenum Press, New York.

*Molecular Pharmacology of Neurotransmitter Receptors*, edited by T. Segawa et al.
Raven Press, New York © 1983.

# Recent Advances in Muscarinic Receptor Heterogeneity and Regulation

*†William R. Roeske, †Frederick J. Ehlert, †Diana S. Barritt, *†Kyozo Yamanaka, *†Lois B. Rosenberger, *†Shizuo Yamada, †Susan Yamamura, and †**Henry I. Yamamura

*Departments of *Internal Medicine, †Pharmacology, **Biochemistry, and **Psychiatry, The University of Arizona Health Sciences Center, Tucson, Arizona 85724*

In this chapter we will present portions of our recent work in muscarinic receptor regulation. Additional reviews of the biochemical approaches to the study of the muscarinic receptor are available (7,9,14,15,18,37,39,44,46).

The first demonstration of [$^3$H]antagonist binding to muscarinic receptors was made by Paton and Rang (32), who measured the binding of [$^3$H]atropine to the longitudinal muscle layer of the guinea pig ileum. Since these studies, the binding of several [$^3$H]antagonists to muscarinic receptors has been demonstrated (18). From the initial results of the binding of [$^3$H]antagonists, a reasonably consistent picture of the nature of antagonist interaction with the muscarinic receptor has emerged: The binding of antagonists is saturable and consistent with the law of mass action for a single class of receptors. The binding is stereospecific and sensitive to inhibition by muscarinic drugs, but not by drugs that lack direct muscarinic cholinergic effects (2,20,21,32,53,54). The distribution of [$^3$H]antagonist binding is consistent with cholinergic innervation, and there is agreement between the values of antagonist affinity constants determined by binding measurements and by pharmacological antagonism of smooth muscle contraction (5,54).

However, complexities in the nature of antagonist binding have been noted recently. Analysis of pirenzepine/[$^3$H]N-methylscopolamine competition curves revealed deviations from simple mass action behavior, which could be explained on the basis of multiple antagonist receptor subtypes (23). Antagonist receptor heterogeneity has also been detected with classical muscarinic antagonists under unusual assay conditions, depending primarily on the ionic composition of the incubation medium (16,24). Thus, the interaction of antagonists with the muscarinic receptor is more complicated than originally thought. Our recent data on the detection and

---

Present address of Dr. Rosenberger: Mead Johnson Corporation, Evansville, Indiana 47721.
Present address of Dr. Yamada: Department of Pharmacology, Shizuoka College of Pharmaceutical Sciences, 2-2-1 Oshika, Shizuoka 422, Japan.

regulation of the different antagonist affinity states of the muscarinic receptor will be discussed below.

In contrast to antagonist binding, agonist binding has long been recognized as complex, deviating significantly from mass action behavior. This heterogeneity is manifested by agonist/[³H]antagonist competition curves which extend over 3 to 4 log concentration units of the agonist; the Hill coefficients are less than one (6,7,19). Figure 1 illustrates the competitive inhibition of [³H]quinuclidinyl benzilate (QNB) binding by the antagonist atropine and the agonist carbachol in the longitudinal muscle of the ileum. The carbachol competition curve is shallow compared with the mass action curve (dotted line). In contrast, the atropine competition curve is consistent with the law of mass action. Birdsall and co-workers (6) first formulated the concept that the complexities of agonist/[³H]antagonist competition curves are the result of receptor heterogeneity. Their data were sufficiently described by the contribution of three populations of muscarinic receptors, superhigh, high, and low affinity (SH, H and L), each having different affinities for agonists and equal affinity for antagonists.

The complexities of agonist binding observed in agonist/[³H]antagonist competition experiments have been verified by direct measurements of the binding of radiolabeled agonists. Typically, Scatchard analysis of the [³H]agonist binding isotherm indicates more than one population of labeled muscarinic sites (6,11,13). Studies of the competitive inhibition of [³H]agonist binding by nonlabeled agonists have provided further evidence for agonist receptor heterogeneity, since the potency of nonlabeled agonists is generally much greater than that determined by measurement of [³H]antagonist displacement (6,11,13). This behavior would be expected

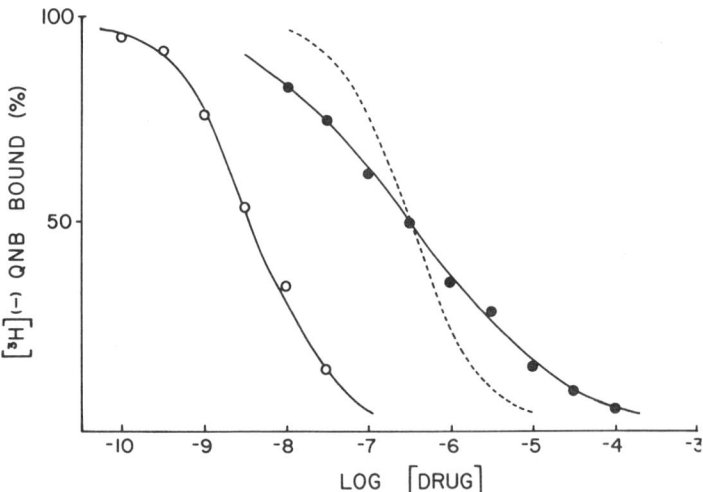

**FIG. 1.** Competitive inhibition of [³H](−)QNB binding to the longitudinal muscle of the rat ileum by atropine *(open cirlces)* and carbachol *(closed circles)*. The *dotted line* represents a mass action curve intersecting the carbachol competition curve at the $IC_{50}$ point. The radiolabeled ligand concentration was 0.4 nM. (From Ehlert et al., ref. 18, with permission.)

if [$^3$H]agonists selectively label the SH and H receptors at the low ligand concentrations usually employed in binding assays.

The existence of multiple agonist binding sites poses fundamental questions concerning the significance of muscarinic receptor heterogeneity. The inability of classical muscarinic antagonists to distinguish between the multiple classes of agonist binding sites might be rationalized on the basis of a lack of complementarity between antagonists and the agonist binding region of the receptor (18). A theory proposed by Birdsall et al. (5) contends that the three different classes of agonist binding sites represent independent states of the same receptor molecule, and that the differences in affinity arise as the result of conformational constraints imposed by the environment or coupling state of the receptor. This model predicts that antagonists should have equal affinity for the different classes of agonist binding sites, that pure and partial agonists should have a constant ratio ($K_{SH}/K_H$) of affinity constants for the SH and H sites and that $K_H/K_L$ should be proportional to efficacy. These predictions have been fulfilled by several agonists (5,6,8). The existence of mutliple agonist affinity binding states (three or more) might also be construed as evidence for the existence of different effector systems with which the various agonist receptors (SH, H, and L) are coupled (39). However, comparison of agonist dissociation constants ($K_{SH}$, $K_H$, and $K_L$) with ED$_{50}$ values for pharmacological responses is complicated by the diversity of pharmacological responses that are thought to be mediated by muscarinic receptors and by the complex (often nonlinear) relationship between receptor occupancy and pharmacological response. In the next four sections, we will demonstrate several experimental approaches to the detection and regulation of both multiple agonist affinity states and multiple antagonist affinity states.

## GUANINE NUCLEOTIDE REGULATION OF MUSCARINIC RECEPTORS

Following the original demonstration that guanine nucleotides modify the binding properties of glucagon (34) several additional systems were also noted to have a similar modulation (18,26,28,29,33,51). Muscarinic receptors are regulated by guanine nucleotides (3,12,22,40,41,45,48). The modulation by guanine nucleotides is characterized by a selective reduction in agonist potency. In studies of several adenylate cyclase systems, guanosine triphosphate (GTP) has been shown to be a requirement for neurotransmitter and hormonal activation. Accordingly, the results of studies of the regulation of muscarinic receptor binding by guanine nucleotides may have important implications for the relationship between agonist receptor heterogeneity and receptor-effector coupling. Since carbachol had been shown to inhibit the GTP-stimulated adenylate cyclase activity in myocardial homogenates (31,47), initial studies of the influence of guanine nucleotides on the binding properties of muscarinic receptors used homogenates of the rat myocardium (3,40,41). When measured by competitive inhibition of [$^3$H]antagonist binding, the IC$_{50}$ values of the agonists oxotremorine and carbachol increased by a factor of 10 to 20 in the presence of GTP or its nonhydrolyzable analogue, Gpp(NH)p (3,40,41). In contrast, only small or insignificant effects of guanine nucleotides on the binding properties of antagonists were reported in these initial studies. The effects of various concentrations of Gpp(NH)p on the competitive inhibition of cardiac [$^3$H]QNB binding by oxotremorine are shown in Figure 2. It can be seen that Gpp(NH)p caused a dose-dependent reduction in the potency of oxotremorine and that the $ED_{50}$ of Gpp(NH)p for this effect was in the $10^{-8}$ to $10^{-7}$ M range.

Although the effects of guanine nucleotides on agonist binding in myocardial homogenates are readily demonstrable in the absence of added $Mg^{2+}$ ions, the effect certainly requires $Mg^{2+}$. This $Mg^{2+}$ requirement was demonstrated in a study in which microsomal preparations of the rat atria were treated with EDTA and washed by centrifugation (49). These $Mg^{2+}$ free homogenates caused only a twofold increase in the $IC_{50}$ of carbachol in the presence of GTP ($10^{-3}$ M), whereas an elevenfold increase in the $IC_{50}$ of carbachol was observed when similar experiments were carried out in the presence of both $MgCl_2$ ($10^{-3}$ M) and GTP. Similar results have been obtained in left ventricular homogenates (Rosenberger et al., *unpublished results*).

Guanine nucleotides have also been shown to modulate the binding of agonists to muscarinic receptors in smooth muscle and various brain regions (12,45), al-

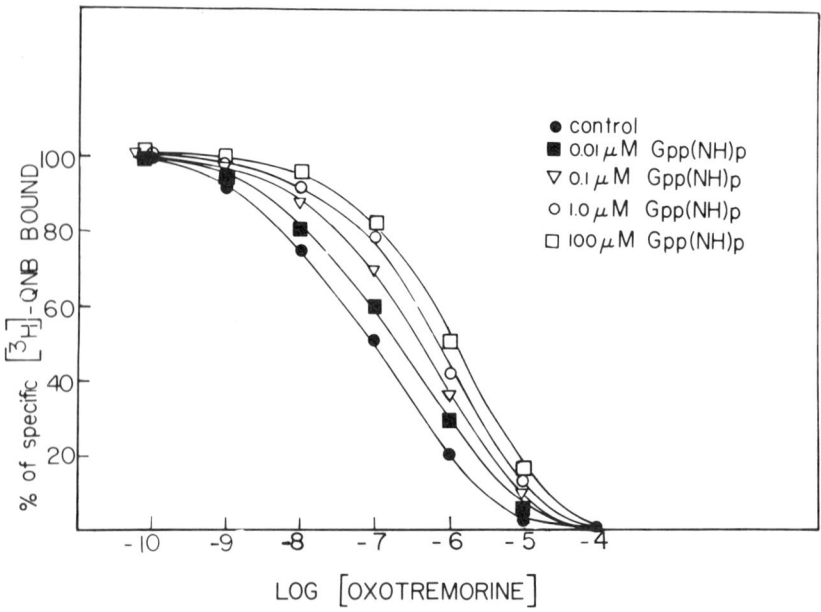

**FIG. 2.** Effect of Gpp(NH)p on the competitive inhibition of [$^3$H](−)QNB binding to myocardial homogenates by oxotremorine. Assays were done in the absence *(closed circles)* and presence of various concentrations of Gpp(NH)p: 0.01 μM *(closed squares)*, 0.1 μM *(triangles)*, 1.0 μM *(open circles)*, and 100 μM *(open squares)*. The radiolabeled ligand concentration was 0.12 nM. (The data are replotted from ref. 41 and the figure is reprinted from Ehlert et al., ref. 18, with permission.)

though the magnitude of the effect in these tissues is not as great as that observed in the heart.

The selective inhibitory effects of Gpp(NH)p on the binding of agonists have also been detected by direct measurement of [$^3$H]agonist binding in the presence of Gpp(NH)p (13,14,19). A guanine nucleotide-induced shift in an agonist/[$^3$H]antagonist competition curve may result in a small percentage difference between binding values in the competition curve. In contrast, the same effect may be manifested by a relatively larger percentage difference between direct measurements of [$^3$H]agonist binding to H and SH receptors.

Using the agonist ligand [$^3$H]CD, we have screened several brain regions and tissues of the rat to determine the regional sensitivity of muscarinic receptors to the effects of Gpp(NH)p (100 μM) (14). We found the largest effects of guanine nucleotides were measured in the heart, ileum, and cerebellum. We have also determined the sensitivity of [$^3$H]agonist binding to the effects of guanine nucleotides by measuring [$^3$H]CD binding in the presence of various concentrations of Gpp(NH)p. The results of these experiments are shown in Fig. 3 which illustrates that the potency of inhibition of [$^3$H]CD binding by Gpp(NH)p varies in the heart, longitudinal muscle of the ileum, corpus striatum, and cerebral cortex of the rat. The $ED_{50}$ values of this Gpp(NH)p effect are 0.18, 1.8, 20, and 22 μM in the heart, ileum, corpus striatum, and cerebral cortex, respectively. Consequently, the guanine nucleotide regulation of muscarinic receptors differs in both absolute magnitude

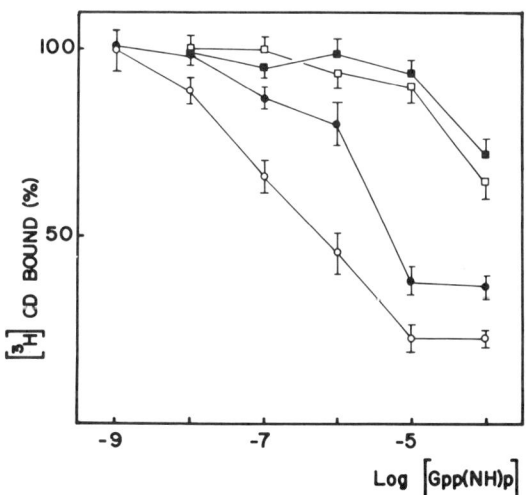

**FIG. 3.** Effect of Gpp(NH)p on [$^3$H]agonist binding in various tissues of the rat. [$^3$H]CD binding was measured at a concentration of 5.0 nM in homogenates of the heart *(open circles)*, longitudinal muscle of the ileum *(closed circles)*, corpus striatum *(open squares)*, and cerebral cortex *(closed squares)* in the presence of various concentrations of Gpp(NH)p. Binding assays were run in 50 mM Tris citrate buffer, pH 7.4 at 0°C, containing 10 mM $MgCl_2$. Incubations were carried out for 15 min at 37°C followed by 1 hr at 0°C. Mean binding values ± SEM of at least four experiments are shown. (Experimental details are similar to those described in ref. 11 and the figure is reprinted from Ehlert et al., ref. 18, with permission.)

and sensitivity in various tissues. This interesting result is compatible with differing proportions of guanine regulated muscarinic receptors or differences in the guanine regulatory site in these tissues.

Recently, we have used [$^3$H]CD binding to study the development of both the high affinity muscarinic receptors in the heart and the appearance of ionic and guanine nucleotide regulation (1). We have previously studied cardiac muscarinic receptor development using the ligand [$^3$H]QNB (35,37,38). Figure 4 clearly indicates that there is a postnatal peak of high affinity muscarinic receptors (18-day neonates) and that guanine regulation and ionic regulation were seen at all ages. These data are compatible with the development of muscarinic receptor recognition sites in the presence of an excess of guanine regulatory sites or alternatively the guanine regulatory site could be closely linked with the recognition site and appear simultaneously during development.

Interestingly, the muscarinic receptor can demonstrate guanine nucleotide regulation of both agonists and antagonists. Unlike the modulation of agonist binding, the binding of classical antagonists is enhanced by guanine nucleotides (13,14,24). The magnitude of this guanine nucleotide effect is much less than that of the inhibitory effect observed with pure agonists, and it appears to be more demonstrable in buffers of low ionic strength which lack inorganic ions. Among the tissues that have been examined, the largest effects were noted in the heart and ileum in which

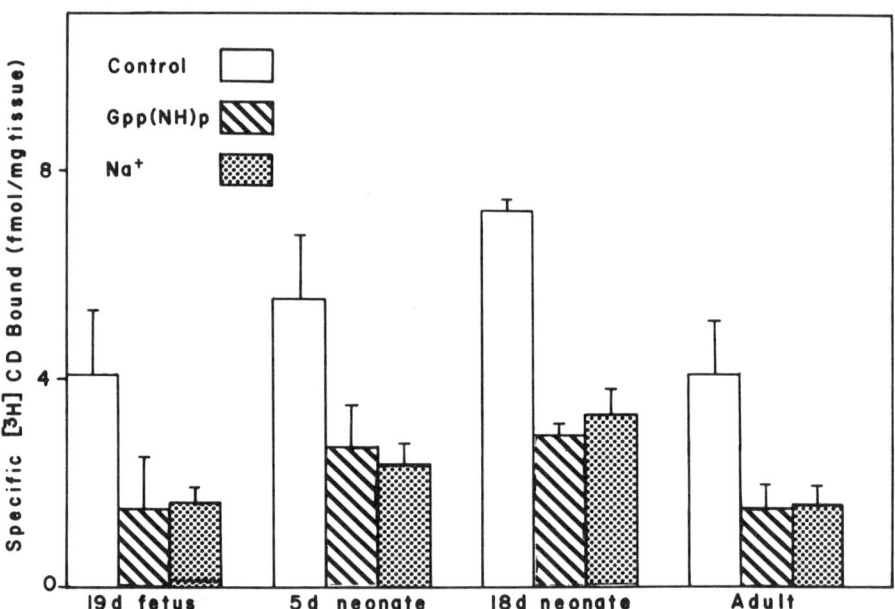

**FIG. 4.** Gpp(NH)p and Na$^+$ inhibition of [$^3$H]CD binding in mouse heart homogenates at various stages of development. The [$^3$H]CD concentration was 16 nM and each bar graph represents the mean (and SEM) of three to eight experiments done in duplicate. Assays were done in the presence or absence of 30 μM Gpp(NH)p, 50 mM NaCl, in a 50 mM Tris-HCl buffer, pH 7.4, at 0°C for 90 min, using an assay similar to that described in ref. 11.

the binding of [³H](−)QNB at a concentration of 0.05 nM was stimulated by 73 and 50%, respectively, in the presence of 10 μM Gpp(NH)p (14). Guanine nucleotides enhance [³H]QNB binding by increasing the affinity of muscarinic receptors without a significant change in their number (13). In general, the potency of guanine nucleotides for enhancement of antagonist binding in the heart and ileum is greater than that for inhibition of agonist binding (13,14,24). This relationship is illustrated by the data in Fig. 5 which show the effect of Gpp(NH)p on the binding of [³H](−)QNB and [³H]CD to the rat ileum under identical assay conditions. Gpp(NH)p caused a maximal 65% stimulation of [³H](−)QNB binding and a maximal inhibition of [³H]CD binding of at least 60%. The $ED_{50}$'s for these effects were approximately 0.4 and 5.6 μM, respectively. Accordingly, the potency of Gpp(NH)p for perturbation of agonist and antagonist binding in the ileum differs by a factor of 14, suggesting that different GTP-regulatory proteins may be involved in these processes. Alternatively, the same GTP binding site may mediate an allosteric enhancement of antagonist binding and inhibition of agonist binding (18). Although the functional significance of the guanine nucleotide regulation of antagonist binding is not known, it demonstrates that the ground state of the muscarinic receptor can exist in different conformations which might not have been predicted on the basis of classical theories of drug action.

Of potential significance in developing biochemical tests for biological muscarinic drug efficacy, is the finding that the magnitude of the effect of guanine nucleotides on the binding of agonists to the muscarinic receptor depends upon the efficacy of the drug. In a study of the influence of guanine nucleotides on the competitive inhibition of ileal [³H](−)QNB binding by cholinergic agonists (13), it was noted that Gpp(NH), ($10^{-4}$ M) caused a relatively large reduction in the potency of efficacious agonists like carbachol and oxotremorine whereas Gpp(NH)p only caused a small reduction in the potency of partial agonists such as pilocarpine and pentyltrimethylammonium. These results are consistent with the idea that guanine

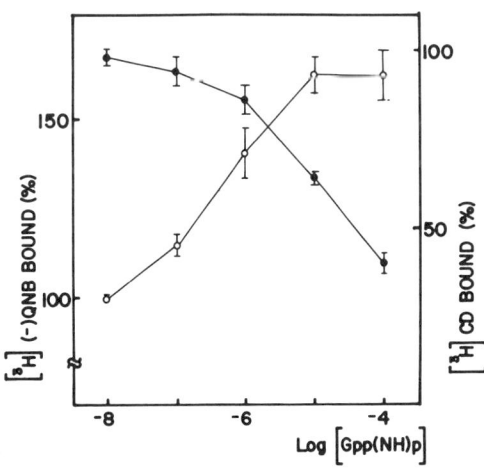

FIG. 5. Effects of Gpp(NH)p on the binding of [³H](−)QNB and [³H]CD to homogenates of the longitudinal muscle of the rat ileum. The binding of [³H]QNB *(open circles)* and [³H]CD *(closed circles)* was measured under identical conditions in the presence of various concentrations of Gpp(NH)p. Incubations lasted 2 hr at 25°C in Tris HCl buffer containing 1 mM $MgCl_2$. (The details of the assay are given in ref. 13 and the figure is reprinted from Ehlert et al., ref. 18, with permission.)

nucleotides cause a selective conversion of H to L sites. For highly efficacious agonists, which have a large geometric difference between the values of $K_H$ and $K_L$ ($K_L/K_H >> 1$), a guanine nucleotide-induced conversion of H to L would cause a relatively large increase in the $IC_{50}$ value. In contrast, the $IC_{50}$ values of partial agonists, which have relatively smaller $K_L/K_H$ ratios, would not be expected to change much in the presence of guanine nucleotides. The relationship between the guanine nucleotide effect and efficacy is illustrated in Fig. 6.

## MECHANISMS OF ADRENERGIC–CHOLINERGIC INTERACTION IN CARDIAC TISSUE

A role for muscarinic receptor-mediated inhibition of adenylate cyclase activity has been established in several tissue preparations. Muscarinic agonists inhibit $PGE_1$ and adenosine-stimulated adenylate cyclase activity in neuroblastoma glial cells (10,30), and GTP-stimulated cyclase activity in myocardial homogenates (4,27,47). In all cases in which the question has been investigated, GTP has been shown to be a requirement for muscarinic cholinergic inhibition of adenylate cyclase. Thus, GTP-induced perturbations in the binding of agonists to muscarinic receptors may represent an activation of the linkage or a "functional" inverse coupling of the

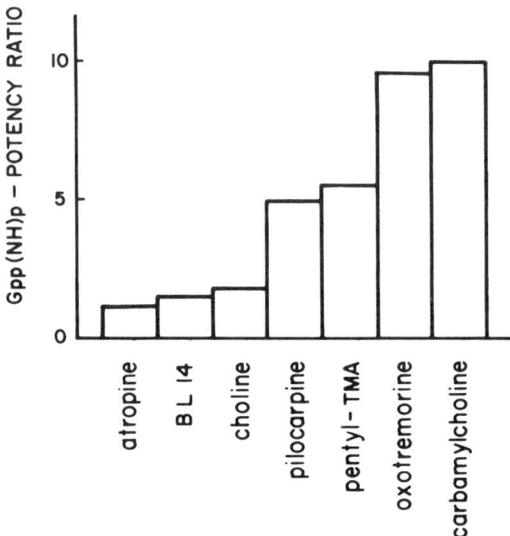

**FIG. 6.** Effect of Gpp(NH)p on the binding of a series of cholinergic analogs to the longitudinal muscle of the rat ileum. The competitive inhibition of [³H]QNB binding by a series of cholinergic analogs was determined in the rat ileum in the presence and absence of 100 μM Gpp(NH)p. $IC_{50}$'s for each drug were determined from 5 to 9 point competition curves, and the ratio of $IC_{50}$ values of a given drug, determined in the presence and absence of Gpp(NH)p, were calculated. The ordinate [Gpp(NH)p–potency ratio] refers to the magnitude of these ratios. The various cholinergic analogs are listed generally in the order of their efficacy starting on the left with the antagonist atropine and ending on the right with the highly efficacious agonist carbachol. Abbreviations used: BL14, N-(5-pyrrolidino-3-pentynyl)-succinimide; pentyl-TMA, N-pentyl-N,N,N-trimethylammonium. (The data are from Ehlert et al., ref. 13, and the figure is reprinted from Ehlert et al., ref. 18, with permission.)

muscarinic receptor with adenylate cyclase (3,40,41). In cardiac homogenates, muscarinic agonists reverse the GTP-induced reduction in the potency of isoproterenol for inhibition of [$^3$H]dihydroalprenolol binding to β-adrenergic receptors, and this effect was correlated with a muscarinic receptor-mediated inhibition of isoproterenol-stimulated cyclase activity (47). Both of these muscarinic effects were blocked by atropine. Interestingly, a similar adrenergic-cholinergic receptor interaction has been described with regard to $\alpha_1$-adrenergic receptor binding in the heart (52). The selective effects of muscarinic agonists on the binding of β-adrenergic agonists suggests that a complementary interaction may function for muscarinic receptors in the heart. Such an interaction was detected in this laboratory during a study of the effects of ( − )isoproterenol on oxotremorine/[$^3$H]( − )QNB competition curves in the heart (39,42). It was noted that isoproterenol ($10^{-6}$ M) caused a reduction in the proportion and affinity of high affinity sites in the rat heart. Figure 7 shows clearly that a small population (24.4%) of high affinity (19.8 nM) sites are converted to lower affinity by ( − )isoproterenol and that this effect can be blocked by ( − )propranolol. $Mg^{2+}$ is an essential component of the buffer system. In the absence of the ion (when all other conditions are the same), there are significant changes in both the $K_H$ and the $K_L$ change as well as the proportion of high affinity sites recognized by oxotremorine: $K_H$ 20 to 77 nM; $K_L$ 2074 to 4224 nM; and percentage of high affinity sites from 24.4 to 46.1. Furthermore, in the absence of $Mg^{2+}$ no regulatory effect of ( − )isoproterenol can be detected. The effect of ( − )isoproterenol also cannot be detected if the membranes are treated with Gpp(NH)p.

Recently, we have studied membranes of rat heart homogenates for the presence of an inversely coupled adenylate cyclase system. Using a standard membrane

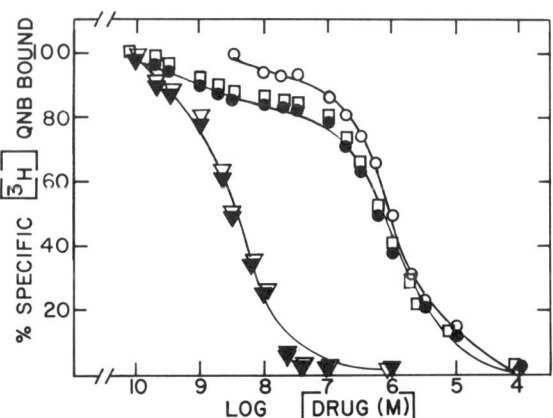

**FIG. 7.** The effect of isoproterenol and/or propranolol on the binding parameters of oxotremorine sesquifumarate or atropine sulfate in competition with [$^3$H]( − )QNB. Drug concentrations range from 0.1 nM to 100 μM. *Closed circles,* oxotremorine; *open circles,* oxotremorine + ( − )isoproterenol (1 μM); *open squares,* oxotremorine + ( − )isoproterenol (1 μM) + ( − )propranolol (1 μM); *open triangles,* atropine sulfate; *closed triangles,* atropine sulfate + ( − )isoproterenol (1 μM). Each point represents the mean of 8 to 10 experiments performed in duplicate. Assay conditions are specified in ref. 42.

preparation and a measurement of cyclic adenosine monophosphate (cAMP) performed by a radioimmunoassay, we have confirmed the presence of such a system in membranes that are similar to our source for the receptor studies outlined above. Specifically, we have noted that oxotremorine sesquifumarate (1 μM) can elicit a 40 percent decrease in the cAMP generated in the presence of 1 μM (−)isoproterenol, 90 mM NaCl, and 30 μM GTP (Rosenberger et al., *in preparation*). Both sodium ion and GTP are important in eliciting the maximal effect in agreement with Jakobs et al. (27). The interactions among adenylate cyclase, GTP regulatory proteins, $Mg^{2+}$, $Na^+$ β-adrenergic receptors, and muscarinic receptors illustrate a "functional" coupling between these macromolecules. Muscarinic receptor-mediated inhibition of adenylate cyclase in the heart is proportional to receptor occupancy of the low affinity agonist state of the receptor ($K_L \simeq K_i$ (4,27). This relationship suggests that the GTP-induced low affinity agonist state of the muscarinic receptor is directly coupled to the catalytic site (C). A possible reaction scheme is given below:

$$\text{high affinity} \quad \text{HRN} + \text{GTP} \rightleftharpoons \text{HRN-GTP} \quad \text{low affinity} \quad (1)$$

$$\begin{array}{c} \text{HRN} + \text{C} \rightleftharpoons \text{HRNC} \\ | \quad\quad\quad\quad\quad + \\ \text{GTP} \quad\quad\quad\quad \text{GTP} \end{array} \quad (2)$$

in which the GTP-bound HRNC complex represents a low affinity agonist state of the muscarinic receptor and an inactive form of the cyclase. Although this model is incomplete, since it does not describe the equilibrium between the various macromolecular components of the system (R, N, and C) or its relationship to ions or the β-adrenergic receptor, it does predict that the dissociation of GTP from the HRNC complex should result in a simultaneous reversal of the effects of GTP on agonist binding and adenylate cyclase inhibition. In contrast, the effects of guanine nucleotides on the binding of agonists to receptors that stimulate adenylate cyclase are readily reversible as compared with the duration of cyclase activation by guanine nucleotides (43,50).

## REGULATION OF ANTAGONIST BINDING BY DOPAMINERGIC AGONISTS

Under conditions in which antagonist receptor heterogeneity is readily demonstrable, dopaminergic agonists enhance the binding of [$^3$H](−)QNB by an apparent conversion of low to high affinity antagonist sites (16,17). This phenomenon is illustrated by the data in Fig. 8, which shows the effects of 1 μM apomorphine on [$^3$H](−)QNB binding in 50 mM NaHEPES buffer containing 10 mM $Mg^{2+}$ and 10 μM Gpp(NH)p. The control binding isotherm deviates from a simple Langmuir isotherm. The Hill coefficient is approximately 0.69. Weighted nonlinear regression analysis showed that these data were consistent with the presence of two binding sites with 57% of the sites having a high affinity dissociation constant of 0.03 nM

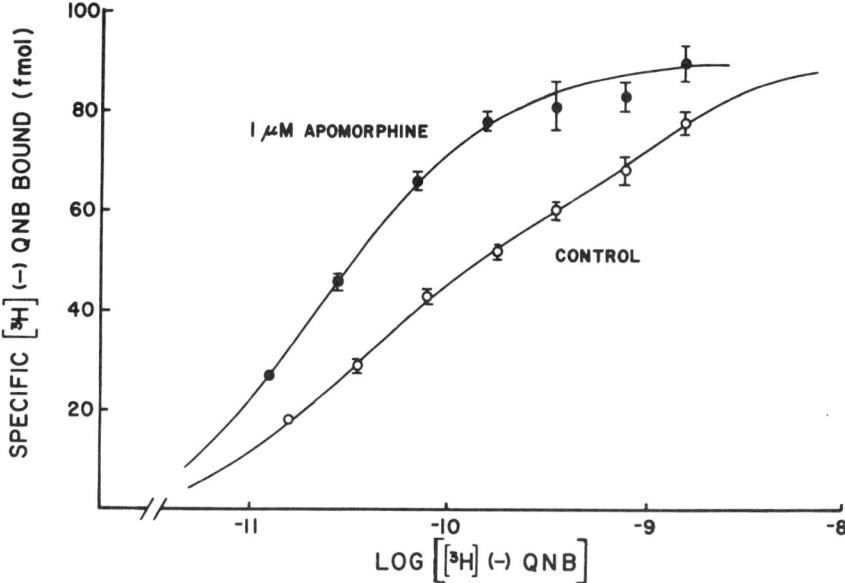

**FIG. 8.** Effect of apomorphine on [$^3$H](−)QNB binding to homogenates of the rat striatium. The binding of [$^3$H](−)QNB was measured in the presence *(closed circles)* and absence *(open circles)* of 1 μM apomorphine. Incubations were carried for 2 hr at 25°C in 50 mM Na HEPES, pH 7.4, containing 10 mM MgCl$_2$ and 10 μM Gpp(NH)p. Mean binding values ± SEM of four individual experiments are shown. (The data are from ref. 16 and the figure is reprinted from Ehlert et al., ref. 18, with permission.)

and the remaining sites having a low affinity dissociation constant of 0.64 nM. Under the assay conditions described above, this manifestation of antagonist receptor heterogeneity required Mg$^{2+}$. Inclusion of 1 μM apomorphine into the incubation media caused an enhancement of [$^3$H](−)QNB binding by an apparent conversion of low to high affinity sites. The resulting data were entirely consistent with that predicted for a single population of high affinity sites having a dissociation constant ($K_D$ = 0.025 nM) that is not significantly different from the value for the subpopulation of high affinity sites shown in the control curve. Although the implications of the dopaminergic regulation of muscarinic receptor binding are not readily apparent, the effect appears to be primarily specific for dopaminergic agonists since, of all the drugs tested, apomorphine, *N*-propylnorapomorphine, and dopamine were the most potent.

## IONIC EFFECTS ON MUSCARINIC RECEPTOR BINDING

The complex effects of ions on the muscarinic receptor have been recently reviewed (18). As noted above, Mg$^{2+}$ is extremely important in the demonstration of the guanine effect, the apomorphine effect, and the isoproterenol effect on antagonist binding. Interestingly, multiple antagonist affinity states can be seen best in conditions of low ionic strength with Mg$^{2+}$ present. The effect of sodium ion on the inversely coupled response of the adenylate cyclase has been discussed above and an apparently selective effect for sodium ion in cardiac membranes has been described (41).

We have noticed that under certain conditions we can apparently shift the multiple agonist affinity states into a single population of homogenous, low affinity sites. Figure 9 demonstrates the effect of 1 μM Gpp(NH)p and of 10 mM NaF on oxotremorine sesquifumarate displacement of [$^3$H]( − )QNB in a buffer containing $Mg^{2+}$ (the same assay conditions as in Fig. 7 and specified in ref. 42). Under basal conditions, there were 16% high affinity sites with a $K_H$ of 14.5 nM which is similar to previous experiments (Fig. 7, ref. 42). Gpp(NH)p, 1 μM, reduced the percent of high affinity sites to 4.5% and shifted the $K_H$ to 2285 nM while also shifting the $K_L$ to 3734 nM (all significantly different from control, $p < 0.01$). NaF alone, 10 mM, shifted the high affinity population ($K_H = 85.6$ nM). However, with both 1 μM Gpp(NH)p and 10 mM NaF, the high affinity population was essentially abolished and a single population (Hill coefficient = 0.98) of low affinity ($K_L = 3850$ nM) sites were obtained.

## FUTURE DIRECTIONS

We have demonstrated clearly that biochemical methods can identify a relevant muscarinic receptor in a wide variety of tissues and species. Useful probes such as [$^3$H]( − )QNB are also supplemented by other ligands (18) and by new ligands, such as [$^3$H]( − )NMQNB ([$^3$H]( − )N-methyl-3-quinuclidinyl benzilate), which we have recently shown to bind specifically to muscarinic receptors (Fig. 10).

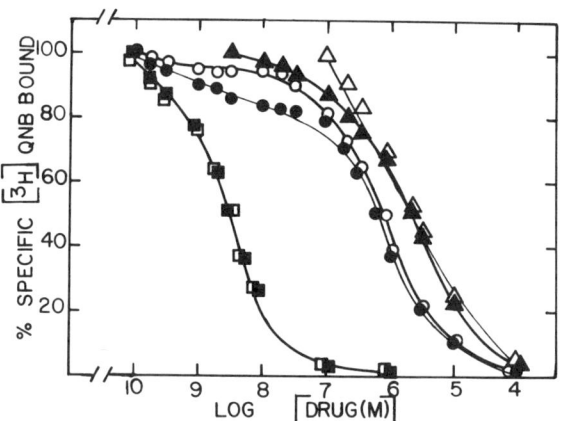

**FIG. 9.** The effect of Gpp(NH)p and NaF on the binding parameters of oxotremorine sesquifumarate and atropine sulfate in competition with [$^3$H]( − )QNB. Drug concentrations range from 0.1 nM to 100 μM. *Closed circles,* oxotremorine sesquifumarate; *open circles,* oxotremorine sesquifumarate + 10 mM NaF; *closed triangles,* oxotremorine sesquifumarate + 1 μM Gpp(NH)p; *open triangles,* oxotremorine sesquifumarate + 1 μM Gpp(NH)p + 10 mM NaF; *open squares,* atropine sulfate; *closed squares,* atropine sulfate + 10 mM NaF. Each point represents the mean of 5 to 10 experiments performed in duplicate. The assay and buffer conditions are the same as in Fig. 7.

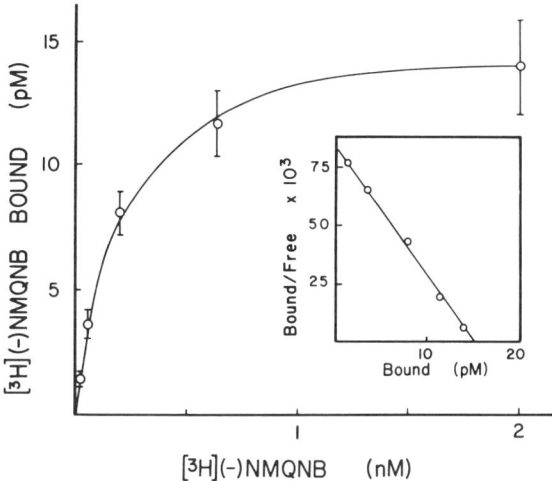

**FIG. 10.** The binding of [$^3$H](−)N-methyl-3-quinuclidinyl benzilate ([$^3$H](−)NMQNB) to the muscarinic receptors of homogenates of the forebrains of rats. Specific binding was defined by 10 μM atropine sulfate. The incubation was 1 hr at 37°C in a volume of 2 ml containing 50 mM NaK phosphate buffer, pH 7.4. The receptor concentration in the assay was 15 pM. Each point represents the mean ± SEM of three experiments each done in triplicate. The inset shows a Scatchard plot of the data. ($K_d$ = 0.18 mM and a $B_{max}$ of 15 pM which is equivalent to 60 fmoles/mg tissue or 0.77 pmoles/mg protein.)

The diversity of agonist and antagonist heterogeneity and regulation suggests that muscarinic recognition sites are coupled in differing proportions to several effectors in different tissues (18,39). A major challenge is to separate these effector systems from their regulatory systems and recognition sites. When this is achieved and when reconstituted membrane receptor-regulatory-effector systems are obtained, then we will finally understand the true meaning of the multiple agonist and antagonist affinity states as described in this chapter.

## ACKNOWLEDGMENTS

We thank Isabelle Preiss, Cheryl Bahrychuk, and Patricia Johnson for secretarial assistance. The work was supported by United States Public Health Service Grants MH-27257, MH-30626, and Program Project Grant HL-20984. William R. Roeske is a recipient of a United States Public Health Service Research Scientist Development Award (HL-00776) from the National Heart, Lung and Blood Institute, and Henry I. Yamamura is a recipient of a United States Public Health Service Research Scientist Development Award, Type II (MH-00095), from the National Institute of Mental Health.

## REFERENCES

1. Barritt, D., Roeske, W. R., Yamamura, S., and Yamamura, H. I. (1981): Postnatal development and regulation of the muscarinic receptor in the mouse heart using the agonist [$^3$H]cis methyldioxolane. *Fed. Proc.*, 40:488.

2. Beld, A. J., and Ariens, E. J. (1974): Stereospecific binding as a tool in attempts to localize and isolate muscarinic receptors. II. Binding of (+)benzetimide, (-)benzetimide and atropine to a fraction from bovine tracheal smooth muscle and to bovine caudate nucleus. *Eur. J. Pharmacol.*, 25:203–209.
3. Berrie, C. P., Birdsall, N. J. M., Burgen, A. S. V., and Hulme, E. C. (1979): Guanine nucleotides modulate muscarinic receptor binding in the heart. *Biochem. Biophys. Res. Commun.*, 87: 1000–1005.
4. Birdsall, N. J. M., Berrie, C. P., Burgen, A. S. V., and Hulme, E. C. (1980): Modulation of the binding properties of muscarinic receptors: evidence for receptor-effector coupling. In: *Receptors for Neurotransmitters and Peptide Hormones*, edited by G. Pepeu, M. J. Kuhar, and S. J. Enna, pp. 107–116. Raven Press, New York.
5. Birdsall, N. J. M., Burgen, A. S. V., and Hulme, E. C. (1977): Correlation between the binding properties and pharmacological responses of muscarinic receptors. In: *Cholinergic Mechanisms and Psychopharmacology*, edited by D. J. Jenden, pp. 25–33. Plenum Press, New York.
6. Birdsall, N. J. M., Burgen, A. S. V., and Hulme, E. C. (1978): The binding of agonists to brain muscarinic receptors. *Mol. Pharmacol.*, 14:723–736.
7. Birdsall, N. J. M., Hulme, E. C., (1976): Biochemical studies on muscarinic acetylcholine receptors. *J. Neurochem.*, 27:7–16.
8. Birdsall, N. J. M., Hulme, E. C., and Burgen, A. S. V. (1980): The character of muscarinic receptors in different regions of the rat brain. *Proc. R. Soc. Lond.*, 207:1–12.
9. Birdsall, N. J. M., Hulme, E. C., Hammer, R., and Stockton, J. S. (1980): Subclasses of muscarinic receptors. In: *Psychopharmacology and Biochemistry of Neurotransmitter Receptors*, edited by H. I. Yamamura, R. W. Olsen, and E. Usdin, pp. 97–100. Elsevier/North-Holland, New York.
10. Blume, A. J., Chen, C., and Foster, C. J. (1977): Muscarinic regulation of cAMP in mouse neuroblastoma. *J. Neurochem.*, 29:625–632.
11. Ehlert, F. J., Dumont, Y., Roeske, W. R., and Yamamura, H. I. (1980): Muscarinic receptor binding in rat brain using the agonist, [$^3$H]*cis* methyldioxolane. *Life Sci.*, 26:961–967.
12. Ehlert, F. J., Roeske, W. R., Rosenberger, L. B., and Yamamura, H. I. (1980): The influence of guanyl-5'-yl imidodiphosphate and sodium on muscarinic receptor binding in the rat brain and longitudinal muscle of the rat ileum. *Life Sci.*, 26:245–252.
13. Ehlert, F. J., Roeske, W. R., and Yamamura, H. I. (1980): Regulation of muscarinic receptor binding by guanine nucleotides and N-ethylmaleimide. *J. Supramol. Struct.*, 14:149–162.
14. Ehlert, F. J., Roeske, W. R., and Yamamura, H. I. (1981): Muscarinic receptor: Regulation by guanine nucleotides, ions and N-ethylmaleimide. *Fed. Proc.*, 40:153–159.
15. Ehlert, F. J., Roeske, W. R., and Yamamura, H. I. (1983): The regulation of the muscarinic receptor by guanine nucleotides, ions and dopaminergic agonists. In: *Pharmacologic and Biochemical Aspects of Neurotransmitter Receptors*, edited by H. Yoshida, and H. I. Yamamura, pp. 27–42. Wiley, New York.
16. Ehlert, F. J., Roeske, W. R., and Yamamura, H. I. (1981): Striatal muscarinic receptors: regulation by dopaminergic agonists. *Life Sci.*, 28:2441–2448.
17. Ehlert, F. J., Roeske, W. R., and Yamamura, H. I. (1981): Dopaminergic regulation of muscarinic receptor binding in the corpus striatum. *Proc. West. Pharmacol. Soc.*, 24:93–95.
18. Ehlert, F. J., Roeske, W. R., and Yamamura, H. I. (1983): The nature of muscarinic receptor binding. In: *Handbook of Psychopharmacology*, Vol. 17, edited by L. Iversen, S. Iversen, and S. Snyder, pp.241–283. Plenum Press, New York.
19. Ehlert, F. J., Yamamura, H. I., Triggle, D. J., and Roeske, W. R. (1980): The influence of guanyl-5'-yl imidodiphosphate and sodium chloride on the binding of the muscarinic agonist, [$^3$H]*cis* methyldioxolane. *Eur. J. Pharmacol.*, 61:317–318.
20. Fields, J. Z., Roeske, W. R., Morkin, E., and Yamamura, H. I. (1978): Cardiac cholinergic receptors. *J. Biol. Chem.*, 253:3251–3258.
21. Galper, J. B., Klein, W., and Catterall, W. A. (1977): Muscarinic acetylcholine receptors in developing chick heart. *J. Biol. Chem.*, 252:8692–8699.
22. Galper, J. B., and Smith, T. W. (1980): Agonist and guanine nucleotide modulation of muscarinic cholinergic receptors in cultured heart cells. *J. Biol. Chem.*, 255:9571–9579.
23. Hammer, R., Berrie, C. P., Birdsall, N. J. M., Burgen, A. S. V., and Hulme, E. C. (1980): Pirenzepine distinguishes between different subclasses of muscarinic receptors. *Nature*, 283: 90–92.
24. Hulme, E. C., Berrie, C. P., Birdsall, N. J. M., and Burgen, A. S. V. (1980): Interactions of muscarinic receptors with guanine nucleotides and adenylate cyclase. In: *Drug Receptors and Their Effectors*, edited by N. J. M. Birdsall, pp. 23–34. MacMillan, London.

25. Hulme, E. C., Birdsall, N. J. M., Burgen, A. S. V., and Mehta, P. (1978): The binding of antagonists to brain muscarinic receptors. *Mol. Pharmacol.*, 14:737–750.
26. Jakobs, K. H. (1979): Inhibition of adenylate cyclase by hormones and neurotransmitters. *Mol. Cell. Endocrinol.*, 16:147–156.
27. Jakobs, K. H., Aktories, K., and Schultz, G. (1979): GTP-dependent inhibition of cardiac adenylate cyclase by muscarinic cholinergic agonists. *Naynyn-Schmiedebergs Arch. Pharmacol.*, 310:113–119.
28. Jakobs, K. H., Saur, W., and Schultz, G. (1976): Reduction of adenylate cyclase activity in lysates of human platelets by the alpha-adrenergic component of epinephrine. *J. Cyclic Nucleotide Res.*, 2:381–392.
29. Jakobs, K. H., Saur, W., and Schultz, G. (1978): Inhibition of platelet adenyl cyclase by epinephrine requires GTP. *FEBS Lett.*, 85:167–170.
30. Lichtshtein, D., Boone, G., and Blume, A. (1979): Muscarinic receptor regulation of NG108–15 adenylate cyclase: requirement for $Na^+$ and GTP. *J. Cyclic Nucleotide Res.*, 367–375.
31. Murad, F., Chi, Y. M., Rall, T. W., and Sutherland, E. W. (1962): The effect of catecholamines and choline esters on the formation of adenosine $3'$-$5'$-phosphate by preparations from cardiac muscle and liver. *J. Biol. Chem.*, 237:1233–1238.
32. Paton, W. D., and Rang, H. P. (1965): The uptake of atropine and related drugs by intestinal smooth muscle of the guinea pig in relation to acetylcholine receptors. *Proc. R. Soc. London*, 163B:1–44.
33. Rodbell, M. (1980): The role of hormone receptors and GTP-regulatory proteins in membrane transduction. *Nature*, 284:17–22.
34. Rodbell, M., Krans, H. M. S., Pohl, S. L., and Birnbaumer, L. (1971): The glucagon-sensitive adenylate cyclase system in plasma membranes of rat liver. *J. Biol. Chem.*, 246:1861–1871.
35. Roeske, W. R., Chen, F. M., and Yamamura, H. I. (1979): Development of autonomic receptors in the fetal mouse heart. In: *Catecholamines: Basic and Clinical Frontiers, Vol. I*, edited by E. Usdin, I. Kopin, and J. Barchas, pp. 779–781. Pergamon Press, New York.
36. Roeske, W. R., Yamamura, H. I., and Yamada, S.(1981): Post-synaptic β-adrenergic receptors increase and pre-synaptic muscarinic receptors decrease in splenic tissue after 6-hydroxydopamine treatment. *Fed. Proc.*, 40:260.
37. Roeske, W. R., and Wildenthal, K. (1981): Responsiveness to drugs and hormones in the murine model of ontogenesis. *Pharm. Ther.*, 14:55–66.
38. Roeske, W. R., and Yamamura, H. I. (1978): Maturation of mammalian myocardial muscarinic receptors. *Life Sci.*, 23:127–132.
39. Roeske, W. R., and Yamamura, H. I. (1980): Muscarinic cholinergic receptor regulation. In: *Psychopharmacology and Biochemistry of Neurotransmitter Receptors*, edited by H. I. Yamamura, R. W. Olsen, and E. Usdin, pp. 101–114. Elsevier/North-Holland Biomedical Press, New York.
40. Rosenberger, L. B., Roeske, W. R., and Yamamura, H. I. (1979): The regulation of muscarinic cholinergic receptors by guanine nucleotides in cardiac tissue. *Eur. J. Pharmacol.*, 56:179–180.
41. Rosenberger, L. B., Yamamura, H. I., and Roeske, W. R. (1980): Cardiac muscarinic cholinergic receptor binding is regulated by $Na^+$ and guanyl nucleotides. *J. Biol. Chem.*, 255:820–823.
42. Rosenberger, L. B., Yamamura, H. I., and Roeske, W. R. (1980): The regulation of cardiac muscarinic cholinergic receptors by isoproterenol. *Eur. J. Pharmacol.*, 65:129–130.
43. Ross, E. M., Maguire, M. E., Sturgill, T. W., Biltonen, R. L., and Gilman, A. G. (1977): Relationship between the β-adrenergic receptor and adenylate cyclase. *J. Biol. Chem.*, 252:5761–5775.
44. Snyder, S. H., Chang, K. J., Kuhar, M. J., and Yamamura, H. I. (1975): Biochemical identification of the mammalian muscarinic cholinergic receptor. *Fed. Proc.*, 34:1915–1921.
45. Sokolovsky, M., Gurwitz, D., and Galron, R. (1980): Muscarinic receptor binding in mouse brain: regulation of guanine nucleotides. *Biochem. Biophys. Res. Commun.*, 94:487–492.
46. Triggle, D. J. (1979): The muscarinic receptor: structural, ionic and biochemical implications. In: *Recent Advances in Receptor Chemistry*, edited by F. Gualtieri, M. Giannella, and C. Melchiorre, pp. 127–146. Elsevier/North-Holland, New York.
47. Watanabe, A. M., McConnaughey, M. M., Strawbridge, R. A., Fleming, J. W., Jones, L. R., and Besch, H. R. (1978): Muscarinic cholinergic receptor modulation of β-adrenergic receptor affinity for catecholamines. *J. Biol. Chem.*, 253:4833–4836.
48. Wei, J. W., and Sulakhe, P. V. (1979): Agonist-antagonist interactions with rat atrial muscarinic cholinergic receptor sites: Differential regulation by guanine nucleotides. *Eur. J. Pharmacol.*, 58:91–92.

49. Wei, J. W., and Sulakhe, P. V. (1980): Cardiac muscarinic cholinergic receptor sites: opposing regulation by divalent cations and guanine nucleotides of receptor-agonist interaction. *Eur. J. Pharmacol.*, 62:345–347.
50. Welton, A. F., Lad, P. M., Newby, A. C., Yamamura, H., Nicosia, S., and Rodbell, M. (1977): Solubilization and separation of the glucagon receptor and adenylate cyclase in guanine nucleotide-sensitive states. *J. Biol. Chem.*, 252:5947–5950.
51. Wilkening, D., Sabol, S. L., and Nirenberg, M. (1980): Control of opiate receptor-adenylate cyclase interactions by calcium ions and guanosine-5'-triphosphate. *Brain Res.*, 189:459–466.
52. Yamada, S., Yamamura, H. I., and Roeske, W. R. (1980): The regulation of cardiac $\alpha_1$-adrenergic receptors by guanine nucleotides and muscarinic cholinergic agonists. *Eur. J. Pharmacol.*, 63:239–241.
53. Yamamura, H. I., and Snyder, S. H. (1974): Muscarinic cholinergic binding in rat brain. *Proc. Natl. Acad. Sci. USA*, 71:1725–1729.
54. Yamamura, H. I., and Snyder, S. H. (1974): Muscarinic cholinergic receptor binding in the longitudinal muscle of the guinea pig ileum with [$^3$H]quinuclidinyl benzilate. *Mol. Pharmacol.*, 10:861–867.

Molecular Pharmacology of Neurotransmitter
Receptors, edited by T. Segawa et al.
Raven Press, New York © 1983.

# Muscarinic Acetylcholine Receptors in Smooth Muscles: Regulation of Contraction and Molecular Nature

### Shuji Uchida, Kunio Takeyasu, Hiroshi Higuchi, Kazuo Matsumoto, and Hiroshi Yoshida

*Department of Pharmacology I, Osaka University School of Medicine, Osaka 530, Japan*

In tissues under the control of neurotransmitters and hormones, cells adapt to persistent or repetitive stimulation by a transient decrease in reactivity to stimulation—a phenomenon known as "desensitization." Two types of desensitization have been recognized. One is short-term desensitization, in which the decrease of reactivity occurs within minutes and the reactivity is restored immediately after the stimulation is stopped. The other is long-term desensitization, in which the onsent and restoration of reactivity occur over periods of hours or days. The former type is thought to be caused by conformational change of the receptor molecule, and latter by change in the number of receptors or amount of some protein concerned in coupling between the receptor and its reaction.

We studied the mechanism of long-term desensitization of muscarinic acetylcholine receptors (mAChR) in smooth muscle and brain. We found that a change in the number of mAChR was paralleled with that of contraction to cholinergic stimulation of smooth muscle in general and that long-term desensitization of the muscarinic cholinergic system was mainly due to a decrease in the number of mAChR (7,8,13,14,15,16).

The molecular nature of short-term desensitization is still unknown. However, it may involve the effect of guanine nucleotides on binding of the agonist to the receptors, since guanine nucleotides are known to reduce the affinity of agonists, but not antagonists, to many receptors, such as α-adrenergic, β-adrenergic, dopaminergic, muscarinic, and opiate receptors. Moreover, mAChR in heart (1), ileum (3), and brain (11) are regulated by guanine nucleotides.

This chapter describes studies on the different mechanisms of long-term desensitization of muscarinic and α-adrenergic systems. The specific inactivation of the effect of a guanine nucleotide by γ-ray irradiation or trypsin treatment and the role of guanine nucleotide binding protein in the muscarinic system are also discussed.

## CHANGES IN MUSCARINIC AND α-ADRENERGIC SYSTEMS DURING LONG-TERM DESENSITIZATION OF GUINEA PIG VAS DEFERENS IN ORGAN CULTURE

### Effects of Drugs on the Decrease of mAChR and the Contractile Response

In guinea pig vas deferens in organ culture, the number of mAChR, measured by the binding of 3-quinuclidinyl benzilate (QNB), was specifically decreased by addition of a muscarinic agonist to the culture medium. This change was associated with simultaneous decrease of the contraction to ACh as seen in Fig. 1. The long-term desensitization was very specific to the muscarinic system and the contractions by α-adrenergic agonists and high K$^+$ solution were not affected. The extent of this long-term desensitization depended on the doses and efficacies of the muscarinic agonists, indicating that the desensitization was caused through activation of mAChR (8). These changes in the receptor and contraction were due to stimulated degradation of mAChR (14). Therefore, we examined the effects of drugs that are thought to act on the degradation of membranous proteins.

As shown in Table 1, change in the number of mAChR was affected by drugs that inhibit clustering and endocytosis of membrane proteins and lysosomal functions. Dansylcadaverine, methylamine, ethylamine, and paraformaldehyde, which are all known to inhibit clustering and endocytosis of membrane receptors, prevented the decrease of mAChR induced by ACh in the culture medium. The antimicro-

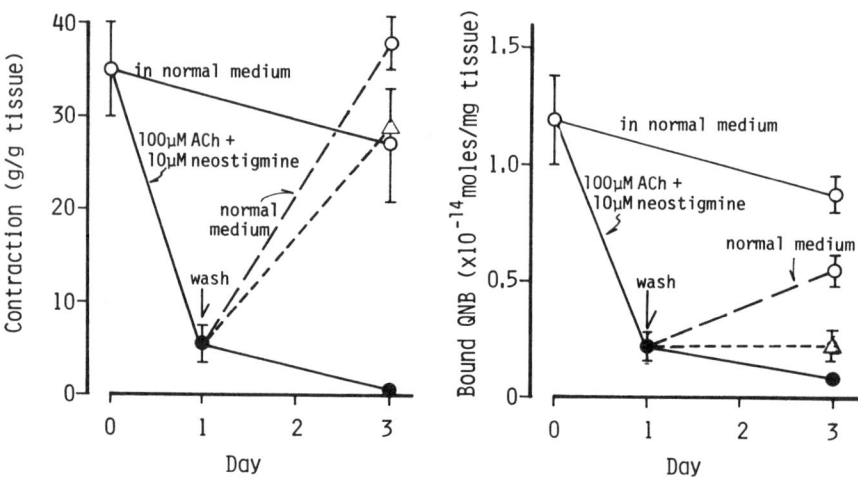

**FIG. 1.** Long-term desensitization and recovery of the muscarinic cholinergic system of guinea pig vas deferens in organ culture. **Left:** Contractions by 5 × 10$^{-5}$ M ACh at 20°C before and after organ culture. **Right:** Number of QNB binding sites (fmoles/mg tissue) in vas deferens used for measurements of contraction in A. Cultured in control medium (○—○); cultured with 10$^{-4}$ M ACh and 10$^{-5}$ M neostigmine (●—●); recovery after washing (○---○); recovery in the presence of cycloheximide (△---△). *Points* and *bars* are means ± SDM for eight measurements.

TABLE 1. Effects of various agents on the accelerated degradation of mAChR by ACh

| Agent | $B_{max}$ of [$^3$H]-QNB (pmoles/g tissue) | |
|---|---|---|
| Control | 11.2 ± 2.0 | (7) |
| ACh (27 μM) (24 hr) | 2.2 ± 0.6 | (8) |
| ACh (27 μM) + DMSO (1%) | 2.6 ± 0.8 | (8) |
| ACh (27 μM) + DC[a] (100 μM) + DMSO | 3.3 ± 0.8 | (4) |
| ACh (27 μM) + DC (500 μM) + DMSO | 6.0 ± 1.8 | (7) |
| ACh (27 μM) + methylamine (20 mM) | 7.7 ± 2.2 | (4) |
| ACh (27 μM) + ethylamine (20 mM) | 7.5 ± 2.6 | (4) |
| DC (500 μM) + DMSO | 11.1 ± 1.5 | (4) |
| Methylamine (20 mM) | 11.1 ± 0.6 | (4) |
| Ethylamine (20 mM) | 8.4 ± 1.4 | (4) |
| 1% Paraformaldehyde (10 min 37°C) | 12.1 ± 1.1 | (4) |
| ACh + 1% paraformaldehyde | 8.5 ± 2.8 | (8) |
| ACh (27 μM) + 2 × 10$^{-4}$ M chloroquine | 14.5 ± 3.5 | (4) |
| ACh (27 μM) + 10 mM NH$_4$Cl | 2.8 ± 0.8 | (3) |
| ACh (27 μM) + 10$^{-4}$ M vinblastine | 8.5 ± 3.4 | (6) |
| ACh (27 μM) + 5 mM colchicine | 8.8 ± 1.0 | (4) |
| ACh (27 μM) + 20 μM cytochalasin B | 3.7 ± 1.2 | (4) |
| ACh (9 hr) | 3.79 ± 1.08 | (8) |
| ACh + leupeptin (4.8 × 10$^{-5}$ M) | 3.62 ± 0.37 | (4) |
| ACh + antipain (1.7 × 10$^{-5}$ M) | 5.48 ± 1.11 | (8) |
| Chymostatin (1.7 × 10$^{-5}$ M) | 5.48 ± 1.11 | (8) |
| Pepstatin A (1.8 × 10$^{-5}$ M) | 5.48 ± 1.11 | (8) |

[a] DC: dansylcadaverine.
Guinea pig vasa deferentia were cultured with the compounds indicated in Eagle's MEM with 5% calf serum being loaded tension passively. Incubation was carried out at 37°C under 95% $O_2$ and 5% $CO_2$ for 24 hr, except with the last group of compounds (9 hr).

tubular agents vinblastine and colchicine also blocked the decrease of mAChR. A lysosomotropic agent, chloroquine, strongly inhibited the accelerated degradation of mAChR.

These results indicate that the main pathway for decrease of mAChR is their disappearance from the membrane by endocytosis and degradation in lysosomes. However, another pathway may also be involved because even high doses of these drugs did not inhibit receptor degradation completely.

As stated above, change in the number of mAChR was usually paralleled with that of the contractile response in long-term desensitization. However, when chloroquine was added to the medium for desensitization, there was a large discrepancy between the number of mAChR and the contractile response, as shown in Fig. 2: Although chloroquine prevented ACh-induced decrease in the number of mAChR, it did not affect a decrease in the contraction by ACh. Moreover, the contractions induced by high K$^+$ and norepinephrine were not decreased under these conditions,

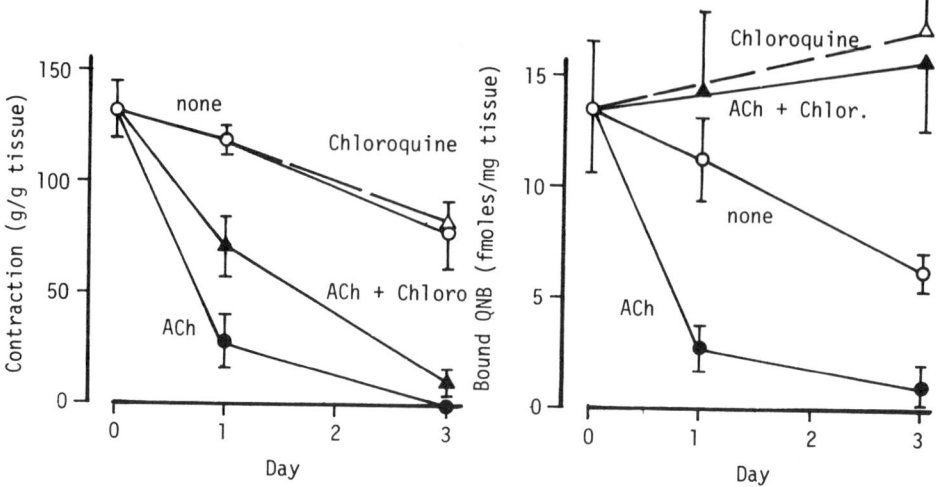

**FIG. 2.** Effect of chloroquine on long-term desensitization of the muscarinic system. Tissues were cultured with $2.7 \times 10^{-5}$ M ACh and $2 \times 10^{-4}$ M chloroquine. After measurement of the contraction (**left**), the binding of QNB was assayed (**right**). *Open circles*, control; *filled circles*, cultured with $2.7 \times 10^{-5}$ M ACh; *filled triangles*, ACh + $2 \times 10^{-4}$ M chloroquine; *open triangles*, chloroquine.

indicating that decreased contraction was not due to nonspecific inactivation of smooth muscle by chloroquine. Vinblastine had a similar effect to chloroquine.

These data suggest that, in addition to control of the number of mAChR, another factor between the receptor and contractile protein is involved in adaptation of smooth muscle to overstimulation of the cholinergic system. The presence of two systems of regulation may keep the safety level high and may cooperate in producing a suitable response to nervous activity.

## Difference in Long-Term Desensitizations of Muscarinic and α-Adrenergic Contractions

In guinea pig vas deferens, α-adrenergic stimulation as well as muscarinic stimulation causes contraction. Short-term and long-term desensitization also occur in the α-adrenergic system in this tissue. When tissue was cultured in medium containing norepinephrine it lost sensitivity to norepinephrine and the time course of this desensitization was similar to that of muscarinic desensitization. However, unlike muscarinic desensitization, α-adrenergic receptors measured by assay of binding of $^3$H-WB4101 did not change during the desensitization, as shown in Fig. 3. Norepinephrine caused some heterologous desensitization of the muscarinic system in which mAChR was also not changed. High $K^+$ (100 mM)-induced contraction was not affected in the above condition, indicating no change in the system from depolarization of membranes to contractile proteins.

The involvement of protein synthesis in the development of this desensitization was suggested by the fact that cycloheximide and puromycin in the culture medium prevented the desensitization by norepinephrine.

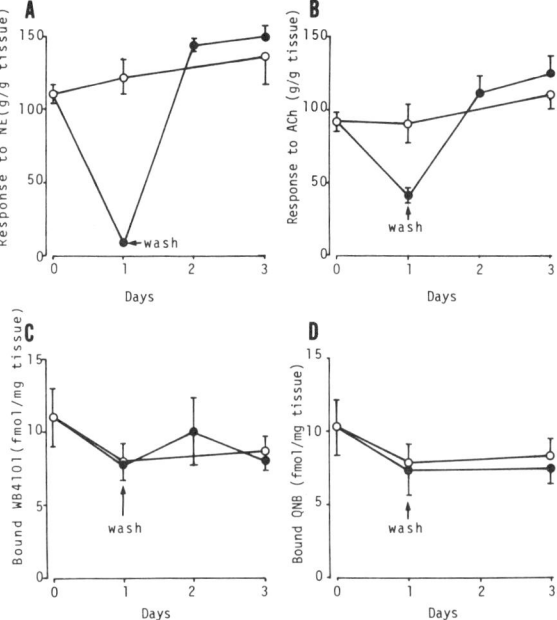

**FIG. 3.** Long-term desensitization of guinea pig vas deferens induced by norepinephrine. **A:** Maximal contraction induced by $5 \times 10^{-5}$ M norepinephrine. **B:** Maximal contraction induced by $5 \times 10^{-5}$ M ACh. **C:** Number of α-adrenergic receptors measured by binding of WB4101. **D:** Number of mAChR measured by binding of QNB.

The above data indicate that there are at least two different types of long-term desensitization. One is caused by a change in the number of receptors, as seen in the muscarinic system, and the other by a change in the amount of a protein other than the receptor which is a part of a coupling system between receptor excitation and membrane depolarization.

## EFFECTS OF GUANINE NUCLEOTIDE ON mACHR

### Effect of Guanyl-5'-yl-imidodiphosphate on mAChR in Guinea Pig Ileum

As in many other tissues, binding of agonists to mAChR in microsomal fractions of smooth muscle in guinea pig ileum was affected by guanyl-5'-yl-imidodiphosphate [Gpp(NH)p]. As shown in Fig. 4, Gpp(NH)p reduced the affinity of carbachol, measured by determining inhibition of $^3$H-QNB binding, but had no effect on the antagonist, atropine, or the $K_D$ value of QNB binding. The Hill coefficient of the inhibition by carbachol was increased dose-dependently by Gpp(NH)p.

Guanine nucleotide should have an important role in the muscarinic cholinergic system. Several possible roles of this compound are as follows: (a) control of the transition between the sensitized and desensitized states of receptor molecule, namely the regulation of short-term desensitization; (b) negative coupling between mAChR and adenylate cyclase; (c) as a carrier of the signal from mAChR to an effector

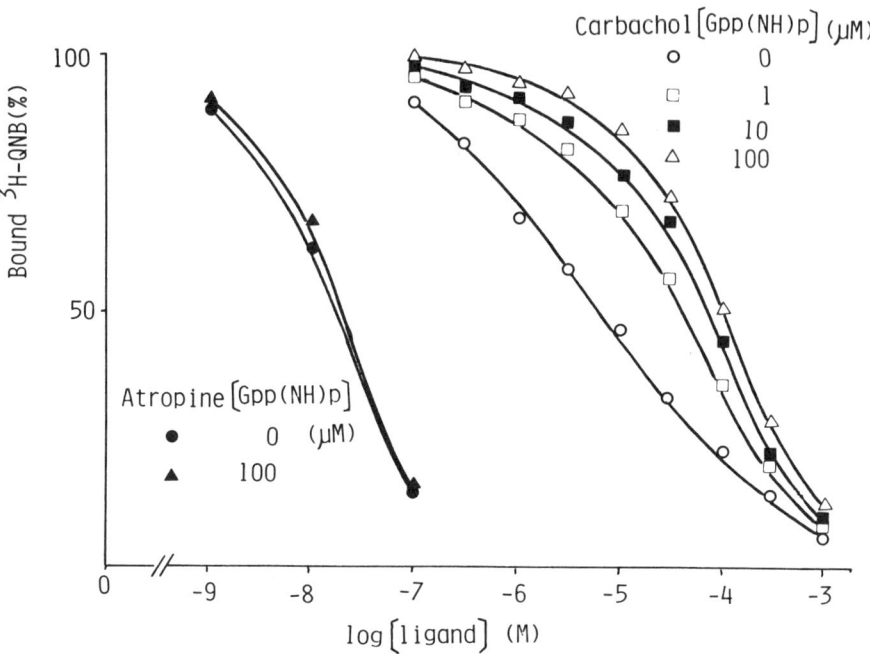

**FIG. 4.** Effect of Gpp(NH)p on inhibition of QNB binding by carbachol and atropine. Microsomal fractions of guinea pig ileum were preincubated with Gpp(NH)p in medium containing 100 mM NaCl, 50 mM Tris-HCl (pH 7.4) and 1 mM MgCl$_2$ at 37°C for 10 min and then binding of QNB was started by addition of $^3$H-QNB (0.7 nM) at 37°C for 15 min. Bound QNB was measured by the filtration method using a GF/F filter (Whatman). All points after this figure indicate means of 3 to 5 measurements within 5% deviation.

other than adenylate cyclase. We tried to clarify the molecular nature of the effect of guanine nucleotide on mAChR in smooth muscles.

## Radiation Inactivation of mAChR

In the β-adrenergic system, it is well known that a guanosine triphosphate (GTP)-binding protein acts as a mediator of the signal from the β-adrenergic receptor to adenylate cyclase. A GTP-binding protein on the disc membrane in the rod outer segment of retina also acts as a carrier of the signal from rhodopsin to phosphodiesterase and has been named transducin (4,17). In the mutant cell line of lymphoma cells, which is thought to lack the GTP-binding protein, guanine nucleotides did not affect the affinity of β-agonists for the receptor or activation of adenylate cyclase. Addition of an extract of wild-type lymphoma cells to these cell membranes restored the effect of guanine nucleotides on β-adrenergic receptor, suggesting that GTP binding protein regulates β-adrenergic receptors (12).

To determine whether guanine nucleotide acts directly on the ligand binding subunit in mAChR or indirectly through the GTP binding subunit, we used radiation inactivation by γ-rays of $^{60}$Co. The radiation inactivation method has been well established and used for determination of the molecular sizes of many proteins (9) including β-adrenergic receptor (10). The advantage of this method is that the functional molecular size can be determined without any purification procedure.

Figure 5 shows radiation inactivation curves of QNB binding and Gpp(NH)p effect at $10^{-6}$ M and $5 \times 10^{-6}$ M carbachol on the inhibition of QNB binding in guinea pig ileum. Both curves were linear on a semilogarithmic scale, suggesting that in each case the molecular size was homogeneous. The calculated molecular size for QNB binding was 75,800 ± 2,000 and that of the effect of Gpp(NH)p on the inhibition of QNB binding by carbachol was 179,000 ± 8,000. The molecular size for QNB binding was very similar to that reported by Birdsall et al. (2) (77,600 for guinea pig ileum), but smaller than those in other tissues reported by Birdsall et al. (2) and Haga (6).

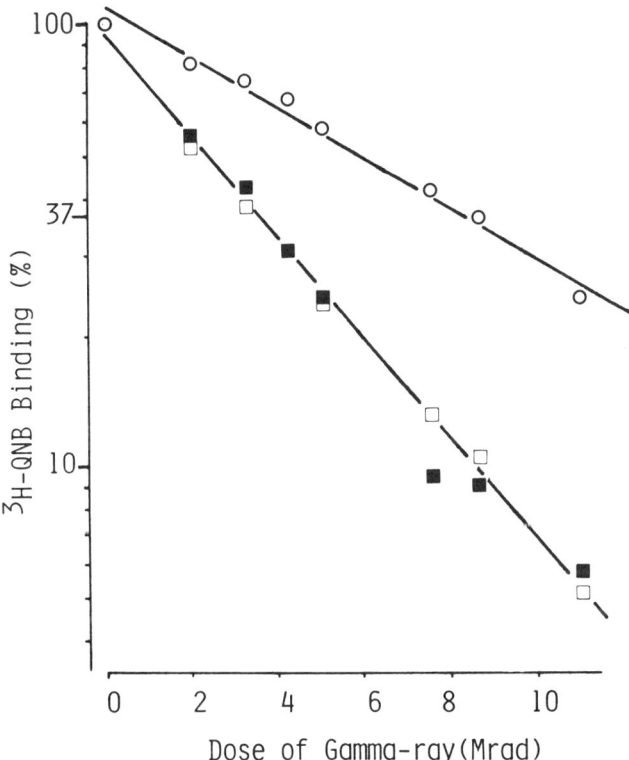

**FIG. 5.** Radiation inactivation of QNB binding and the effect of Gpp(NH)p on carbachol. Lyophilized microsomal fractions were irradiated *in vacuo* at room temperature from a $^{60}$Co source (200 Ci) for 50 hr. Samples were then suspended in 10 mM Tris-HCl (pH 7.4) and stored at −40°C until use. The effect of Gpp(NH)p was calculated from the difference between QNB binding with and without 100 μM Gpp(NH)p at $10^{-6}$ M and $5 \times 10^{-6}$ M carbachol. *Circles*, QNB binding; *filled squares*, Gpp(NH)p effect at $10^{-6}$ M carbachol; *open squares*, Gpp(NH)p effect at $5 \times 10^{-6}$ M carbachol.

On the other hand, the molecular size for the Gpp(NH)p effect was much greater than those for ligand bindings. This indicates that the binding site for guanine nucleotide is on another subunit than the ligand binding subunit. However, we could not calculate the size of the actual binding subunit for Gpp(NH)p from the difference between the two values because we did not know how many subunits were included in this phenomenon and what type of interaction there was among the subunits, i.e., tight coupling or so-called collision coupling.

We compared the shape of the inhibition curves of QNB binding by carbachol at various doses of γ-rays, as shown in Fig. 6. The affinities of carbachol became lower and Hill coefficients became higher with increase in the radiation dose. Therefore, with increase in the irradiation the shape of the curves became closer to that in the presence of Gpp(NH)p. These results indicate that damage of the subunit that binds guanine nucleotides by irradiation has the same effect as the binding of a guanine nucleotide to this subunit. These findings suggest that the ligand-binding subunit is released from control of the guanine nucleotide-binding subunit when guanine nucleotide binds to the subunit. This mechanism seems similar to that in the β-adrenergic system reported by Sternweis and Gilman (12).

Early studies on bindings to receptors raised the problem of why inhibition by agonists of binding of a radiolabeled antagonist was not simply competitive for the receptor and why the Hill coefficients of their curves were far less than unity. Now

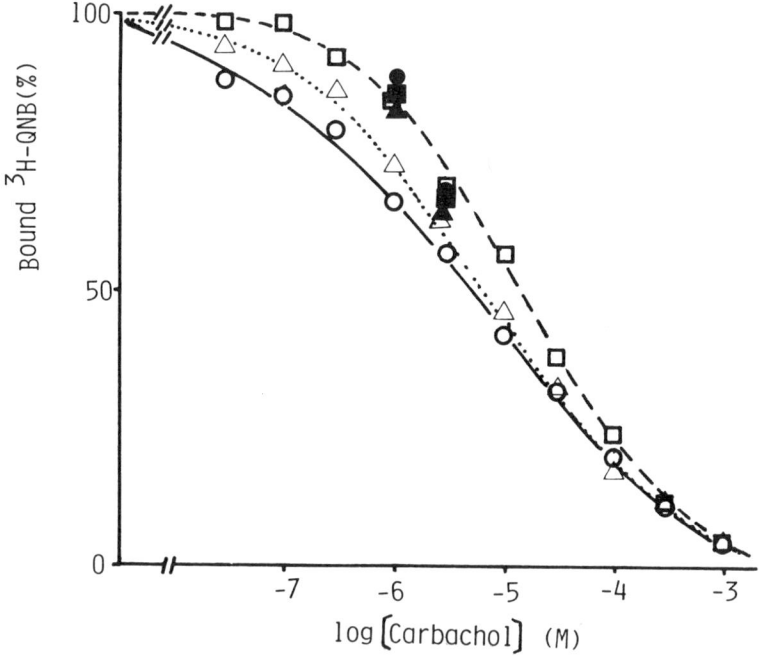

**FIG. 6.** Effect of irradiation on inhibition of QNB binding by carbachol. *Open circles*, 0 Mrad; *open triangles*, 5 Mrad; *open squares*, 8.7 Mrad. *Solid symbols* show QNB binding with 100 μM Gpp(NH)p.

this phenomenon can be explained by supposing that mAChR is a mixture of at least two subtypes or states which have different affinities for agonists, but the same affinities for antagonists.

On the basis of this hypothesis, the data in Fig. 6 were examined by nonlinear regression analysis. The results showed that the change in shape of the inhibition curve, namely change in the Hill coefficient, with the radiation dose, was mainly due to decrease in the ratio of the high affinity state (subtype) of mAChR, not to change in the affinity of either state. Further studies on the interactions of agonist and antagonist on mAChR are necessary to explain this finding.

### Specific Inactivation by Trypsin of the Effect of Guanine Nucleotide

In α-adrenergic receptors, proteolysis by trypsin specifically cancels the effect of guanine nucleotide (5). Trypsin had a similar effect on the muscarinic system.

As shown in Fig. 7, trypsin decreased the effect of Gpp(NH)p, without changing the affinity or amount of QNB binding. The affinity of carbachol for mAChR was decreased from an $IC_{50}$ value of 6.31 to 34.3 μM at 0.75 μM QNB and the Hill coefficient was increased from 0.47 to 0.64. As a result, in trypsin-treated membranes the inhibition curve of QNB binding by carbachol became similar to that of control membranes at the presence of Gpp(NH)p.

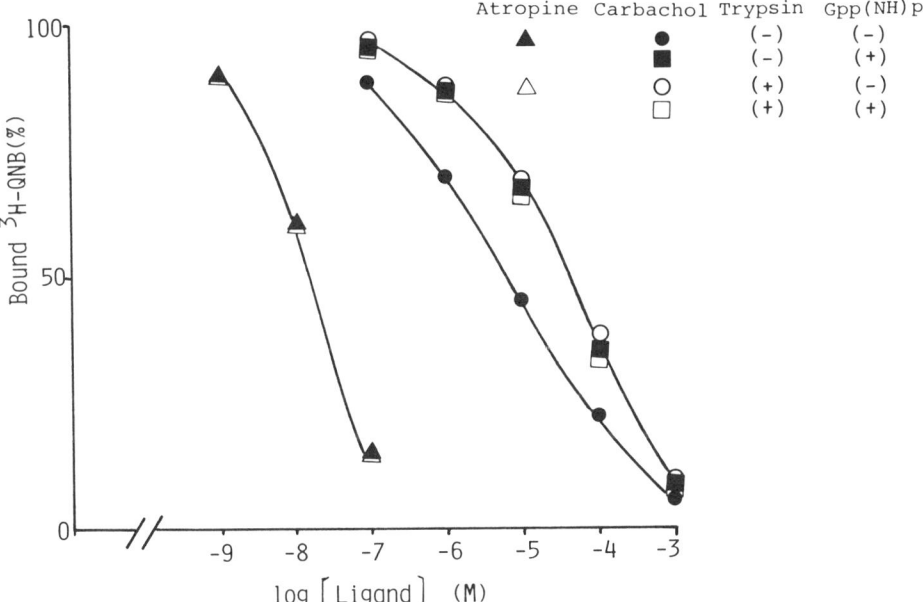

**FIG. 7.** Effect of trypsin treatment on inhibition of QNB binding by carbachol and atropine. Microsomal fractions were treated with trypsin (40 μg/mg protein) at 30°C for 20 min. Then trypsin inhibitor was added and assay of QNB binding was started by adding QNB. Inhibition by atropine *(open and filled triangles)*; inhibition by carbachol with *(open and filled circles)* or without *(open and filled squares)* Gpp(NH)p. *Open symbols* indicate trypsin treatment.

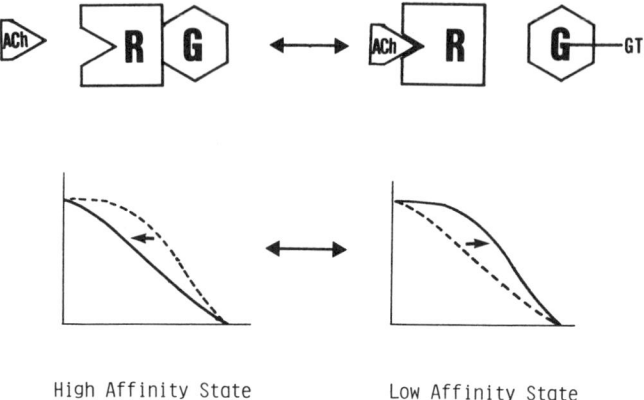

**FIG. 8.** Model of the effect of guanine nucleotide on mAChR.

This result indicates that proteolysis by trypsin-like radiation inactivation destroys some subunit that is involved in the guanine nucleotide effect or a part of the receptor subunit that functions in attachment to guanine nucleotide binding subunit.

Our work did not provide any information on the physiological role of the guanine nucleotide binding subunit. For information on this, more studies are required on the nature of the binding of guanine nucleotide and the interaction between mAChR and its direct reactions such as adenylate cyclase and phospholipid metabolism.

Figure 8 summarizes results on the effect of guanine nucleotides. In this scheme, the ligand binding subunit attached to the guanine nucleotide-binding subunit is in a high affinity state for agonist or in a condition with a high ratio of high affinity state. When a guanine nucleotide occupies this site, the ligand binding subunit is dissociated from the guanine nucleotide-binding subunit and takes a low affinity state or a condition with a low ratio of high affinity state. In this figure, the ACh molecule is drawn by analogy with the β-adrenergic system and rhodopsin–phosphodiesterase coupling system in eye. However, further studies are required on this interaction.

## ACKNOWLEDGMENTS

We thank Dr. Juzo Ohkuma and Mr. Toshiji Ikeda for technical assistance and helpful suggestions on γ-ray radiation, Mrs. M. Takano for programming of data analysis, and Mrs. Mieko Nakamura for help in preparation of this manuscript. This work was supported in part by a Grant-in-Aid for Scientific Research from the Ministry of Education, Science and Culture of Japan.

## REFERENCES

1. Berrie, C. P., Birdsall, N. J., Burgen, A. S., and Hulme, E. C. (1979): Guanine nucleotides modulate muscarinic receptor binding in the heart. *Biochem. Biophys. Res. Commun.*, 87: 1000–1005.

2. Birdsall, N. J. M., Burgen, A. S. V., and Hulme, E. C. (1979): A study of the muscarinic receptor by gel electrophoresis. *Br. J. Pharmacol.*, 66:337–342.
3. Ehlert, F., Rosenberger, L., Roeske, W., and Yamamura, H. I. (1979): The influence of sodium chloride and guanyl-5'-yl imidodiphosphate on muscarinic receptor binding. *Soc. Neurosci. Abstr.*, 5:401.
4. Fung, B. K.-K., Hurley, J. B., and Stryer, L. (1981): Flow information in the light-triggered cyclic nucleotide cascade of vision. *Proc. Natl. Acad. Sci. USA*, 78:152–156.
5. Geynet, P., Borsodi, A., Ferry, N., and Hanoune, J. (1980): Proteolysis of rat liver plasma membranes cancels the guanine nucleotide sensitivity of agonist binding to the alpha-adrenoceptor. *Biochem. Biophys. Res. Commun.*, 97:949–954.
6. Haga, T. (1980): Molecular size of muscarinic acetylcholine receptors of rat brain. *FEBS Lett.*, 113:68–72.
7. Hata, F., Takeyasu, K., Morikawa, Y., Lai, R.-T., Ishida, H., and Yoshida, H. (1980): Specific changes in cholinergic system in guinea pig vas deferens after denervation. *J. Pharmacol. Exp. Ther.*, 215:716–722.
8. Higuchi, H., Takeyasu, K., Uchida, S., and Yoshida, H. (1981): Receptor-activated and energy-dependent decrease of muscarinic cholinergic receptors in guinea-pig vas deferens. *Eur. J. Pharmacol. (in press)*.
9. Kempner, E. S., and Schlegel, W. (1979): Size determination of enzymes by radiation inactivation. *Anal. Biochem.*, 92:2–10.
10. Nielsen, T. B., Lad, R. M., Preston, M. S., Kempner, E., Schlegel, W., and Rodbell, M. (1981): Structure of the turkey erythrocyte adenylate cyclase system. *Proc. Natl. Acad. Sci. USA*, 78: 722–726.
11. Sokolovsky, M., Gurwitz, D., and Galron, R. (1980): Muscarinic receptor binding in mouse brain: Regulation by guanine nucleotides. *Biochem. Biophys. Res. Commun.*, 94:487–492.
12. Sternweis, P. C., and Gilman, A. G. (1979): Reconstitution of catecholamine-sensitive adenylate cyclase. *J. Biol. Chem.*, 254:3333–3340.
13. Takeyasu, K., Hata, F., Uchida, S., Higuchi, H., and Yoshida, H. (1981): Action of colchicine on cholinergic and adrenergic mechanisms in guinea pig vas deferens. *Life Sci.*, 28:851–861.
14. Takeyasu, K., Uchida, S., Lai, R.-T., Higuchi, H., Noguchi, Y., and Yoshida, H. (1981): Regulation of muscarinic acetylcholine receptors and contractility of guinea pig vas deferens. *Life Sci.*, 28:527–540.
15. Uchida, S., Takeyasu, K., Higuchi, H., and Yoshida, H. (1981): Muscarinic acetylcholine receptors and contractile responses in smooth muscle. In: *Neurotransmitter Receptors: Biochemical Aspect and Physiological Significance*, edited by H. I. Yamamura and H. Yoshida. Wiley, New York *(in press)*.
16. Uchida, S., Takeyasu, K., Matsuda, T., and Yoshida, H. (1979): Changes in muscarinic acetylcholine receptors of mice by chronic administration of diisopropylfluorophosphate and papaverine. *Life Sci.*, 24:1805–1812.
17. Uchida, S., Wheeler, G. L., Yamazaki, A., and Bitensky, M. W. (1981): A GTP-protein activator of phosphodiesterase which forms in response to bleached rhodopsin. *J. Cyclic Nucleotide Res. (in press)*.

*Molecular Pharmacology of Neurotransmitter Receptors*, edited by T. Segawa et al.
Raven Press, New York © 1983.

# Presynaptic Muscarinic Cholinergic and Postsynaptic β-Adrenergic Receptors in Splenic Tissue

Shizuo Yamada, Eiichi Hayashi, *Henry I. Yamamura, and *William R. Roeske

*Department of Pharmacology, Shizuoka College of Pharmaceutical Sciences, Shizuoka 422, Japan; *Departments of Internal Medicine, Pharmacology, Biochemistry, and Psychiatry, The University of Arizona Health Sciences Center, Tucson, Arizona 85724*

Presynaptic mechanisms appear to be involved in the autoregulation of norepinephrine (NE) release during sympathetic nerve stimulation. The presynaptic α-adrenoceptors and muscarinic cholinoceptors mediate a negative feedback mechanism which leads to an inhibition of transmitter release, while the presynaptic β-adrenoceptors mediate a positive feedback mechanism which increases transmitter release (14,15,27). Biochemical approaches to the study of the neurotransmitter receptor localization using radioligand binding technique have been reported (19,20,21,22,28,29). However, direct binding measurements with [$^3$H]quinuclidinyl benzilate (QNB) on sympathetically denervated rat heart indicate certain discrepancies concerning the alteration of cardiac muscarinic receptors (20,21,22,28,30), which may be due to some major differences in tissue preparation, the dosage of 6-hydroxydopamine (6-OHDA) injected, and the [$^3$H]QNB binding assay itself. The fact that [$^3$H]QNB nonselectively labels both presynaptic and postsynaptic muscarinic receptors complicates the interpretation of the results obtained with the sympathetically denervated tissue. Thus the alteration in [$^3$H]QNB binding sites of denervated tissues may depend on the relative proportion of presynaptic to postsynaptic muscarinic receptor density of the tissue. Since the development of presynaptic and postsynaptic supersensitivity in physiological response following sympathetic denervation demonstrated a different time course (7,18,24), and since there was a significant recovery in the NE concentration of sympathectomized tissues (6,23,33), a time course study should be important for the analysis of receptor alteration following sympathetic denervation (28,29). In this chapter we will present our recent work in the localization of muscarinic and β-adrenergic receptors in the rat spleen using specific radioligands, [$^3$H](−)QNB and [$^3$H](−)dihydroalprenolol (DHA), in comparison with the cardiac and renal receptors.

## MATERIALS AND METHODS

### Chemical Sympathectomy by 6-OHDA

Chemical sympathectomy by 6-OHDA was performed as described previously (28). Male Sprague-Dawley rats (150–200 g) were divided into two groups of 10 to 12 rats each. Rats of the first group were injected i.v. in the tail vein with 6-OHDA·HBr, at two doses of 50 mg/kg at 24-hr intervals. The control rats received an equivalent volume (0.1 ml/100 g i.v.) of 0.001 N HCl. Three rats from each group were sacrificed 1, 2, 3, and 5 weeks after the first dose of 6-OHDA or 0.001 N HCl. Three separate sets of experiments were performed and the results were averaged. 6-OHDA·HBr was dissolved in 0.001 N HCl saturated with nitrogen gas (23).

### Binding Assays

Rats were killed by decapitation and the viscera were perfused with 0.9% saline. The spleen was removed and homogenized with a polytron in 39 vol of cold 50 mM Tris-HCl buffer (pH 7.7 at 25°C). The homogenates were centrifuged at 50,000 × $g$ for 15 min at 4°C. [$^3$H](−)QNB binding was performed in the twiced washed splenic homogenates as described previously (28). The homogenates containing 5 and 7.5 mg wet weight tissues were incubated with [$^3$H](−)DHA (0.15 to 1.2 nM) and [$^3$H](−)QNB (20 to 430 pM) in a total volume of 2 ml in 50 mM Tris-HCl buffer. The incubation was carried out for 30 min at 25°C in [$^3$H](−)DHA binding and 60 min at 37°C in [$^3$H](−)QNB binding. Reactions were terminated by rapid filtration under vacuum through Whatman GF/B glass fiber filters. Filters were immediately washed four times with 4 ml of cold buffer. Tissue-bound radioactivity was extracted from the filters overnight in 8 ml of scintillation fluid and counted. Every binding experiment was performed using fresh tissue. Specific binding for each ligand was defined as the difference in binding determined in the absence and presence of the following drugs: 0.1 μM (−)propranolol in [$^3$H](−)DHA assays and 1 μM atropine in [$^3$H](−)QNB assays. The protein concentration was determined by the method of Lowry et al. (17) using bovine serum albumin as a standard.

### NE Determination

The concentration of norepinephrine in the spleen was determined by a sensitive radioenzymatic assay procedure (8).

### Analysis of Data

The analysis of binding data was performed as described previously (1). Statistical analysis of the data was performed using either a double tailed Student's $t$-test or a hierarchical single factor analysis of variance (ANOVA) (34).

## RESULTS

### Reciprocal Alterations of Splenic β-Adrenergic and Muscarinic Cholinergic Receptors Following Chemical Sympathectomy with 6-OHDA

The specific binding of [$^3$H](−)DHA and [$^3$H](−)QNB to the splenic homogenates was saturable and stereospecific (Table 1). (−)Propranolol inhibited the specific [$^3$H](−)DHA binding with the greater (180 times) affinity than (+)propranolol, and dexetimide was 10,000 times more potent than its stereoisomer levetimide in inhibiting specific [$^3$H](−)QNB binding. Scatchard analysis in control rat splenic homogenates demonstrated a $K_D$ of 0.33 ± 0.03 nM and a $B_{max}$ of 6.17 ± 0.20 fmoles/mg tissue (124.9 ± 5.5 fmoles/mg protein) ($N = 19$) for [$^3$H](−)DHA binding, and a $K_D$ of 0.06 ± 0.01 nM and a $B_{max}$ of 1.75 ± 0.07 fmoles/mg tissue (30.1 ± 1.2 fmoles/mg protein) ($N = 8$) for [$^3$H](−)QNB binding. These data are compatible with our previously published assay conditions for the β-adrenergic and muscarinic cholinergic receptors (3,5,28,32).

Saturation isotherms for [$^3$H](−)DHA and [$^3$H](−)QNB binding and Scatchard analysis were carried out in the splenic homogenates from control and 6-OHDA treated rats. As shown in Fig. 1, the number of [$^3$H](−)DHA binding sites ($B_{max}$) in the rat spleen was significantly increased by 26% at 2 weeks and by 22% at 3 weeks, after 6-OHDA treatment. Since the $K_D$ values for splenic [$^3$H](−)DHA binding were not significantly changed by the 6-OHDA treatment, the increase in the specific [$^3$H](−)DHA binding of the 6-OHDA treated spleen may be due to a significant alteration in the receptor density of the splenic β-adrenoceptors. There was no significant alteration in the density of [$^3$H](−)DHA binding sites at 1 and 5 weeks after 6-OHDA treatment (Fig. 1).

In contrast, chemical sympathectomy with 6-OHDA caused a significant decrease in the $B_{max}$ values for specific [$^3$H](−)QNB binding to the rat spleen at all the times

TABLE 1. *Inihibition of [$^3$H](−)DHA and [$^3$H](−)QNB binding by adrenergic and cholinergic antagonists in the rat spleen*

| Binding/antagonists | $K_i$ values (nM) |
|---|---|
| Specific [$^3$H](−)DHA binding | |
| (−)propranolol | 0.24 ± 0.01 |
| (+)propranolol | 43.5 ± 3.2 |
| phentolamine | 6390 ± 2660 |
| Specific [$^3$H](−)QNB binding | |
| QNB | 0.08 ± 0.02 |
| atropine | 2.27 ± 0.25 |
| dexetimide | 0.15 ± 0.012 |
| levetimide | 1550 ± 283 |

A value for the inhibition constant, $K_i$, was calculated from the equation, $K_i = IC_{50}/[1 + (H)_T/K_D]$ where $K_D$ and $H_T$ are the dissociation constant and free ligand concentration, respectively. The experiments were conducted 3 to 6 times and values represent the means ± SEM.

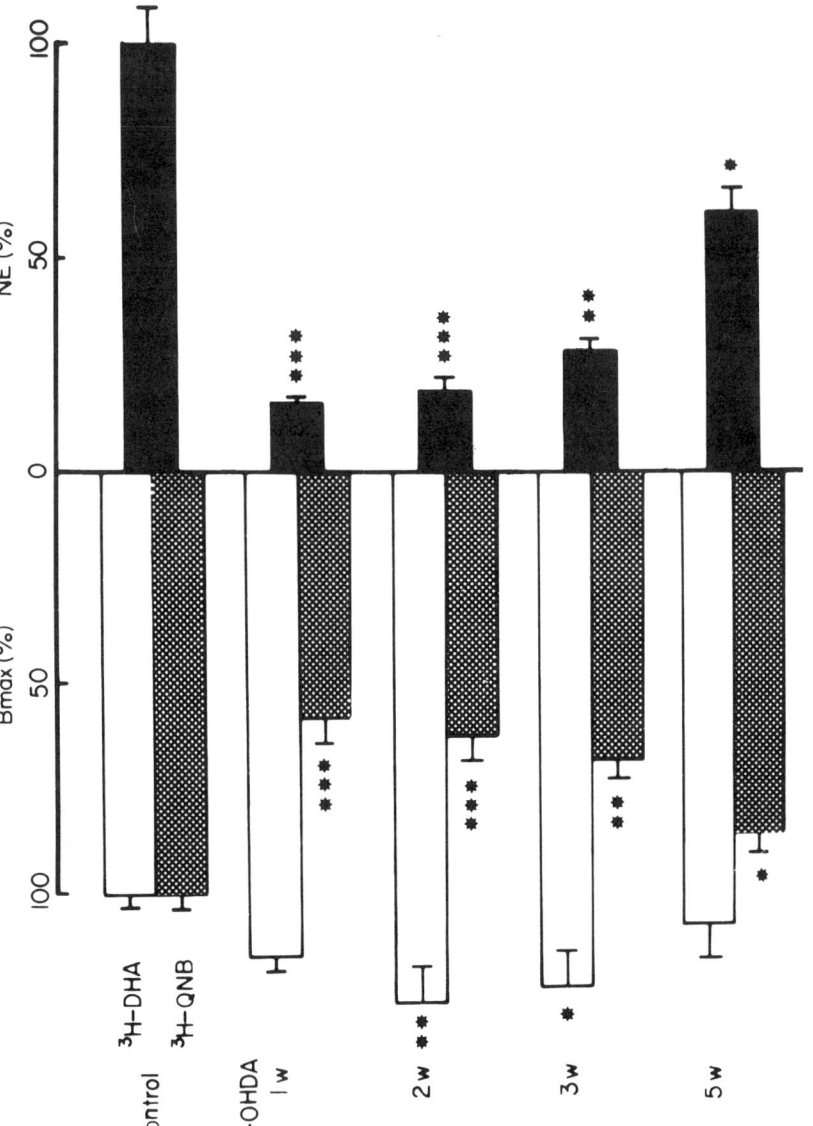

**FIG. 1.** Alteration of [$^3$H](−)DHA and [$^3$H](−)QNB binding sites ($B_{max}$) and NE concentration in the 6-OHDA treated spleen. Each column represents the percentage (means ± SEM) of control value ($N$ = 5–14). The data were analyzed by a hierarchical single factor analysis of variance (ANOVA). Asterisks show a significant difference from control value, * $p < 0.05$, ** $p < 0.01$, *** $p < 0.001$.

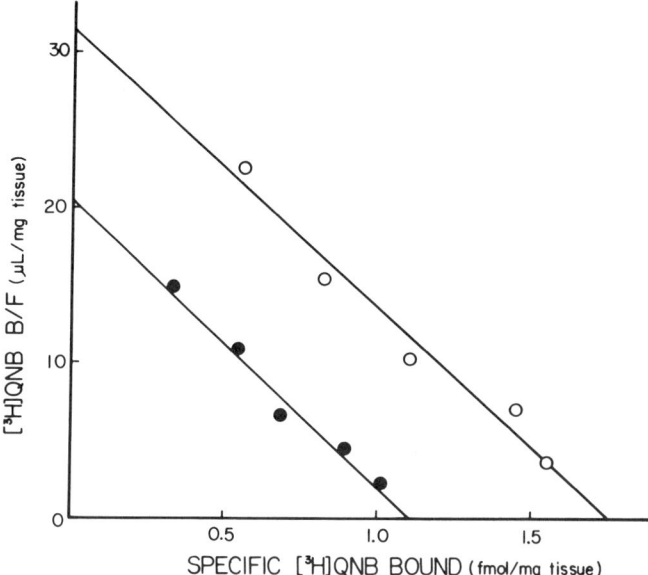

**FIG. 2.** Scatchard plot of [³H](−)QNB binding to splenic homogenates from control *(open circles)* and 6-OHDA treated *(solid circles)* rats. The apparent $K_D$ and receptor density ($B_{max}$) are: 0.06 ± 0.01 nM and 1.75 ± 0.07 fmoles/mg tissue for the control, correlation coefficient, $r = 0.98$ and 0.05 ± 0.01 nM and 1.09 ± 0.10 fmoles/mg tissue after 6-OHDA treatment (2 weeks), $r = 0.99$. Each point represents the average of duplicate determinations from 8 (control) and 6 (treated) animals.

(1 to 5 weeks) (Fig. 1). Figure 2 illustrates Scatchard plots for [³H](−)QNB binding in the control and 6-OHDA treated (2 weeks) rat spleen. Since the $K_D$ values were unchanged by the 6-OHDA treatment, these data revealed a significant reduction in the density of [³H](−)QNB binding sites following 6-OHDA treatment. The $B_{max}$ value at 5 weeks was significantly ($p < 0.01$, $p < 0.05$) greater than that at 2 or 3 weeks in the treated tissues, suggesting a substantial recovery of splenic [³H](−)QNB binding sites in the 6-OHDA treated (5 weeks) spleen.

### Reduction of Splenic NE Concentration Following 6-OHDA Treatment

The NE concentration in control rat spleen was 0.67 ± 0.06 µg/g fresh wet weight ($N = 14$) which was similar to the value previously reported (8). Following 6-OHDA treatment, there was 84, 81, and 72% reduction in the splenic NE concentration at 1, 2, and 3 weeks, respectively (Fig. 1). Splenic NE concentration at 3 weeks was significantly ($p < 0.05$) greater than the value at 1 and 2 weeks, which suggests a significant recovery of endogenous NE following 6-OHDA treatment, as we and others previously found in rat tissues (23,28). At 5 weeks following 6-OHDA treatment, there was further recovery in the splenic NE concentration since NE concentration in the treated spleen was about 61% of the control value (Fig. 1). Similar recovery of splenic NE following 6-OHDA treatment was previously reported (23,33).

## DISCUSSION

The present study presents a direct biochemical demonstration of postsynaptic β-adrenergic and presynaptic muscarinic receptors in the rat spleen. There was a reciprocal alteration in the splenic β-adrenergic (increase) and muscarcinic (decrease) receptors by chemical sympathectomy of rats with 6-OHDA, which closely correlated with a change in the splenic NE concentration.

Splenic tissues are innervated by the both sympathetic and parasympathetic nerves (4). Physiological studies have suggested presynaptic localization of β-adrenergic and muscarinic cholinergic receptors on splenic sympathetic nerves in addition to postsynaptic localization of these receptors on the smooth muscles (4,10,11,15). Recently, Nahorski et al. (19) have characterized the β-adrenergic receptors in the rat spleen using [$^3$H](−)DHA assays with different conditions. In the present study, specific binding of [$^3$H](−)DHA and [$^3$H](−)QNB in the rat spleen was saturable and of high affinity. There was a relatively greater density of [$^3$H](−)DHA binding sites as compared with [$^3$H](−)QNB binding sites. The specific binding of [$^3$H](−)DHA and [$^3$H](−)QNB showed a pharmacological drug profile compatible with β-adrenergic and muscarinic cholinergic receptors, respectively.

To characterize autonomic receptors using direct binding measurements, we extensively studied the alteration of NE levels, α-adrenergic, β-adrenergic, and muscarinic receptors in peripheral tissues from chemically sympathectomized rats. Table 2 summarizes the data concerning alteration of these receptors as well as NE concentration in spleen, heart (left ventricle; see refs. 28 and 29 for other cardiac regions), and kidney (Yamada et al., *in preparation*) at various times following the

TABLE 2. *Alteration of autonomic receptor density ($B_{max}$) and NE concentration in spleen, heart, and kidney of 6-OHDA treated rats*

| Organs | Change following 6-OHDA treatment (% of control values) | | | | Absolute control values[a] |
|---|---|---|---|---|---|
| | 1 w | 2 w | 3 w | 5 w | |
| Spleen | | | | | |
| β-Adrenoceptors | +14.9 | +26.3 | +22.2 | + 7.1 | 6.17 |
| muscarinic receptors | −39.6 | −37.7 | −32.1 | −14.3 | 1.75 |
| NE concentration | −83.6 | −80.6 | −71.6 | −38.8 | 0.67 |
| Heart (left ventricle)[b] | | | | | |
| α-Adrenoceptors | +47.5 | +26.5 | +17.5 | ND[c] | 2.57 |
| β-Adrenoceptors | +31.8 | +37.5 | +16.9 | ND | 2.96 |
| muscarinic receptors | +16.3 | +18.4 | + 3.9 | ND | 15.2 |
| NE concentration | −78.7 | −76.6 | −70.2 | ND | 0.47 |
| Kidney | | | | | |
| α-Adrenoceptors | +23.4 | +31.0 | + 2.2 | ND | 4.06 |
| β-Adrenoceptors | +26.3 | +29.9 | +13.4 | ND | 2.24 |
| muscarinic receptors | − 7.9 | + 5.7 | − 9.9 | ND | 3.53 |
| NE concentration | −72.7 | −72.7 | −63.6 | ND | 0.11 |

[a] $B_{max}$, fmoles/mg tissue or NE, μg/g tissue.
[b] Revised from refs. 28 and 29, with permission.
[c] ND = not determined.

treatment of rats with 6-OHDA. In all the tissues of chemically sympathectomized rats, as determined by a marked reduction of NE concentration, α- and β-adrenoceptors showed the largest (20 to 40%) increase in the density at 1 and 2 weeks. The increased density of these adrenoceptors, which may be partly responsible for postsynaptic supersensitivity to catecholamines (2,7,18), suggests that the majority of α- and β-adrenoceptors in spleen, heart, and kidney is localized on postsynaptic cells and regulated by the sympathetic nervous system. Although experiments in intact splenic preparations suggest that a portion of the β-adrenoceptors is presynaptic in this tissue (15), Nahorski (19) and we did not find a significant decrease in splenic [$^3$H]( − )DHA binding sites at any time after 6-OHDA treatment.

Physiological evidence that presynaptic muscarinic receptors participate in the regulation of NE release has been presented for heart and blood vessels (14,15, 16,25,26) and also for the spleen (10,11). Interestingly, we found a consistent decrease in the density of muscarinic receptors at all periods examined (1 to 5 weeks) in the 6-OHDA treated rat spleen (Table 2), which is in contrast to the alteration (increase) of β-adrenoceptors. The largest part of the decrease (about 40%) was present at 1 and 2 weeks, and thus appeared to coincide with the loss of sympathetic nerve terminals (6,23) as shown by an 80% reduction in the NE concentration and by a significantly increased density of the β-adrenoceptors. At 5 weeks when there was no longer an increase in splenic β-adrenoceptors, the density of muscarinic receptors in the sympathectomized spleen recovered as compared with that at 1, 2, and 3 weeks (Table 2). The recovery of muscarinic receptors appears to correlate closely with the marked recovery in splenic NE. This suggests the process of regeneration of adrenergic nerve terminals (6,23,33). The reversible loss of splenic muscarinic receptors following 6-OHDA treatment is consistent with the presence of presynaptic receptors on the sympathetic terminals. Our finding is supported by the following two observations in the spleen. Kirpekar et al. (10,11) found that muscarinic inhibition of splenic nerve stimulation evoked release of NE by acetylcholine and carbachol in the perfused cat spleen. Recently, Laduron (13) measured the stereospecific [$^3$H]dexetimide binding in the different segments of dog splenic nerves ligature and found a rapid accumulation of the [$^3$H]dexetimide binding sites on either sides of a ligature, which demonstrates bidirectional axonal flow for [$^3$H]dexetimide binding sites in the dog splenic nerves. Thus, their observation provides biochemical evidence for the presence of muscarinic cholinergic receptors on sympathetic nerves in the dog spleen.

In spite of some physiological evidence for presynaptic muscarinic receptors in cardiac tissues (16,26), we failed to demonstrate any significant loss of muscarinic receptors in five cardiac regions of 6-OHDA treated rats at all periods (Table 2) (28). In these animals, there was a simultaneous increase in the density of α-adrenergic and β-adrenoceptors and a marked reduction of the NE concentration. [$^3$H]QNB appears to label nonselectively both presynaptic and postsynaptic muscarinic receptors. Since there is a significant variation in the density of sympathetic and parasympathetic innervation to each tissue (4,9,12) and in the number of muscarinic receptors (28,29), the relative proportion of presynaptic to postsynaptic receptors should differ among spleen, heart, and kidney. In fact, muscarinic cholinergic receptors in the spleen have a much lower density compared with other tissues such as heart, kidney, intestine, and the brain of rats (28,31). On the basis of tissue weight, the $B_{max}$ value of [$^3$H](−)QNB binding sites in the rat spleen was 10 and 66 times lower than the $B_{max}$ values in the left ventricles and cerebral cortex, respectively (28,31). Our data indicate that there may be much greater proportion of presynaptic muscarinic receptors in the rat spleen than in the heart. Thus we conclude that the majority of cardiac and renal muscarinic receptors is located on the postsynaptic cells. In contrast, a substantial number of muscarinic receptors in the rat spleen may be located presynaptically on the adrenergic terminals.

## ACKNOWLEDGMENTS

We thank Terry Austin for secretarial assistance. This work was supported by the United States Public Health Service Grants MH-30626 and Program Project Grant HL-20984. Henry I. Yamamura is a recipient of a United States Public Health Service Research Scientist Development Award, Type II(MH-00095), from the National Institute of Mental Health, and William R. Roeske is a recipient of a United States Public Health Service Research Scientist Development Award (HL-00776) from the National Heart, Lung, and Blood Institute.

## REFERENCES

1. Bennett, J. P. (1978): Methods in binding studies. In: *Neurotransmitter Receptor Binding*, edited by H. I. Yamamura, S. J. Enna, and M. J. Kuhar, pp. 57–90. Raven Press, New York.
2. Burn, J. H., and Rand, M. J. (1959): The cause of the supersensitivity of smooth muscle to noradrenaline after sympathetic degeneration. *J. Physiol.*, 147:135–143.
3. Chen, F. M., Yamamura, H. I., and Roeske, W. R. (1979): Ontogeny of mammalian myocardial β-adrenergic receptors. *Eur. J. Pharmacol.*, 58:255–264.
4. Davies, B. N., and Withrington, P. G. (1973): The actions of drugs on the smooth muscle of the capsule and blood vessels of the spleen. *Pharmacol. Rev.*, 25:373–413.
5. Fields, J. Z., Roeske, W. R., Morkin, E., and Yamamura, H. I. (1978): Cardiac muscarinic cholinergic receptors: Biochemical identification and characterization. *J. Biol. Chem.*, 253:3251–3258.
6. Goldman, H., and Jacobowitz, D. (1971): Correlation of norepinephrine content with observations of adrenergic nerves after a single dose of 6-hydroxydopamine in the rat. *J. Pharmacol. Exp. Ther.*, 176:119–133.
7. Haeusler, G., Haefely, W. D., and Thoenen, H. J. (1969): Chemical sympathectomy of the cat with 6-hydroxydopamine. *J. Pharmacol. Exp. Ther.*, 170:60–61.
8. Henry, D. P., Staman, B. J., Johnson, D. G., and Williams, R. H. (1975): A sensitive radioenzymatic assay for norepinephrine in tissue and plasma. *Life Sci.*, 16:375–384.
9. Higgins, C. B., Vatner, S. F., and Braunwald, E. (1973): Parasympathetic control of the heart. *Pharmacol. Rev.*, 25:119–155.
10. Kirpekar, S. M., Prat, J. C., Puig, M., and Wakade, A. R. (1972): Modification of the evoked release of noradrenaline from the perfused cat spleen by various ions and agents. *J. Physiol.*, 221:601–615.
11. Kirpekar, S. M., Prat, J. C., and Wakade, A. R. (1975): Effect of calcium on the relationship between frequency of stimulation and release of noradrenaline from the perfused spleen of the cat. *Naunyn Schmiedebergs Arch. Pharmacol. Exp. Pathol.*, 287:205–212.
12. Kostrzewa, R. M., and Jacobowitz, D. M. (1974): Pharmacological actions of 6-hydroxydopamine. *Pharmacol. Rev.*, 26:199–288.
13. Laduron, P. (1980): Axoplasmic transport of muscarinic receptors. *Nature (Lond.)*, 286:287–288.

14. Langer, S. Z. (1974): Presynaptic regulation of catecholamine release. *Biochem. Pharmacol.*, 23:1793–1800.
15. Langer, S. Z. (1977): Presynaptic receptors and their role in the regulation of transmitter release. *Br. J. Pharmacol.*, 60:481–497.
16. Loffelholz, K., and Muscholl, E. (1969): A muscarinic inhibition of the noradrenaline release evoked by postganglionic sympathetic nerve stimulation. *Naunyn Schmiedebergs Arch. Pharmacol. Exp. Pathol.*, 265:1–15.
17. Lowry, O. H., Rosebrough, H. J., Farr, A. L., and Randall, R. J. (1951): Protein measurement with the Folin phenol reagent. *J. Biol. Chem.*, 193:265–275.
18. Nadeau, R. A., DeChamplain, J., and Tremblay, D. M. (1971): Supersensitivity of the isolated rat heart after chemical sympathectomy with 6-hydroxydopamine. *Can. J. Physiol. Pharmacol.*, 49:36–44.
19. Nahorski, S. R., Barnett, D. B., Howlett, D. R., and Rugg, E. L. (1979): Pharmacological characteristics of β-adrenoceptor binding sites in intact and sympathectomized rat spleen. *Naunyn Schmiedebergs Arch. Pharmacol. Exp. Pathol.*, 307:227–233.
20. Sharma, V. K., and Banerjee, S. P. (1978): Presynaptic muscarinic cholinergic receptors. *Nature (Lond.)*, 27:276–278.
21. Story, D. F., Briley, M. S., and Langer, S. Z. (1979): The effects of chemical sympathectomy with 6-hydroxydopamine on β-adrenoceptor and muscarinic cholinoceptor binding in rat heart ventricle. *Eur. J. Pharmacol.*, 57:423–426.
22. Story, D. F., Briley, M. S., and Langer, S. Z. (1979): The effects of 6-hydroxydopamine treatment on the binding of [$^3$H]quinuclidinyl benzilate, [$^3$H]dihydroergocryptine and [$^3$H]WB4101 to rat ventricular membrane. In: *Advances in Biosciences, Vol. 18, Presynaptic Receptors*, edited by S. Z. Langer, K. Starke, and M. L. Dubocovich, pp. 105–109. Pergamon Press, London, New York.
23. Thoenen, H., and Tranzer, J. P. (1968): Chemical sympathectomy by selective destruction of adrenergic nerve endings with 6-hydroxydopamine. *Naunyn Schmiedebergs Arch. Pharmacol. Exp. Pathol.*, 261:271–288.
24. Trendelenburg, U. (1966): Mechanisms of supersensitivity and subsensitivity to sympathomimetic amines. *Pharmacol. Rev.*, 18:629–640.
25. Vanhoutte, P. M. (1977): Cholinergic inhibition of adrenergic transmission. *Fed. Proc.*, 36:2444–2449.
26. Vanhoutte, P. M., and Levy, M. N. (1980): Prejunctional cholinergic modulation of adrenergic neurotransmission in the cardiovascular system. *AM. J. Physiol.*, 238, H275–H281.
27. Vizi, E. S. (1980): Presynaptic modulation of neurochemical transmission. *Prog. Neurobiol.*, 12:181–290.
28. Yamada, S., Yamamura, H. I., and Roeske, W. R. (1980): Alterations in cardiac autonomic receptors following 6-hydroxydopamine treatment in rats. *Mol. Pharmacol.*, 18:185–192.
29. Yamada, S., Yamamura, H. I., and Roeske, W. R. (1980): Characterization of alpha-1 adrenergic receptors in the heart using [$^3$H]WB4101: Effect of 6-hydroxydopamine treatment. *J. Pharmacol. Exp. Ther.*, 215:176–185.
30. Yamada, S., Yamamura, H. I., and Roeske, W. R. (1980): Regional distribution of cardiac autonomic receptors and alteration following chemical sympathectomy. In: *Psychopharmacology and Biochemistry of Neurotransmitter Receptors*, edited by H. I. Yamamura, R. W. Olsen, and E. Usdin, pp. 135–146. Elsevier/North-Holland, New York.
31. Yamada, S., Yamamura, H. I., and Roeske, W. R. (1980): Alteration in central and peripheral adrenergic receptors in deoxycorticosterone/salt hypertensive rats. *Life Sci.*, 27:2405–2416.
32. Yamamura, H. I., and Synder, S. H. (1974): Muscarinic cholinergic binding in rat brain. *Proc. Natl. Acad. Sci. USA*, 71:1725–1729.
33. Yamori, Y., Yamabe, H., De Jong, W., Lovenberg, W., and Sjoerdsma, A. (1972): Effect of tissue norepinephrine depletion by 6-hydroxydopamine on blood pressure in spontaneously hypertensive rats. *Eur. J. Pharmacol.*, 17:135–140.
34. Zar, J. H. (1974): *Biostatistical Analysis*. Prentice-Hall, Englewood Cliffs.

ms
# The $\alpha_2$-Adrenergic Receptor: Multiple Affinity States and Regulation of a Receptor Inversely Coupled to Adenylate Cyclase

David C. U'Prichard, Joan C. Mitrius, Deborah J. Kahn, and Bruce D. Perry

*Departments of Pharmacology, Neurobiology, and Physiology, Northwestern University Medical School, Chicago, Illinois 60611, and College of Arts and Sciences, Evanston, Illinois 60201*

The $\alpha_2$-adrenergic receptor mediates inhibition of norepinephrine (NE) release from central and peripheral noradrenergic terminals (20), and in several tissues, such as adipocytes and platelets, also mediates inhibition of adenylate cyclase (6,32). Altered $\alpha_2$-receptor function in brain and vascular tissue has been implicated in the pathogenesis of depression (7) and hypertension, and it is therefore important to understand the mechanisms by which $\alpha_2$-receptors are coupled to effector systems in neurons and smooth muscle cells, as a prelude to determining the ways in which function of this receptor may be altered. While a generalized hypothesis that $\alpha_2$-receptors in all tissues are inversely coupled to adenylate cyclase is appealing, there is as yet no direct evidence for this in brain and vascular tissue, although activation of $\alpha_2$-receptors has been shown to inhibit adenylate cyclase activity in a hybrid clonal neuroblastoma $\times$ glioma (NG 108–15) cell line (29).

$\alpha_2$-Receptors have been labeled with the antagonist radioligands $^3$H-dihydro-$\alpha$-ergocryptine (DHEC) (9,26,47) and $^3$H-yohimbine (YOH) (4,25). From extensive studies of the interaction of DHEC with human platelet and rat hepatocyte $\alpha_2$-receptors, Lefkowitz and co-workers (3) have concluded that this receptor, like the erythrocyte $\beta$-receptor (19) can exist in two conformations differentiated by high and low affinity, respectively, for agonists, and designated $\alpha_2$(H) and $\alpha_2$(L). More recently, it has been shown that agonists interact at platelet YOH sites in a similarly heterogeneous manner (4,25). According to the general model derived by this group for $\alpha_2$- and $\beta$-receptors (4), antagonists exhibit the same affinity for R(H) and R(L). Guanine nucleotides and monovalent cations reduce the affinity of agonists at radioantagonist sites and increase the Hill slope ($n_H$) for competition by agonists (38,39). Using computer modeling techniques, Lefkowitz et al. have demonstrated that nucleotides shift the equilibrium between the different affinity states in favor of R(L) for both frog erythrocyte $\beta$-receptors (19) and human platelet $\alpha_2$-receptors (3). Limbird and co-workers have solubilized $\beta$- and $\alpha_2$-receptors and have provided evidence that R(H) is equivalent to a ternary hormone (agonist)-receptor-guanine nucleotide binding regulatory protein (H.R.N.) complex (23,34). Guanosine triphosphate (GTP) is obligatory for both β-receptor mediated stimulation and $\alpha_2$-receptor mediated inhibition of adenylate cyclase (18,24), and the formal kinetic models that have been presented to account for β- and $\alpha_2$-receptor coupling are essentially identical (4). There is, however, no explanation as yet for the ultimate difference of β- and $\alpha_2$-effects on adenylate cyclase, although different types of N proteins mediating stimulation and inhibition have been invoked (35).

In several tissues, such as rat heart, muscarinic cholinergic (MACh) receptors are also inversely coupled to adenylate cyclase in a GTP-dependent manner (17), and GTP modulates agonist affinities at MACh receptors in a manner analogous to effects at adrenergic receptors (5,45). Several groups have postulated the existence of three affinity states of the MACh receptor (2,5), including a state with very high affinity for agonists, or "superhigh" (SH), as well as R(H) and R(L). However, the significance of R(SH) in terms of receptor-cyclase coupling has not yet been demonstrated.

$\alpha_2$-Receptors have also been labeled with agonist radioligands such as $^3$H-catecholamines in brain, platelets, and liver (6,27,42), and $^3$H-imidazolines in brain, platelets, and ileum (33,36,41). These sites, in general, exhibit high affinity for agonist competitors and are directly sensitive to inhibition by guanine nucleotides, suggesting that the R(H) form of the $\alpha_2$-receptor is being labeled (43,44). With the exception of a comparison by Hoffman et al. (6) of DHEC and $^3$H-epinephrine (EPI) binding to platelet $\alpha_2$-receptors, there has been little rigorous analysis of the interactions of radioagonist and radioantagonist binding to $\alpha_2$-receptors in the same tissue, as has been done for β-receptors (12). A related question also unexplored in detail is to what extent the interactions of labeled ligands, which are partial agonists such as $^3$H-clonidine (CLO) or $^3$H-p-aminoclonidine (PAC), differ from the interactions of full agonists such as EPI at the $\alpha_2$-receptor. The studies presented here attempt to address the following questions: (a) are neural $\alpha_2$-receptors coupled to adenylate cyclase in the same manner as platelet $\alpha_2$-receptors? (b) do brain and vascular $\alpha_2$-receptors also occur in multiple affinity states and show GTP sensitivity, suggesting they are coupled to adenylate cyclase? (c) is there evidence for more than two affinity states of the $\alpha_2$-receptor? (d) is the process of agonist-induced desensitization similar for the β- and the $\alpha_2$-receptor? To examine these questions, the binding of radioligands of different efficacy to $\alpha_2$-receptors in human platelets, NG 108–15 cells, rat and bovine cerebral cortex, and tunica media of bovine aorta has been compared. The ligands used were the full agonist EPI (40–80 Ci/mmole), the partial agonist PAC (40–50 Ci/mmole), and the antagonists YOH (80–90 Ci/mmole) and $^3$H-rauwolscine (RAUW, 80 Ci/mmole), which is a more selective $\alpha_2$-blocker than YOH (11,37).

## METHODS

Human platelet membranes were prepared by a modification of the method of Newman et al. (26) as described previously (4). Most experiments were performed using discarded platelets (no more than 3 days old) from blood banks, but binding was also compared in platelet membranes prepared from freshly drawn blood samples from volunteers. Binding to intact platelets was performed using platelets originally centrifuged in isotonic Tris-saline, and then washed and resuspended in Hank's physiological buffer. NG 108–15 (108CC15) cells were cultured as monolayers in Dulbecco's modified MEM supplemented with newborn calf serum (10%) and HAT. For binding studies, cells were removed by agitation, homogenized in 50 mM Tris-HCl buffer, and membranes washed three times by centrifugation. Rat and bovine cortex membranes were prepared as described previously (41,42). Bovine aortas were obtained from a local slaughterhouse, tunica media was dissected free and minced finely, then homogenized in 50 mM Tris-HCl using a Polytron PT-10. The supernatant from an initial 1000 × $g$ centrifugation was centrifuged at 50,000 × $g$, and the resulting pellet washed twice by centrifugation before final resuspension.

Binding assays for EPI, PAC, and YOH (platelets and NG 108–15 cells) were conducted at 25°C, with equilibrium binding being reached by 40 to 60 min, in 50 mM Tris-HCl buffers. EPI and PAC assays routinely included 1.0 mM $MgCl_2$, and in the case of EPI, 1.0 mM pyrocatechol and antioxidants (42). YOH and RAUW binding to brain and aorta membranes was performed at 4°C for 90 to 120 min in 50 mM Na-K phosphate buffer, since in these conditions the ligands exhibited the highest affinity, although $B_{max}$ values were the same in either buffer. Assay volumes were 1.0 to 2.0 ml, and generally contained 0.4 to 1.0 mg protein. Nonspecific binding for each ligand was defined by parallel incubations containing 1.0 μM oxymetazoline (EPI), 10 μM (−)-NE or 1.0 μM phentolamine (PAC), and 100 μM (−)-NE (YOH and RAUW). Assays were performed in duplicate or triplicate and were terminated by filtration under reduced pressure over Whatman GF/B filters. All ligands were obtained from New England Nuclear.

Adenylate cyclase activity in NG 108–15 and platelet membranes was assayed by the method of Salomon (31), with some modifications. Substrate [adenosine triphosphate (ATP)] concentration was 0.05 to 0.2 mM, and 10 μM GTP was routinely included. Incubations were at 25, 30, or 37°C.

## RESULTS

### Platelets

In confirmation of other observations (25), no binding of $^3$H-prazosin to $\alpha_1$-receptors in human platelet membranes could be observed. YOH labeled a single set of sites in platelet membranes in kinetic and saturation experiments with a $K_D$ of about 1.0 nM (4). The presence of 1.0 mM or 5.0 mM $Mg^{2+}$ in the assay increased the $K_D$ of YOH two-fold, indicating that divalent cations may modify the affinity of antagonists at the $\alpha_2$-receptor. Competition studies showed that YOH labeled an $\alpha_2$-receptor in platelet membranes since, in addition to the expected rank order of catecholamine potencies, prazosin was much less potent than YOH (Table 1).

TABLE 1. *Inhibition of (−)-³H-EPI, ³H-PAC, and ³H-YOH binding to $\alpha_2$-adrenergic receptors on human platelet membranes*

| Drug | ³H-EPI | | ³H-PAC | | ³H-YOH | |
|---|---|---|---|---|---|---|
| | $IC_{50}$ | $n_H$ | $IC_{50}$ | $n_H$ | $IC_{50}$ | $n_H$ |
| | nM | | | | | |
| Agonists | | | | | | |
| (−)-EP | 3.3 | 0.80 | 2.4 | 0.82 | 87 | 0.72 |
| (−)-NE | 14 | 0.80 | 6.5 | 0.78 | 420 | 0.71 |
| (+)-NE | 410 | 0.65 | 250 | 0.63 | 6,800 | 0.80 |
| (−)-isoproterenol | 1,500 | 0.48 | 800 | 0.83 | 29,000 | 0.66 |
| Imidazolines | | | | | | |
| PAC | — | — | 3.4 | 0.64 | 34 | 0.94 |
| CLO | 3.3 | 0.82 | 3.1 | 0.70 | 60 | 1.01 |
| Antagonists | | | | | | |
| phentolamine | 3.8 | 0.91 | 2.9 | 0.80 | 4.3 | 0.98 |
| YOH | 11 | 0.81 | 17 | 0.76 | 1.0 | 0.95 |
| WB-4101 | 19 | 0.82 | 26 | 0.66 | 2.8 | 0.98 |
| prazosin | 20,000 | 0.44 | 29,000 | 0.94 | 430 | 0.93 |

Assays were performed on membranes from discarded platelets, as described in text, at 25°C. 1.0 mM $MgCl_2$ was present in EPI and PAC assays. Ligand concentrations were EPI 1.0 nM; PAC 0.6 nM; YOH 0.2 nM. $IC_{50}$ values were determined from Hill plots and are the mean of individual values from four to eight experiments. $n_H$ values are from averaged competition curves.

Interactions of agonists and antagonists at platelet YOH sites were similar to those previously described at DHEC $\alpha_2$-receptor sites in platelets (3), in that full agonists inhibited binding with shallow slopes ($n_H$ 0.6–0.8) whereas antagonist competition curves had $n_H$ values of about 1.0, and imidazolines such as CLO and PAC, which were observed by us and others (22) to have a partial agonist action in inhibiting platelet adenylate cyclase, had competition curves with intermediate slopes ($n_H$ 0.85–1.0) (Table 1; Fig. 1, left panels). By analogy to the model derived from similar platelet DHEC binding data by Lefkowitz and co-workers (4), the data suggest that YOH labels two conformations of the platelet receptor, $\alpha_2(H)$ and $\alpha_2(L)$, at which agonists, but not antagonists, have different affinities. The slope for the competition curve of the partial agonist PAC may be steeper because it induces the formation of fewer $\alpha_2(H)$ states (Fig. 1B). The effects of $Mg^{2+}$ and GTP on competitor affinities at platelet YOH sites were very similar to those previously reported for platelet DHEC binding (38,39). $MgCl_2$, 5.0 mM, increased the affinity of (−)-EPI and PAC and reduced the $n_H$ values for these competitors (Fig. 1, right panels), suggesting that $Mg^{2+}$ promotes the formation of $\alpha_2(H)$. $Mg^{2+}$ also slightly reduced the affinity of phentolamine at YOH sites, in line with the reduction in the affinity of YOH itself. In other experiments, 1.0 mM $MgCl_2$ caused a twofold reduction in the affinity of prazosin at platelet YOH sites. A similar reduction in the affinity of prazosin induced by $Mg^{2+}$ has been reported at rat brain $\alpha_2$-receptor sites labeled with CLO (8).

These data suggest that the $\alpha_2(H)$ form of the receptor may have lower affinity for antagonists, as well as higher affinity for agonists. GTP reduced the affinity of

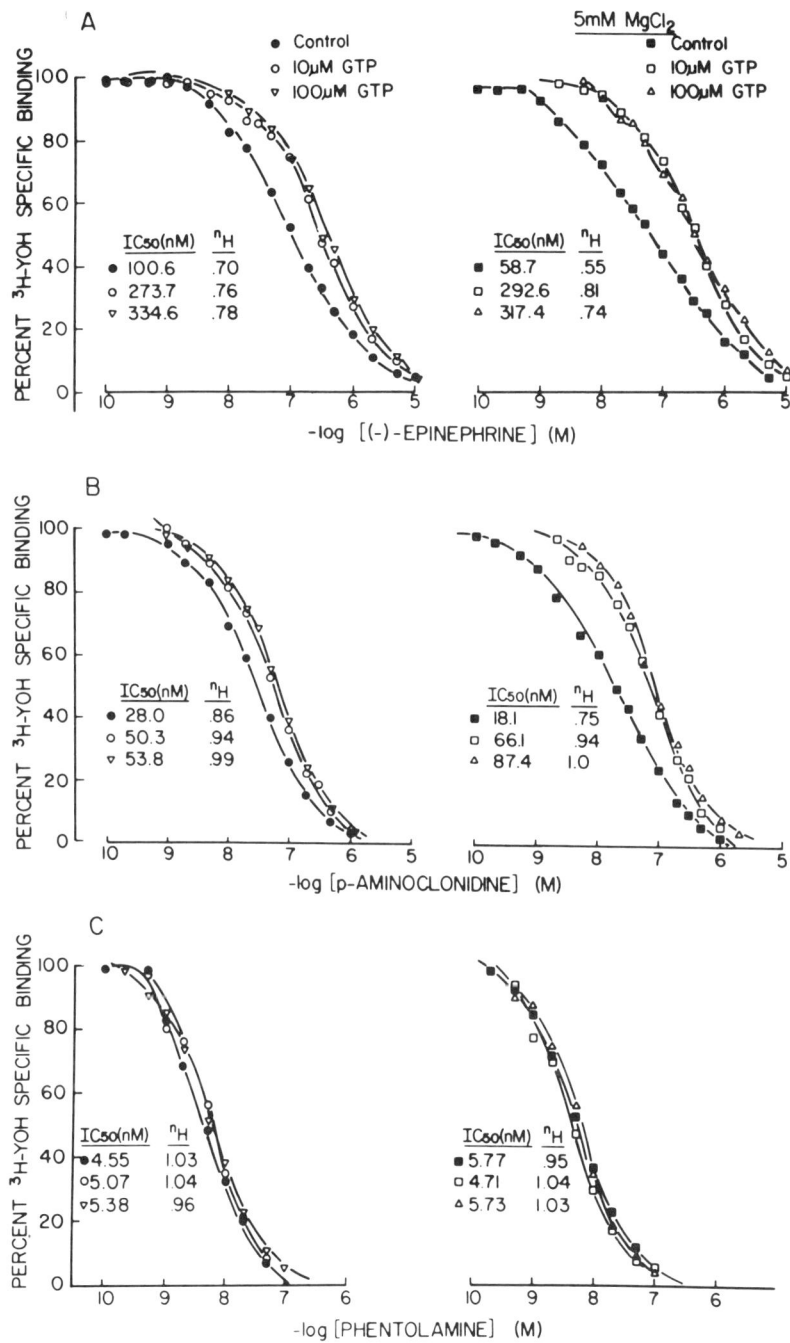

**FIG. 1.** Inhibition of 0.2 nM $^3$H-YOH binding to platelet membranes at 25°C (60 min) by (−)-EPI, p-aminoclonidine, and phentolamine in the presence or absence of GTP and $MgCl_2$. Points represent mean data from four to six experiments.

(−)-EPI and PAC and steepened the competition curves (Fig. 1), suggesting that in the presence of GTP, most of the receptors are in the $\alpha_2(L)$ form. However, even in the presence of 100 μM GTP, the $n_H$ value for (−)-EPI competition is significantly less than 1.0.

EPI binding to platelet membranes with 1.0 mM $MgCl_2$ present was saturable and high affinity (Fig. 2). Unlike YOH binding, the Scatchard plot of EPI binding was distinctly curvilinear, even over a restricted ligand concentration range, as would be expected if EPI exhibited different affinities for various states of the platelet $\alpha_2$-receptor. The mean $K_D$ value for EPI in these experiments was about 7.0 nM. More precise estimates of the $K_D$ values for EPI were obtained from kinetic experiments. Dissociation of EPI (1.5 nM) was biphasic (see Fig. 5) and $K_D$ values determined from $k_{-1}/k_1$ ratios were 2.0 nM and 40 nM, neither of which corresponds to the affinity of (−)-EPI ($IC_{50}$ about 350 nM) at YOH sites in the presence of GTP when most of the receptors would be in the $\alpha_2(L)$ state. Scatchard plots of platelet PAC binding with 1.0 mM $MgCl_2$ present were more markedly biphasic, as was PAC dissociation (see Fig. 5). Two PAC sites with $K_D$ values of 0.7 and 9.0 nM were observed, again not corresponding to the affinity of PAC at YOH

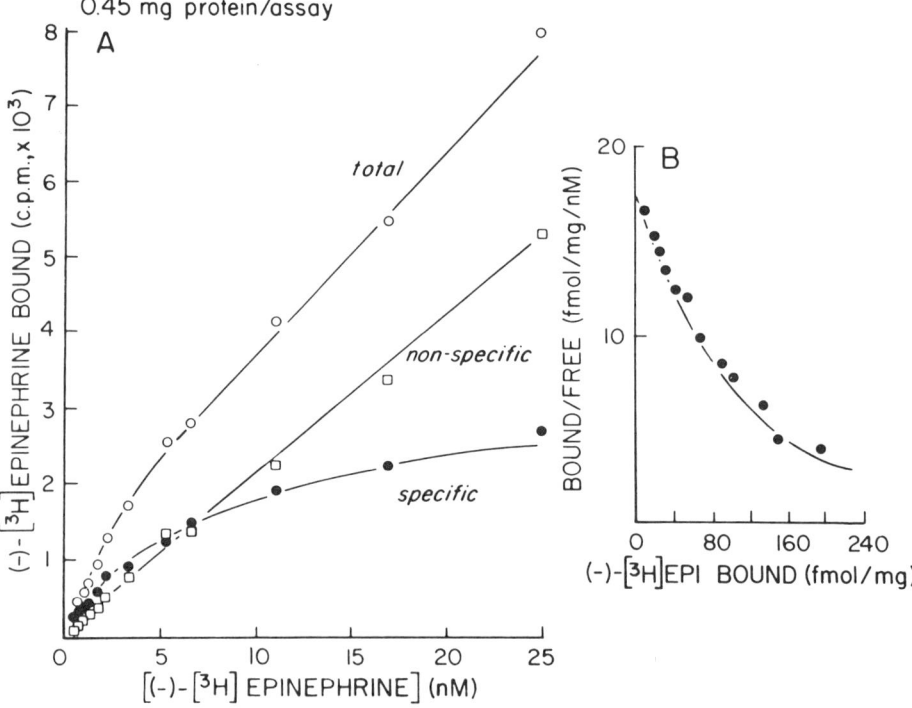

**FIG. 2.** (−)-³H-EPI binding to platelet membranes at 25°C (60 min) in the presence of 1.0 mM $MgCl_2$ as a function of increasing ligand concentration. Nonspecific binding was defined by 1.0 μM oxymetazoline. **A:** Saturation isotherm; **B:** Scatchard plot.

sites in the presence of GTP (Fig. 1B). These data suggest that three affinity states of the platelet $\alpha_2$-receptor may be present: (SH), (H), and (L).

The pharmacologic profiles of platelet EPI and PAC sites were very similar, and indicated $\alpha_2$-receptor interactions. At both sites catecholamine and imidazoline drugs had much higher affinity than they exhibited at YOH sites, suggesting that EPI and PAC at low concentrations predominantly labled high affinity states (Table 1), although the shallow competition curves ($n_H < 1.0$) indicated that even at low EPI and PAC concentrations, more than one state of the receptor is being labeled. Some antagonists were significantly less potent at EPI and PAC sites than at YOH sites, indicating that antagonists have lower affinity at $\alpha_2$(H) and/or $\alpha_2$(SH). In theory, EPI and PAC at high enough concentrations should, like YOH, label the total $\alpha_2$-receptor population. However, over the relatively limited concentration ranges of EPI and PAC that were practicable, the $B_{max}$ values derived from Scatchard analysis would represent predominantly $\alpha_2$(SH) and $\alpha_2$(H), and should therefore be lower than the $B_{max}$ value for YOH. The mean $B_{max}$ values for YOH, EPI, and PAC in platelet membranes were 182, 130, and 109 fmoles/mg protein, respectively; thus with 1.0 mM $MgCl_2$ present, EPI and PAC labeled with high affinity 72 and 60% of the total $\alpha_2$-receptor population. The $B_{max}$ for PAC was routinely lower than the $B_{max}$ for EPI. Since PAC and EPI appeared to label the same high affinity states of the receptor, the steeper competition curve for the partial agonist PAC in inhibiting YOH binding appears to be due to the induction of fewer high affinity states. PAC maximally inhibited basal adenylate cyclase activity in fresh platelet membranes by 15% at 25°C (0.05 mM ATP present), compared to 50% inhibition by ($-$)-EPI. A similar correlation between efficacy and induction of high affinity states has been proposed for the erythrocyte $\beta$-receptor (19).

Omission of $MgCl_2$ reduced the number of high affinity platelet sites labeled by EPI and increased the $K_D$ (Fig. 3). Similar results were obtained with PAC, and in the absence of $Mg^{2+}$, both phases of PAC dissociation were accelerated (data not shown). These data parallel the $Mg^{2+}$-induced increases in the affinity of these two drugs at platelet YOH sites (Fig. 1). On the other hand, pretreatment of platelet membranes with 5.0 mM EDTA increased the number of sites labeled by EPI and PAC, possibly by chelating endogenous nucleotides (see Table 2).

Nucleotides inhibited the specific binding of 1.5 nM EPI and 0.6 nM PAC to platelet membranes in the following potency order: Gpp(NH)p > GTP > GDP > ITP > ATP = CTP > GMP. Gpp(NH)p and GTP had $ED_{50}$ values of 0.2 and 0.7 μM respectively. In EPI and PAC saturation experiments, the effect of 10 μM GTP was seen as a reduction in affinity, with, in the case of PAC a reduction also in the number of sites labeled (Fig. 4, Table 2). GTP increased the $K_D$ of *observable* EPI binding to 30–40 nM, similar to the $K_D$ of the rapidly dissociating component of binding in the absence of GTP, and increased the $K_D$ of PAC binding to 5–10 nM, similar to the lower affinity component of PAC binding in the absence of nucleotide. These results suggest that GTP either converts $\alpha_2$(SH) to $\alpha_2$(H), or converts $\alpha_2$(SH) to $\alpha_2$(L), which cannot be observed using EPI or PAC. In any case, even with 10 μM GTP present, there were still significant $\alpha_2$(H) interactions,

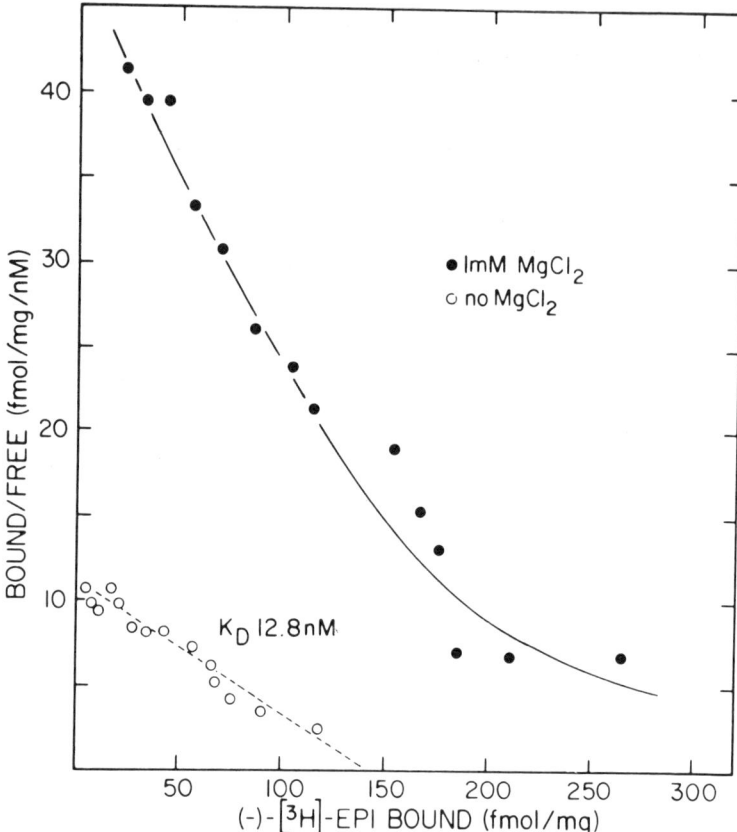

**FIG. 3.** Effect of 1.0 mM MgCl$_2$ on the saturation characteristics of $(-)$-$^3$H-EPI binding to platelet membranes (Scatchard plot).

as also indicated by the data in Fig. 1. Dissociation microconstants ($k_{-1}$) for EPI and PAC were not changed when platelet $\alpha_2$-receptors had been labeled in the presence of 1.0 µM GTP (Fig. 5), which further suggests that the nucleotide alters the ratio of the different affinity states of the receptor, rather than reducing the affinity of agonists at any particular receptor state.

GTP and Gpp(NH)p were less effective in reducing EPI and PAC binding in the absence of Mg$^{2+}$ (not shown), paralleling the less extensive GTP-induced shifts of agonist affinities at YOH sites in the absence of Mg$^{2+}$ (Fig. 1). These data may indicate that $\alpha_2$(SH) is particularly susceptible to GTP. The effects of various agents on EPI and PAC saturation constants are summarized in Table 2.

Another indication of the alteration of the ratio of different affinity states labeled by EPI and PAC in the presence of 1.0 µM GTP is that the affinities of catecholamine and imidazoline competitors were reduced two- to threefold, together with a reduction in $n_H$ values for these drugs (Table 3). On the other hand, 1.0 µM GTP

TABLE 2. *Saturation constants for (−)-³H-EPI and ³H-PAC binding to human platelet membrane α₂-receptors: effects of pretreatment with EDTA, added magnesium, and added GTP*

| Condition | | | ³H-EPI | | ³H-PAC | |
|---|---|---|---|---|---|---|
| EDTA | $Mg^{2+}$ (mM) | GTP (μM) | $K_D$ (nM) | $B_{max}$ (fmol/mg) | $K_D$ (nM) | $B_{max}$ (fmol/mg) |
| − | 1.0 | — | 7.2 ± 0.6 | 130 ± 10 | 1. 0.7 ± 0.03 <br> 2. 9.1 ± 2.0 | 42 ± 13 <br> 109 ± 19 |
| − | 1.0 | 10 | 29.6 ± 2.7 | 144 ± 4 | | |
| + | 1.0 | — | 5.2 ± 0.8 | 252 ± 11 | 1. 0.6 ± 0.09 <br> 2. 8.3 ± 2.1 | 55 ± 11 <br> 134 ± 19 |
| + | 1.0 | 10 | | | 10.7 ± 5.2 | 65 ± 8 |
| + | — | — | 6.7 ± 3.9 | 137 ± 4 | 4.0 ± 0.1 | 103 ± 25 |
| + | — | 10 | 38.1 | 121 | 9.8 | 95 |

All assays were conducted at 25°C using discarded platelet membranes. Platelet membranes were pretreated with EDTA by resuspending them twice in 50 mM Tris-HCl containing 5.0 mM EDTA, with intervening centrifugation at 50,000 × g. Values are mean ± SEM of three to six saturation experiments.

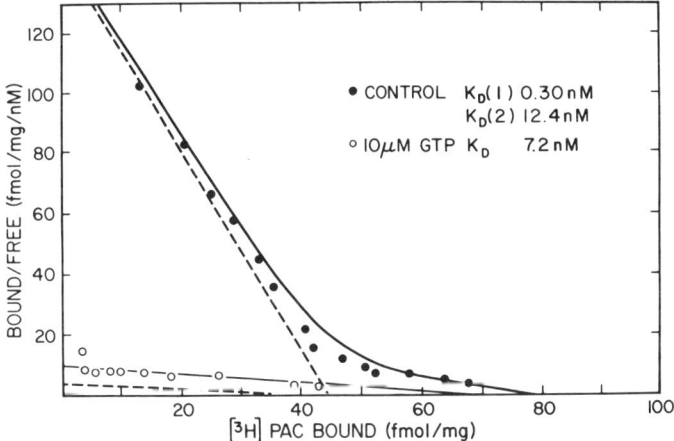

**FIG. 4.** Effect of 10 μM GTP on the saturation characteristics of ³H-*p*-aminoclonidine binding to platelet membranes at 25°C (40 min) in the presence of 1.0 mM $MgCl_2$ (Scatchard plot). Nonspecific binding was defined by 1.0 μM phentolamine.

caused a two- to threefold increase in the affinity of antagonists at sites labeled by EPI and PAC, further evidence that the $α_2$(SH) form of the receptor may have lower affinity for antagonists (Table 3). GTP, 10 μM also reduced the $K_D$ of YOH by 40% (not shown). $MgCl_2$, 1.0 mM, increased the $IC_{50}$ value for prazosin two-fold at platelet PAC sites, similar to the effect of $MgCl_2$ on prazosin interactions at YOH sites mentioned above.

The characteristics of YOH binding to intact platelets at 25°C were compared with the binding in membranes (in Tris-HCl). Association of YOH to intact platelets

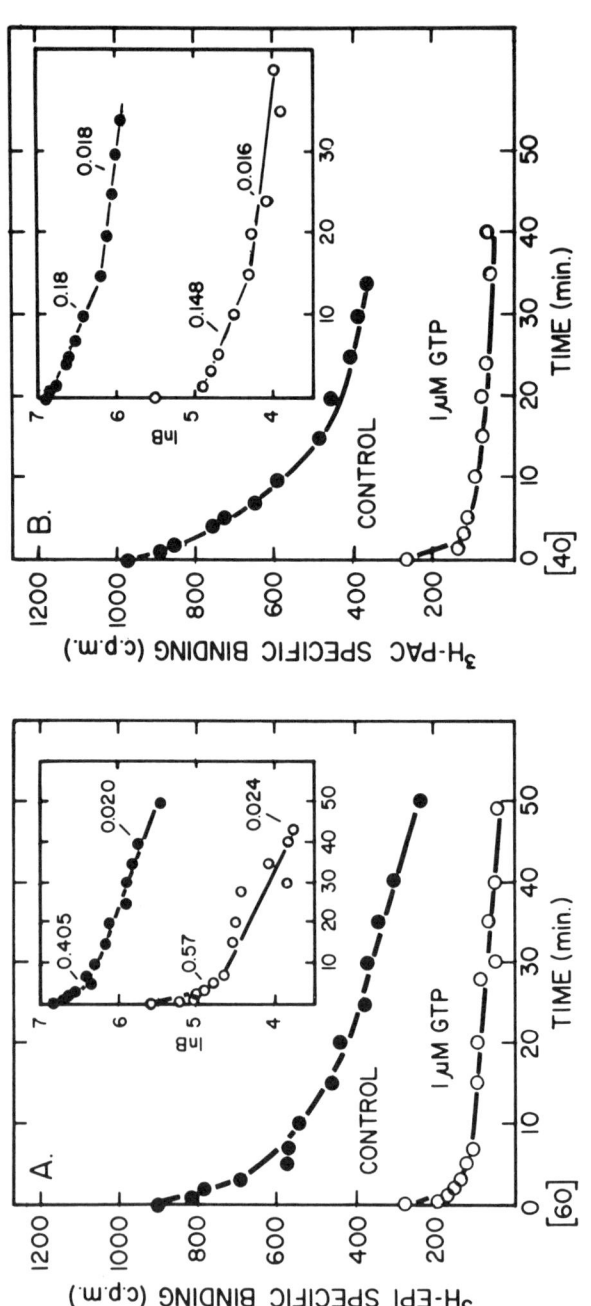

**FIG. 5.** Dissociation of **A**: (−)-³H-EPI and **B**: ³H-p-aminoclonidine specific binding to human platelet membranes at 25°C. Membranes were incubated to equilibrium for 60 min (EPI) or 40 min (p-aminoclonidine), in the absence or presence of 1.0 μM GTP, and binding was then dissociated by addition of 1.0 μM oxymetazoline (EPI) or 10 μM (−)norepinephrine (PAC). *Inserts:* Semilogarithmic plots of dissociation curves. Numbers represent $k_{-1}$ values determined by feathering procedures.

TABLE 3. *Effect of GTP on competitor affinities at platelet $\alpha_2$-receptor sites labeled by (−)-$^3$H- EPI and PAC*

| | $^3$H-EPI | | | | $^3$H-PAC | | | |
|---|---|---|---|---|---|---|---|---|
| | Control | | 1.0 μM GTP | | Control | | 1.0 μM GTP | |
| Drug | IC$_{50}$ (nM) | $n_H$ | IC$_{50}$ (nM) | $n_H$ | IC$_{50}$ (nM) | $n_H$ | IC$_{50}$ (nM) | $n_H$ |
| Catecholamines | | | | | | | | |
| (−)-EPI | 3.3 | 0.80 | 7.1 | 0.67 | 2.4 | 0.82 | 7.8 | 0.74 |
| (−)-NE | 13.6 | 0.80 | 20.2 | 0.69 | 6.5 | 0.78 | 12.7 | 0.64 |
| Imidazolines | | | | | | | | |
| CLO | 3.3 | 0.82 | 12.7 | 0.72 | 3.1 | 0.70 | 5.0 | 0.93 |
| Antagonists | | | | | | | | |
| phentolamine | 3.8 | 0.91 | 1.8 | 1.00 | 2.9 | 0.80 | 1.4 | 0.65 |
| YOH | 10.6 | 0.81 | 6.2 | 1.03 | 16.5 | 0.73 | 5.0 | 0.59 |

See legend to Table 1. Values are means of three to nine experiments.

in Hank's buffer was rapid and monophasic at 25°C. In saturation experiments, YOH labeled a single set of sites with a $K_D$ (1.9 nM) and $B_{max}$ (129 fmol/mg protein; 145 receptors/platelet) similar to binding constants in membranes. Binding was stereospecific and had an $\alpha_2$-receptor profile. CLO (48 nM) and phentolamine (12 nM) had similar $K_I$ values at YOH sites on intact platelets and membranes, but (−)-EPI was seven times less potent in competing at intact cell YOH sites ($K_I$ 520 nM). Interestingly, (−)-EPI competition curves were still shallow ($n_H$ 0.77). Identical results were obtained for YOH binding to platelet membranes in Hank's buffer. However, in Hank's buffer, 100 μM GTP caused a right shift for (−)-EPI inhibition at YOH sites in membranes, but not on intact platelets (Fig. 6). These data indicate both that GTP acts on the inner face of the cell membrane, while Na$^+$ (137 mM) acts on the outer face, and, additionally, that GTP and Na$^+$ effects on agonist affinity are additive. (−)-EPI competition curves at intact platelet sites may be shallow because of the presence of 1.0 mM Mg$^{2+}$ in Hank's buffer, and would indicate the presence of high affinity states of the receptor; specific, saturable binding of PAC to intact platelets at 25°C was observed, with a $K_D$ of 7.0 nM and $B_{max}$ of 27 fmol/mg protein. Thus PAC labeled fewer sites with lower affinity in intact platelets.

## NG 108–15 Cells

The characteristics of radioligand binding to $\alpha_2$-receptors in NG 108–15 cell membranes were quite similar to the above platelet membrane data. Binding of YOH, EPI, and PAC was saturable, and in each case monophasic ($K_D$ values of 7.1, 11.2, and 1.8 nM, respectively), and reversible. Linear dissociation and Scatchard plots for EPI and PAC indicated that the distinction between (H) and (SH) states was not so observable for the NG 108–15 $\alpha_2$-receptor. However, over restricted radioligand concentration ranges, while YOH labeled 22,600 receptors/cell, EPI and PAC labeled only 14,550 (64%) and 8500 (37%) receptors/cell, respectively. Table 4 shows that while competition studies confirmed that all three ligands labeled an $\alpha_2$-receptor, EPI and PAC appeared to bind to a high affinity state of

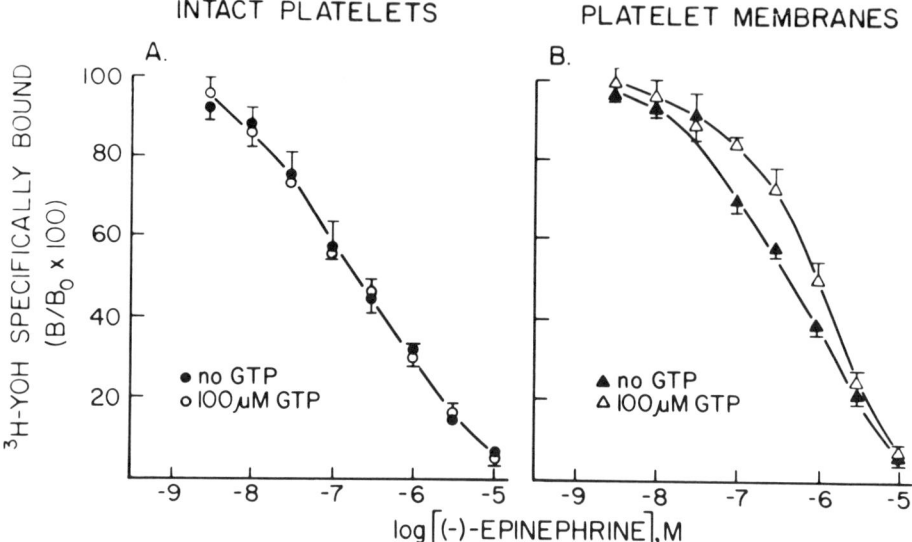

**FIG. 6.** Inhibition of 0.2 nM $^3$H-YOH binding to intact platelets or platelet membranes in Hank's buffer by (−)-EPI, in the presence or absence of 100 μM GTP. Points represent mean data from three experiments.

TABLE 4. *Potencies of $\alpha_2$-receptor agonists and antagonists in inhibiting $^3$H-PAC, (−)-$^3$H-EPI, and $^3$H-YOH binding, and in inhibiting or reversing the inhibition of basal and $PGE_1$-stimulated adenylate cyclase activity in NG 108-15 membranes*

| Drug | $^3$H-EPI | $^3$H-PAC | $^3$H-YOH | Basal | 10 μM $PGE_1$ |
|---|---|---|---|---|---|
| | | | $IC_{50}$ (nM) | | |
| Catecholamines | | | | | |
| (−)-NE | 6.1 | 3.0 | 390 | 510 | 520 |
| (−)-EPI | 11.2 | 5.4 | 250 | 250 | 390 |
| (−)-isoproterenol | 270 | 60 | 29,000 | 24,000 | 28,000 |
| (+)-NE | 32 | 90 | 1900 | 380,000 | 100,000 |
| Imidazolines | | | | | |
| PAC | 4.0 | 1.3 | 52 | 660 | 430 |
| CLO | 32 | 30 | 48 | 470 | 415 |
| oxymetazoline | 5.6 | 3.9 | 270 | 575 | 560 |
| Antagonists | | | | | |
| dihydroergocryptine | 40 | 4.0 | 6.0 | 10 | — |
| phentolamine | 65 | 22 | 39 | 10 | — |
| YOH | 140 | 36 | 7.8 | 40 | — |
| prazosin | 5500 | 2100 | 42 | — | — |

Drug inhibition of specific binding of 0.5 nM PAC, 0.8 nM YOH, and 1.4 nM EPI, using 6 to 8 concentrations of inhibitor, was performed as described in text. Agonist inhibition of basal or $PGE_1$-stimulated adenylate cyclase activity, and antagonist reversal of inhibition caused by 1.0 μM (−)-EPI, was also measured. $IC_{50}$ values were determined by log probit analysis. Values are means of two to six experiments.

the $\alpha_2$-receptor, as in platelets. Similar data have been reported for CLO binding to NG 108–15 $\alpha_2$-receptors (1). As in platelets, the antagonists YOH and prazosin were more potent inhibitors of YOH binding than of EPI and PAC binding.

Further evidence that NG 108–15 $\alpha_2$-receptors occur in at least two affinity states was the shallow nature of competition by agonists, and not antagonists, at YOH sites (Fig. 7). Similar results have been observed for DHEC binding to NG 108–15 $\alpha_2$-receptors (10). In the presence of 1.0 mM $MgCl_2$, GTP and GDP had biphasic effects on EPI and PAC binding, with low concentrations enhancing, and higher concentrations inhibiting specific binding (Fig. 8). Both actions resulted from changes in the $B_{max}$ of EPI and PAC. The biphasic nucleotide actions were different from nucleotide effects at platelet $\alpha_2$-receptors, but similar to GTP and GDP interactions at brain EPI and CLO $\alpha_2$-receptor sites in the presence of divalent cation (28,44). Low Gpp(NH)p concentrations did not increase agonist binding in either NG 108–15 or brain membranes. GTP and Gpp(NH)p (50 μM) caused a two- to threefold decrease in the potencies of (−)-EPI and PAC in competing at YOH sites, while lower GTP concentrations (10 μM) increased agonist potencies.

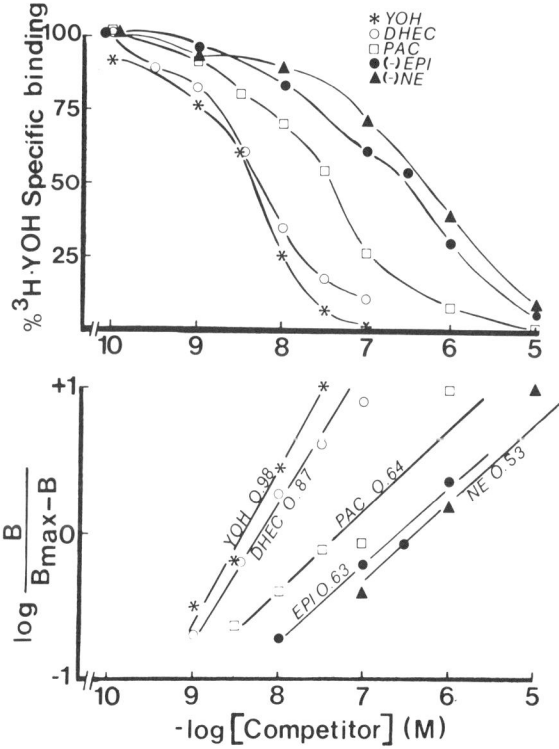

**FIG. 7.** Inhibition of 0.8 nM ³H-YOH binding to NG 108–15 cell membranes at 25°C. Points represent mean data from four experiments. **Above:** Inhibition curves; **Below:** Hill plots.

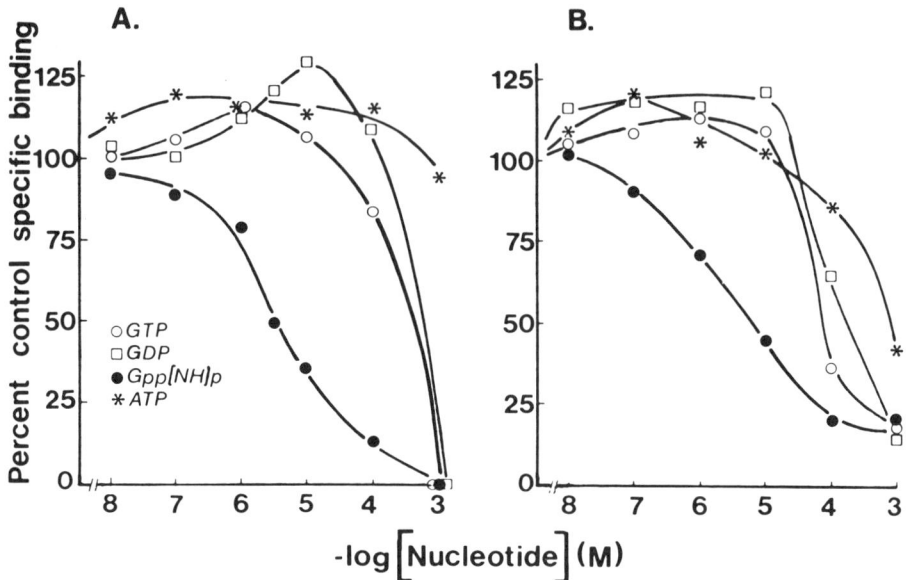

**FIG. 8.** Inhibition of **(A)** 1.4 nM (−)-$^3$H-EPI and **(B)** 0.5 nM $^3$H-$p$-aminoclonidine specific binding to NG 108–15 cell membranes at 25°C by nucleotides. Points are mean data from four experiments.

Catecholamines inhibited basal and prostaglandin $E_1$ (PGE$_1$; 10 μM)-stimulated adenylate cyclase activity to a maximum of 50%, while the imidazolines CLO and PAC inhibited cyclase activity maximally by 25%, and antagonized catecholamine inhibition. CLO and PAC therefore appeared to be partial agonists at NG 108–15 $\alpha_2$-receptors, as reported elsewhere (1). Catecholamines and antagonists had similar potencies at YOH sites and in inhibiting, or reversing the inhibition of, adenylate cyclase activity (Table 4). Therefore, for catecholamines, the binding/cyclase potency ratio, $K_D/K_{INH}$ was about 1.0. However, the $K_D/K_{INH}$ ratio for CLO and PAC was about 0.1, possibly reflecting less efficient coupling due to their partial agonist nature.

Preliminary studies of $\alpha_2$-receptor changes as a result of incubation of NG 108–15 cells with the agonist (−)-EPI (10 μM) showed a reduction in the number of YOH and PAC sites after incubation periods of 2 hr or longer (Table 5). However, maximum inhibition of adenylate cyclase activity by (−)-EPI was not reduced by up to 4 hr of agonist incubation, although the inhibitory potency of (−)-EPI was somewhat lowered. Thus, unlike frog erythrocyte β-receptor desensitization (19), there is not a parallel reduction in binding and maximum response for NG 108–15 $\alpha_2$-receptors. This may reflect the presence of spare receptors on NG 108–15 cells. As reported by Sabol and Nirenberg (30), we observed that incubation of the cells with (−)-EPI increased basal cyclase activity.

TABLE 5. *Effect of (−)-EPI treatment on NG 108-15 $\alpha_2$-receptor sites*

| Treatment | Time (hr) | $K_D$ (nM) | $B_{max}$ (% control) | $K_D$ (nM) | $B_{max}$ (% control) |
|---|---|---|---|---|---|
| | | 3H-YOH | | 3H-PAC | |
| Control | 1.0 | — | — | 3 | |
| EPI | | — | — | 7 | 98 |
| Control | 2.0 | 12 | | 6 | |
| EPI | | 15 | 56 | 13 | 60 |
| Control | 4.0 | 9 | | 4 | |
| EPI | | 13 | 53 | 11 | 54 |
| Control | 8.0 | 8 | | 7 | |
| EPI | | 12 | 63 | 18 | 47 |

Cells in monolayers were incubated with 10 μM (−)-EPI at 37°C for 1–8 hr, then removed by agitation, centrifuged, and lysed by freezing and thawing in hypotonic Tris-HCl buffer. Membranes were incubated in 50 mM Tris-HCl containing 100 μM Gpp (NH)p to remove residual tightly bound EPI, and then washed three times by centrifugation. Seven ligand concentrations were used in saturation experiments. Control $B_{max}$ values (receptors/cell) did not vary as a function of incubation time.

## Bovine Cerebral Cortex and Aorta

Both RAUW- and YOH-labeled $\alpha_2$-receptors in brain and aorta membranes, with RAUW being two to three times more potent, and more $\alpha_2$-selective as judged by the lower affinity of prazosin in competition experiments. In these tissues, binding of both ligands was optimal in 50 mM Na-K buffer at 4°C. $K_D$ values for RAUW were 3.2 nM in cerebral cortex (Fig. 9) and 1.0 nM in aorta. The $B_{max}$ of RAUW binding in cortex was similar to that observed for EPI or CLO binding to high-agonist-affinity, nucleotide-sensitive, bovine cortex $\alpha_2$-receptors. Competition studies in both tissues indicated that RAUW labeled $\alpha_2$-receptors, and the relatively low affinities and low $n_H$ values for catecholamine agonists in both tissues, compared to radioagonist $\alpha_2$-receptor binding, indicated that, as for YOH binding in NG 108–15 cells and platelets, the antagonist ligand RAUW labeled high and low affinity states of the $\alpha_2$-receptor in cerebral cortex and aorta (Table 6).

Catecholamine $K_I$ values at antagonist sites were similar in these tissues and platelets, although 50 mM Na$^+$ was present, which would be expected to produce a right shift. However, the lower incubation temperature may have exerted an effect opposite to that of Na$^+$, by analogy to temperature effects at β-receptor systems (12,46) and bovine cortical EPI binding to $\alpha_2$-receptors (42). GTP, 100 μM, increased catecholamine and imidazoline $K_I$ values two- to threefold and steepened their competition curves at cortex, but not at aorta RAUW sites. These data, together with previous investigations of radioagonist binding, suggest that brain and vascular $\alpha_2$-receptors are similar to platelet and NG 108–15 $\alpha_2$-receptors, in that they occur in two or more affinity states and can be regulated by guanine nucleotides. Brain and vascular $\alpha_2$-receptors are therefore also likely to be inversely coupled to adenylate cyclase.

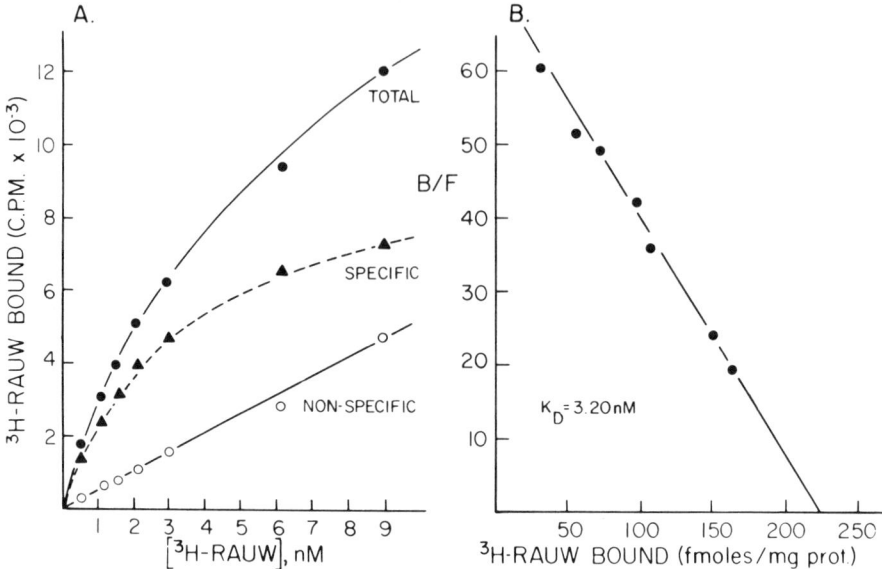

**FIG. 9.** $^3$H-Rauwolscine binding to bovine cortex membranes at 4°C (120 min) in 50 mM Na-K buffer as a function of increasing ligand concentration. Nonspecific binding was defined by 100 μM (−)-NE. **A:** saturation isotherm; **B:** Scatchard plot.

TABLE 6. *Drug competition at bovine cerebral cortex $\alpha_2$-receptors labeled by $^3$H-EPI and $^3$H-rauwolscine*

| Drug | $^3$H-EPI $K_I$ (nM) | $^3$H-RAUW $K_I$ (nM) | $n_H$ |
|---|---|---|---|
| Agonists | | | |
| (−)-EPI | 2[a] | 150 | 0.67 |
| (−)-α-me-NE | 4 | 200 | 0.65 |
| (−)-NE | 6 | 500 | 0.71 |
| (+)-NE | 260 | 4600 | 0.56 |
| (−)-isoproterenol | 1100 | 40,000 | 0.50 |
| Imidazolines | | | |
| p-aminoclonidine | 2 | 2 | 0.55 |
| oxymetazoline | 5 | 2 | 0.75 |
| Antagonists | | | |
| rauwolscine | — | 4 | 1.04 |
| YOH | 40 | 5 | 1.06 |
| dihydroergocryptine | 5 | 7 | 0.91 |
| phentolamine | 2 | 8 | 0.91 |
| WB-4101 | 41 | 1 | 1.04 |
| prazosin | 9000 | 3000 | 0.97 |

Incubations were carried out, as described in text, at 25°C for 60 min for $^3$H-EPI, and at 4°C for 120 min for $^3$H-RAUW. IC$_{50}$ values were determined from Hill plots. Data are mean values from two to five experiments.

[a] All competitors at $^3$H-EPI sites had $n_H$ values of 1.0.

## DISCUSSION

The present investigations of binding of various ligands to human platelet $\alpha_2$-receptors support the notion that this receptor exists in three affiinity states; approximate $K_D$ values at the different affinity states are 2, 40, and 400 nM for ($-$)-EPI, and 0.5, 10, and 100 nM for PAC. Previously, two high affinity binding sites for CLO had been observed in brain membranes, and examined with respect to differences in regional distribution (40) and nucleotide and ion regulation (28). The two brain CLO sites may be equivalent to (SH) and (H) states of the same $\alpha_2$-receptor, rather than two distinct $\alpha_2$-receptor populations, given the similarities between these sites and the two platelets labeled by EPI and PAC. The relationship between the present observations of three $\alpha_2$-receptor states, and the two-state "dynamic receptor affinity" model of $\alpha_2$-receptor function proposed by Hoffman and Lefkowitz (4) is unclear. It is possible that the highest affinity state (SH) labeled by EPI and PAC in discarded platelets represents a "desensitized" or uncoupled form of the receptor (21), since analysis of EPI, PAC and YOH binding in freshly prepared platelet membranes indicates some loss of high affinity ($-$)-EPI and PAC interactions, although the total number of YOH sites is the same in fresh and 3-day old platelets (not shown). The same stimulation of adenylate cyclase by $PGE_1$ is observed in fresh and discarded platelets, but we can observe ($-$)-EPI inhibition of cyclase only in the former tissue.

H.R.N. and H.R.N.$Mg^{2+}$ have been proposed as different states of the $\beta$-receptor (3). The agonist binding data in Figs. 3 and 4, and summarized in Table 2, suggest that $Mg^{2+}$ promotes binding to the (SH) state, which is preferentially sensitive to guanine nucleotides. This would imply that $\alpha_2$(SH) and $\alpha_2$(H) in platelets are equivalent to H.R.N.$Mg^{2+}$ and H.R.N, respectively, and that H.R.N.$Mg^{2+}$ is more readily dissociated by GTP. The labeling of fewer (SH) and (H) by the partial agonist PAC, compared with EPI, and the evidence that guanine nucleotides change equilibria between states rather than alter agonist affinities at any state, complements the $\beta$-receptor model proposed by Lefkowitz et al. (19), but differs from recent data from this group that indicate that guanine nucleotides decrease the affinity of agonists at the platelet $\alpha_2$(H) (5).

The platelet data are very similar to the analysis of another inversely coupled receptor, the MACh receptor, not only in that three states are proposed, but in the evidence that divalent cations and GTP regulate antagonist affinities in a manner opposite to their regulation of agonist affinities (5). If different receptor states do indeed have different affinities for antagonists, then antagonists may alter equilibria between receptor states, with the result that the kinetic model for $\alpha_2$-receptor adenylate cyclase coupling may be significantly more complex than previously proposed.

The NG 108–15 $\alpha_2$-receptor does not appear to possess as many $\alpha_2$(SH) states, supporting the notion that (SH) states may be uncoupled, since the cells were fully functional and not desensitized. The apparent discrepancy between agonist-mediated down-regulation of NG 108–15 $\alpha_2$-receptor sites, and the absence of a decrease in the $\alpha_2$-mediated cyclase response at the same time as there is an increase in basal cyclase activity, needs to be investigated further. Receptor loss in these experiments is not likely to be due to residual tightly bound agonist, since the cell membranes were incubated with Gpp(NH)p and thoroughly washed before assay.

Generally binding data in brain and aorta membranes support the presence in these tissues of multiple $\alpha_2$-receptor affinity states which can be modulated by nucleotides and cations in a manner basically similar to modulation of platelet and NG 108–15 $\alpha_2$-receptors. Thus these receptors are also likely to be adenylate cyclase coupled. The increase in agonist binding seen with low concentrations of GTP and GDP, but not Gpp(NH)p, in the presence of divalent cation at brain and NG 108–15 $\alpha_2$-receptors, but not platelet $\alpha_2$-receptors, may be related to phosphorylation-dephosphorylation reactions specific to neuronal membranes, for which GTP and GDP, but not Gpp(NH)p, are substrates.

## ACKNOWLEDGMENTS

This research was supported in part by USPHS Grants NS 15595 and DA 02763, and a Grant-in-Aid from the American Heart Association. We thank Marina Wolf for her excellent technical assistance.

## REFERENCES

1. Atlas, D., and Sabol, S. L. (1981): Interaction of clonidine and clonidine analogues with α-adrenergic receptors of neuroblastoma × glioma hybrid cells and rat brain. Comparison of ligand binding with inhibition of adenylate cyclase. *Eur. J. Biochem.*, 113:521–529.
2. Birdsall, N. J. M., Burgen, A. S. V., and Hulme, E. C. (1978): The binding of agonists to brain muscarinic receptors. *Mol. Pharmacol.*, 14:723–736.
3. Cech, S. Y., Broaddus, W. C., and Maguire, M. E. (1980): Adenylate cyclase: The role of magnesium and other divalent cations. *Mol. Cell. Biochem.*, 33:67–92.
4. Daiguji, M., Meltzer, H. Y., and U'Prichard, D. C. (1981): Human platelet $\alpha_2$-adrenergic receptors: Labeling with ³H-yohimbine, a selective antagonist ligand. *Life Sci.*, 28:2705–2717.
5. Ehlert, F. J., Roeske, W. R., and Yamamura, H. I. (1980): Regulation of muscarinic receptor binding by guanine nucleotides and N-ethylmaleimide. *J. Supramol. Struc.*, 14:149–162.
6. Garcia-Sainz, J. A., Hoffman, B. B., Li, S.-Y., Lefkowitz, R. J., and Fain, J. N. (1980): Role of alpha₁-adrenoceptors in the turnover of phosphatidylinositol and of alpha₂ adrenoceptors in the regulation of cyclic AMP accumulation in hamster adipocytes. *Life Sci.*, 27:953–961.
7. Garcia-Sevilla, J. A., Zis, A. P., Zelnik, T. C., and Smith, C. B. (1981): Tricyclic antidepressant drug treatment decreases $\alpha_2$-adrenoreceptors in human platelet membranes. *Eur. J. Pharmacol.*, 69:121–123.
8. Glossmann, H., and Hornung, R. (1980): Alpha₂ adrenoceptors in rat brain. The divalent cation site. *Naunyn Schmiedebergs Arch. Pharmacol.*, 314:101–109.
9. Greenberg, D. A., and Snyder, S. H. (1978): Pharmacological properties of [³H]dihydroergokryptine binding sites associated with alpha noradrenergic receptors in rat brain membranes. *Mol. Pharmacol.*, 14:38–49.
10. Haga, T., and Haga, K. (1981): Characterization by [³H]dihydroergocryptine binding of alpha adrenergic receptors in neuroblastoma × glioma hybrid cells. *J. Neurochem.*, 36:1152–1159.
11. Hedler, L., Stamm, G., Weitzell, R., and Starke, K. (1981): Functional characterization of central α-adrenoceptors by yohimbine diastereomers. *Eur. J. Pharmacol.*, 70:43–52.
12. Heidenreich, K. A., Weiland, G. A., and Molinoff, P. B. (1980): Characterization of radiolabeled agonist binding to β-adrenergic receptors in mammalian tissues. *J. Cyclic Nucleotide Res.*, 6:217–230.
13. Hoffman, B. B., Kilpatrick, D. M., and Lefkowitz, R. J. (1980): Heterogeneity of radioligand binding to α-adrenergic receptors. Analysis of guanine nucleotide regulation of agonist binding in relation to receptor subtypes. *J. Biol. Chem.*, 255:4645–4652.

14. Hoffman, B. B., and Lefkowitz, R. J. (1980): Radiolabeled binding studies of adrenergic receptors: new insights into molecular and physiological regulation. *Annu. Rev. Pharmacol. Toxicol.*, 20: 581–608.
15. Hoffman, B. B., Michel, T., Brenneman, T. B., and Lefkowitz, R. J. (1981): Interactions of agonists with platelet alpha$_2$ adrenergic receptors. *Endocrinology*, 110:926–932.
16. Hoffman, B. B., Michel, T., Kilpatrick, D. M., Lefkowitz, R. J., Tolbert, M. E. M., Gilman, H., and Fain, J. N. (1980): Agonist versus antagonist binding to α-adrenergic receptors. *Proc. Natl. Acad. Sci. USA*, 77:4569–4573.
17. Jakobs, K. H., Aktories, K., and Schultz, G. (1979): GTP-dependent inhibition of cardiac adenylate cyclase by muscarinic cholinergic agonists. *Naunyn Schmiedebergs Arch. Pharmacol.*, 310: 113–119.
18. Jakobs, K. H., Saur, W., and Schultz, G. (1978): Inhibition of platelet adenylate cyclase by epinephrine requires GTP. *FEBS Lett.*, 85:167–170.
19. Kent, R. S., De Lean, A., and Lefkowitz, R. J. (1980): A quantitative analysis of beta-adrenergic receptor interactions: Resolution of high and low affinity states of the receptor by computer modeling of ligand binding data. *Mol. Pharmacol.*, 17:14–23.
20. Langer, S. Z. (1974): Presynaptic regulation of catecholamine release. *Biochem. Pharmacol.*, 23:1973–1980.
21. Lefkowitz, R. J., Wessels, M. R., and Stadel, J. M. (1980): Hormones, receptors, and cyclic AMP: Their role in target cell refractoriness. *Curr. Top. Cell. Regul.*, 17:205–229.
22. Lenox, R. H., McMains, C. L., and Van Riper, D. A. (1980): Characterization of alpha adrenergic inhibition of prostacyclin-stimulated adenylate cyclase in the human platelet. *Neurosci. Soc. Abstr.*, 6:252.
23. Limbird, L. E., Gill, D. M., and Lefkowitz, R. J. (1980): Agonist-promoted coupling of the β-adrenergic receptor with the guanine nucleotide regulatory protein of the adenylate cyclase system. *Proc. Natl. Acad. Sci. USA*, 77:775–779.
24. Maguire, M. E., Ross, E. M., and Gilman, A. G. (1977): β-Adrenergic receptor: Ligand binding properties and the interaction with adenylyl cyclase. *Adv. Cyclic Nucleotide Res.*, 8:1–83.
25. Motulsky, H. J., Shattil, S. J., and Insel, P. A. (1980): Characterization of α$_2$-adrenergic receptors on human platelets using [$^3$H]yohimbine. *Biochem. Biophys. Res. Commun.*, 97:1562–1570.
26. Newman, K. D., Williams, L. T., Bishopric, N. H., and Lefkowitz, R. J. (1978): Identification of α-adrenergic receptors in human platelets by $^3$H-dihydroergocryptine binding. *J. Clin. Invest.*, 61:1136–1144.
27. Rouot, B. R., and Snyder, S. H. (1979): [$^3$H]Para-amino-clonidine: A novel ligand which binds with high affinity to α-adrenergic receptors. *Life Sci.*, 25:769–774.
28. Rouot, B. R., U'Prichard, D. C., and Snyder, S. H. (1980): Multiple α$_2$-noradrenergic receptor sites in rat brain: Selective regulation of high-affinity [$^3$H]clonidine binding by guanine nucleotides and divalent cations. *J. Neurochem.*, 34:374–384.
29. Sabol, S. L., and Nirenberg, M. (1979): Regulation of adenylate cyclase of neuroblastoma × glioma hybrid cells by α-adrenergic receptors. I. Inhibition of adenylate cyclase mediated by α-receptors. *J. Biol. Chem.*, 254:1913–1920.
30. Sabol, S. L., and Nirenberg, M. (1979): Regulation of adenylate cyclase of neuroblastoma × glioma hybrid cells by α-adrenergic receptors. II. Long lived increase of adenylate cyclase activity mediated by α-receptors. *J. Biol. Chem.*, 254:1921–1926.
31. Salamon, Y. (1979): Adenylate cyclase assay. *Adv. Cyclic Nucleotide Res.*, 10:35–55.
32. Salzman, E. W., and Neri, L. L. (1969): Cyclic 3′,5′-adenosine monophosphate in human blood platelets. *Nature (Lond.)*, 224:609–612.
33. Shattil, S. J., McDonough, M., Turnbull, J., and Insel, P. A. (1981): Characterization of alpha-adrenergic receptors in human platelets using [$^3$H]clonidine. *Mol. Pharmacol.*, 19:179–183.
34. Smith, S. K., and Limbird, L. E. (1981): Solubilization of human platelet α-adrenergic receptors: Evidence that agonist occupancy of the receptor stabilizes receptor-effector interactions. *Proc. Natl. Acad. Sci. USA*, 78:4026–4030.
35. Steer, M. L., and Wood, A. (1979): Regulation of human platelet adenylate cyclase by epinephrine, prostaglandin E$_1$, and guanine nucleotides. Evidence for separate guanine nucleotide sites mediating stimulation and inhibition. *J. Biol. Chem.*, 254:10791–10797.
36. Tanaka, T., and Starke, K. (1979): Binding of $^3$H-clonidine to an α-adrenoceptor in membranes of guinea-pig ileum. *Naunyn Schmiedebergs Arch. Pharmacol.*, 309:207–215.
37. Tanaka, T., and Starke, K. (1980): Antagonist/agonist-preferring α-adrenoceptors or α$_1$/α$_2$ adrenoceptors? *Eur. J. Pharmacol.*, 63:191–195.

38. Tsai, B. S., and Lefkowitz, R. J. (1978): Agonist-specific effects of monovalent and divalent cations on adenylate cyclase-coupled alpha adrenergic receptors in rabbit platelets. *Mol. Pharmacol.*, 14:540–548.
39. Tsai, B. S., and Lefkowitz, R. J. (1979): Agonist-specific effects of guanine nucleotides on alpha-adrenergic receptors in human platelets. *Mol. Pharmacol.*, 16:61–68.
40. U'Prichard, D. C., Bechtel, W. D., Rouot, B. M., and Snyder, S. H. (1979): Multiple apparent alpha-noradrenergic receptor binding sites in rat brain: Effect of 6-hydroxydopamine. *Mol. Pharmacol.*, 16:47–60.
41. U'Prichard, D. C., Greenberg, D. A., and Snyder, S. H. (1977): Binding characteristics of a radiolabeled agonist and antagonist at central nervous system alpha noradrenergic receptors. *Mol. Pharmacol.*, 13:454–473.
42. U'Prichard, D. C., and Snyder, S. H. (1977): Binding of $^3$H-catecholamines to $\alpha$-noradrenergic receptor sites in calf brain. *J. Biol. Chem.*, 252:6450–6463.
43. U'Prichard, D. C., and Snyder, S. H. (1978): Guanyl nucleotide influences on $^3$H-ligand binding to $\alpha$-noradrenergic receptors in calf brain membranes. *J. Biol. Chem.*, 253:3444–3452.
44. U'Prichard, D. C., and Snyder, S. H. (1980): Interactions of divalent cations and guanine nucleotides at $\alpha_2$-noradrenergic receptor binding sites in bovine brain membranes. *J. Neurochem.*, 34:385–394.
45. Wei, J.-L., and Sulakhe, P. V. (1980): Requirement for sulfhydral groups in the differential effects of magnesium ion and GTP on agonist binding of muscarinic cholinergic receptor sites in rat atrial membrane fraction. *Naunyn Schmiedebergs Arch. Pharmacol.*, 314:51–59.
46. Weiland, G. A., Minneman, K. P., and Molinoff, P. B. (1980): Thermodynamics of agonist and antagonist interactions with mammalian $\beta$-adrenergic receptors. *Mol. Pharmacol.*, 18:341–347.
47. Williams, L. T., and Lefkowitz, R. J. (1976): Alpha-adrenergic receptor identification by [$^3$H]dihydroergocryptine binding. *Science*, 192:791–793.

#  β-Adrenergic Receptor Subtypes in Rat Brain

*Kenneth P. Minneman, Barry B. Wolfe, Randall N. Pittman, and Perry B. Molinoff

*Department of Pharmacology, University of Colorado Health Sciences Center, Denver, Colorado 80262*

The adrenergic catecholamines norepinephrine (NE) and epinephrine (EPI) are thought to function as neurotransmitters in both the peripheral and central nervous system as well as hormones released from the adrenal medulla. These compounds cause their physiological effects by interacting with specific receptor sites on target cells. The adrenergic receptors with which they interact are divided into several classes, with each class having different pharmacological properties. Ahlquist (1) showed that there were at least two types of adrenergic receptors, which he named α and β. Later it became clear that neither α-adrenergic receptors (5) nor β-adrenergic receptors (15,16) had identical properties in all tissues tested, but that both groups were composed of at least two different subtypes, named $\alpha_1$- and $\alpha_2$-receptors and $\beta_1$- and $\beta_2$-receptors.

The major physiological difference between $\beta_1$- and $\beta_2$-receptors is their differential sensitivity to stimulation by NE. $\beta_1$- and $\beta_2$-receptors have approximately equal affinity for EPI, however, $\beta_2$-receptors have a much lower affinity for NE than do $\beta_1$-receptors (15,16). This observation has led to the suggestion that $\beta_1$-receptors may be neuronally stimulated β-adrenergic receptors, responding to NE released from nerve terminals, and that $\beta_2$-receptors may be hormonally stimulated β-adrenergic receptors, responding to circulating EPI released from the adrenal medulla (4,9). It is clear, however, that $\beta_1$-receptors respond equally well to both NE and EPI, and that $\beta_2$-receptors can also be activated by sufficiently high concentrations of NE. Since the concentration of NE in the synaptic cleft is not known, it is yet possible that NE may be the natural agonist at some $\beta_2$-receptors.

## DISTRIBUTION OF β-ADRENERGIC RECEPTOR SUBTYPES IN RAT BRAIN

The use of radioligand binding assays has made it possible to demonstrate that β-adrenergic receptors are present in high concentrations in various rat brain regions

---

*Present address: Department of Pharmacology, Emory University Medical School, Atlanta, Georgia 30322.

(2,7,29). However, the density of β-adrenergic receptors in a particular brain region bears no apparent relationship to the noradrenergic innervation of that tissue. For example, rat cerebellum, which receives a dense noradrenergic innervation from the locus coeruleus, has a lower density of β-adrenergic receptors than rat caudate, which contains only a very small quantity of NE (8,22).

With the development of methods to distinguish between and quantitatively measure $\beta_1$- and $\beta_2$-receptors using radioligand binding (11,18,19,26), it also became clear that there was no apparent relationship between the NE content of a particular brain region and the density of either $\beta_1$- or $\beta_2$-receptors in that brain region. $\beta_2$-Receptors are relatively homogeneously distributed in rat brain, and the density of these receptors varies less than threefold between particular brain regions (18). $\beta_1$-Receptors are more heterogeneously distributed, and vary more than fifteenfold between various brain regions. However, the density of $\beta_1$-receptors is very high in the cerebral cortex and very low in the cerebellum, both brain regions which receive a dense noradrenergic innervation. Furthermore, the density of $\beta_1$-receptors is also very high in the caudate, which contains very little NE (18).

The differences in the distribution of $\beta_1$- and $\beta_2$-receptors in rat brain areas and the apparent lack of correlation with the extent of noradrenergic innervation to the particular brain region led us to examine the factors controlling the density of these receptor subtypes in rat brain, with the hope of obtaining information on the functional roles of $\beta_1$- and $\beta_2$-receptors in discrete brain areas, and the source of the catecholamines to which they respond. Three areas of rat brain with different characteristics were studied in detail: cerebral cortex, cerebellum, and caudate. Rat cerebral cortex contains mainly $\beta_1$-receptors (81%) and a high density of noradrenergic innervation. Rat cerebellum contains mainly $\beta_2$-receptors (95%) and a high density of noradrenergic innervation. Finally, rat caudate contains mainly $\beta_1$-receptors (85%) and little or no noradrenergic innervation (18). To determine whether the $\beta_1$- and $\beta_2$-receptors in each brain region were stimulated by either neuronal or hormonal catecholamines, the effects of chronic drug treatments and adrenalectomy on the density of $\beta_1$- and $\beta_2$-receptors were examined in each brain region.

## REGULATION OF $\beta_1$- OR $\beta_2$-RECEPTOR DENSITY IN RAT CEREBRAL CORTEX

A decrease in the normal afferent input to a tissue is usually associated with an increase in the sensitivity of that tissue to further stimulation (supersensitivity). Conversely, increases in the normal afferent input to a tissue are often associated with decreases in the sensitivity of the tissue to further stimulation (subsensitivity). These changes are often associated with changes in receptor density. Both of these phenomena have been clearly demonstrated in studies of β-adrenergic receptors in rat cerebral cortex. Decreasing neuronal input following chemical denervation with 6-hydroxydopamine (6-OHDA) (28) or following chronic administration of the β-adrenergic receptor antagonist, propranolol (31), resulted in increases in the total density of β-adrenergic receptors in rat cerebral cortex. Conversely, increasing NE availability by chronic administration of the inhibitor of NE reuptake, desmethylimipramine (DMI), or the monoamine oxidase inhibitor, pargyline, resulted in decreases in the total density of β-adrenergic receptors in rat cerebral cortex (31).

In order to determine whether the density of each β-adrenergic receptor subtype was regulated independently, the density of $\beta_1$- and $\beta_2$-receptors in the cerebral cortex were determined following these various drug treatments. Destruction of noradrenergic nerve terminals in the cerebral cortex by neonatal administration of 6-OHDA selectively increased $\beta_1$-receptor density in adult rat cerebral cortex, but had no effect on $\beta_2$-receptor density (17). Conversely, chronic treatment of adult rats with DMI, an inhibitor of NE re-uptake, selectively decreased $\beta_1$-receptor density in rat cerebral cortex, but had no effect on $\beta_2$-receptor density (17). These results suggest that the β-adrenergic receptors in rat cortex involved in noradrenergic neurotransmission are primarily of the $\beta_1$-subtype.

Since both 6-OHDA and DMI treatments relatively selectively affect noradrenergic neurons, we also examined the effects of chronic treatment of rats with the β-adrenergic receptor antagonist, propranolol, or the monoamine oxidase inhibitor, pargyline. Propranolol would be expected to block all β-adrenergic receptor stimulation, regardless of the source of the agonist, and pargyline should inhibit the degradation of all catecholamines. Chronic propranolol treatment caused a selective increase in $\beta_1$-receptor density in the cerebral cortex without affecting $\beta_2$-receptor density (Table 1). These changes were similar to those seen following 6-OHDA treatment. Chronic pargyline treatment caused a selective reduction in the density of $\beta_1$-receptors in the cerebral cortex similar to that seen following chronic DMI treatment, and also did not affect $\beta_2$-receptor density in this tissue (Table 1). Finally, adrenalectomy did not alter either $\beta_1$- or $\beta_2$-receptor density in the cerebral cortex (Table 1).

The results of these studies suggest that the density of $\beta_1$-receptors in rat cerebral cortex is controlled by the activity of the noradrenergic input to this tissue. Decreasing receptor stimulation by treatment of animals with 6-OHDA or propranolol causes an increased $\beta_1$-receptor density, whereas increasing receptor stimulation by treatment of animals with DMI or pargyline causes a decreased $\beta_1$-receptor density. The density of $\beta_2$-receptors in the cerebral cortex does not appear to be controlled either by the noradrenergic neuronal input to the tissue (since 6-OHDA and chronic DMI did not affect these receptors) or by any other input to these receptors (since chronic propranolol, chronic pargyline, and adrenalectomy did not affect these receptors). It is not yet clear whether this means that $\beta_2$-receptors in the cerebral cortex do not receive a neuronal or hormonal input, or whether it simply indicates that the density of these receptors is not subject to alteration when the degree of stimulation is increased or blocked.

## REGULATION OF $\beta_1$- AND $\beta_2$-RECEPTOR DENSITY IN RAT CEREBELLUM

Although the β-adrenergic receptors in most regions of rat central nervous system are mainly of the $\beta_1$-subtype, the β-adrenergic receptors in rat cerebellum are

TABLE 1. *Summary of the effects of chronic drug treatments or adrenalectomy on $\beta_1$- and $\beta_2$-adrenergic receptor density in rat cerebral cortex, cerebellum, and caudate*

| | Cerebral cortex 465 | | Cerebellum 241 | | Caudate <5 | |
|---|---|---|---|---|---|---|
| NE levels (ng/g)[a] | | | | | | |
| Receptor density[b] (fmol/mg prot.) | $\beta_1$ 58 ± 5.8 | $\beta_2$ 13 ± 1.6 | $\beta_1$ 3 ± 0.5 | $\beta_2$ 18 ± 1.9 | $\beta_1$ 41 ± 2.6 | $\beta_2$ 13 ± 0.9 |
| Effect of | | | | | | |
| 6-OHDA | 64% increase[c] | NC[c] | 110% increase[d] | NC[d] | ND | ND |
| Chronic propranolol | 55% increase[g] | NC[f] | 87% increase[d] | NC[d] | 11% increase[e] | NC[e] |
| Adrenalectomy | NC[f] | NC[f] | NC[f] | NC[f] | 30% increase[e] | NC[e] |
| Chronic DMI | 40% decrease[c] | NC[c] | NC[h] | 20% decrease[f] | 22% decrease[e] | NC[e] |
| Chronic pargyline | 19% decrease[g] | NC[g] | NC[h] | 13% decrease[f] | 24% decrease[e] | NC[e] |

[a] Oke et al., 1978; ref. 23.
[b] Minneman et al., 1979; ref. 18.
[c] Minneman et al., 1979; ref. 17.
[d] Wolfe et al., 1981; ref. 32.
[e] Minneman, K. P., Wolfe, B. B., and Molinoff, P.B., *Brain Research* (in press).
[f] Minneman et al., 1981; ref. 20.
[g] Wolfe, B. B., Minneman, K. P., and Molinoff, P. B., *unpublished results*.
[h] Control levels were too low to accurately measure any possible decrease. Levels either remained the same or decreased, but did not increase.
NC, no change; ND, not determined.

predominantly $\beta_2$ (18). In the cerebellum, as in most other brain areas, the major adrenergic neurotransmitter is NE. Since $\beta_2$-receptors have a relatively low affinity for NE (15), it seems unlikely that NE is the natural agonist at these receptors. Some $\beta_1$-receptors do exist in the cerebellum, and depending on the age of the rat comprise 3 to 20% of the total $\beta$-adrenergic receptor population (24,25). In young (3-week-old) rats, $\beta_1$-receptors comprise 20% of the total $\beta$-adrenergic receptor population, whereas in adult (7- to 25-week-old) rats, $\beta_1$-receptors comprise only about 6% of the total $\beta$-adrenergic receptors (24). In very old rats (40- to 60-week-old), the proportion of $\beta_1$-receptors again increases such that 15 to 20% of the $\beta$-adrenergic receptors are $\beta_1$ (25). The functional significance and the factors controlling these fluctuations in cerebellar $\beta_1$-receptor density are not yet understood.

There is a well-defined noradrenergic projection to the cerebellum arising from the locus coeruleus (6) which synapses primarily in the Purkinje and molecular layers of the cerebellum. Using electrophysiological techniques it has been possible to demonstrate that the spontaneous or glutamate-induced firing of cerebellar Purkinje neurons is inhibited by the iontophoretic application of NE (27), and that this effect is mediated through $\beta$-adrenergic receptors. The intracisternal administration of 6-OHDA to adult rats depletes cerebellar NE content and causes an increased responsiveness of cerebellar Purkinje neurons to iontophoretically applied NE (13).

Since the cerebellum contains predominantly $\beta_2$-receptors and only a small proportion of $\beta_1$-receptors, it was of interest to determine whether alterations in the noradrenergic input to this tissue altered the density of either $\beta_1$- or $\beta_2$-receptors. Wolfe et al. (32) showed that depletion of cerebellar NE content by intracisternal administration of 6-OHDA doubled the density of the proportionately small $\beta_1$-receptor population in the cerebellum, without affecting $\beta_2$-receptor density. Similarly, chronic administration of propranolol caused a large increase in $\beta_1$-receptor density in the cerebellum without altering $\beta_2$-receptor density (32). These data suggest that the increased density of $\beta_1$-receptors following 6-OHDA treatment may be responsible for the supersensitive responses of Purkinje cells to iontophoretically applied NE (13). Thus the cerebellar $\beta_1$-receptors, which comprise only 5 to 10% of the total $\beta$-adrenergic receptor population in adult rat cerebellum, may be the receptors mediating the actions of NE in this tissue.

Further evidence suggesting a localization of $\beta_1$-receptors on rat cerebellar Purkinje neurons has come from a study where rat cerebellum was degranulated by neonatal X-irradiation focused on the cerebellum. This procedure destroys the late-maturing cerebellar interneurons, including the granule, basket, and stellate cells; however, the large early-maturing Purkinje neurons are resistant to this treatment (3,33). The remaining Purkinje cells, although having some abnormalities in dendritic orientation, are in many respects normal. There is little or no alteration in intracellular organelles in Purkinje cells in X-irradiated rats; the sustained spiking activity of these cells is similar to that seen in untreated animals, and the chemosensitivity to iontophoretically applied neurotransmitters and drugs is similar to that in untreated controls (33). Examination of $\beta$-adrenergic receptor density in control and X-irradiated cerebella shows that this treatment caused a 70 to 80% loss in the total number of β-adrenergic receptors in the cerebellum; this loss is due almost entirely to a loss of cerebellar $\beta_2$-receptors. The number of $\beta_1$-receptors in an X-irradiated cerebellum is not different from that in a control cerebellum, despite the large (60 to 70%) loss in cerebellar mass caused by this treatment (21; Table 2). The co-survival of Purkinje neurons and $\beta_1$-receptors in the X-irradiated cerebellum suggests that $\beta_1$-receptors may be associated with Purkinje cells in this tissue.

Although this evidence is consistent with the hypothesis that in the cerebellum, as in the cerebral cortex, the β-adrenergic receptors involved in noradrenergic neurotransmission are of the $\beta_1$-subtype, some evidence suggests that cerebellar $\beta_2$-receptors can also be regulated by alterations in NE availability. Harden et al. (12) showed that the rebound increase in rat cerebellar NE content following neonatal 6-OHDA treatment is associated with a substantial decrease in β-adrenergic receptor density which, considering the small number of $\beta_1$-receptors in this tissue, implies that some of the receptors lost must be $\beta_2$-receptors. Similarly, U'Prichard et al. (30) demonstrated that rebound increases in cerebellar NE following lesions of the dorsal noradrenergic bundle selectively decreased $\beta_2$-receptors in rat cerebellum. In addition, chronic treatment of adult rats with DMI or pargyline also decreases the density of $\beta_2$-receptors in the cerebellum (Table 1). The density of $\beta_1$-receptors in the cerebellum may also decrease in these situations; however, the initially low levels of $\beta_1$-receptors in the cerebellum makes accurate measurement of a decrease in density very difficult.

These results suggest that under certain circumstances of increased NE content, the $\beta_2$-receptors in the cerebellum may respond to NE. However, the lack of effect of NE depletion by intracisternal injection of 6-OHDA or β-adrenergic receptor blockade by chronic propranolol treatment on $\beta_2$-receptor density in the cerebellum suggests that under normal conditions these receptors are not tonically activated by

TABLE 2. $\beta_1$- and $\beta_2$-adrenergic receptors in cerebella of rats subjected to neonatal X-irradiation

| Treatment | Total β-adrenergic receptors (fmol/cerebellum) | $\beta_1$-receptors (fmol/cerebellum) | $\beta_2$-receptors (fmol/cerebellum) |
|---|---|---|---|
| 6 weeks old | | | |
| control | 776 ± 39 | 47 ± 17 | 730 ± 40 |
| X-irradiated | 150 ± 18 | 22 ± 4 | 130 ± 16 |
| | (19%) | (47%) | (18%) |
| 12 weeks old | | | |
| control | 805 ± 50 | 21 ± 11 | 780 ± 50 |
| X-irradiated | 178 ± 10 | 18 ± 5 | 160 ± 10 |
| | (22%) | (86%) | (20%) |

Wistar albino rats were subjected to X-irradiation focused on the cerebellum at 93 rads/min starting at birth (day 0). Animals received 200 rads on day 0, 1,250 rads on days 3 and 5, and 200 rads on days 7, 9, 11, 13, and 15 (33). Total β-adrenergic receptors and $\beta_1$- and $\beta_2$-receptors were measured as described previously (18). The weights of control cerebella were 244 ± 6.3 and 291 ± 7.9 mg and the weights of X-irradiated cerebella were 99 ± 8.1 and 95 ± 6.0 mg at 6 and 12 weeks of age, respectively. The number of receptors is expressed as fmol per whole cerebellum. Each value is the mean ± SEM of eight determinations.

NE. The large increases in $\beta_1$-receptor density in rat cerebellum following intracisternal 6-OHDA or chronic propranolol treatment suggests that the small $\beta_1$-receptor population in the cerebellum is actively involved in noradrenergic neurotransmission in this tissue.

## REGULATION OF $\beta_1$- AND $\beta_2$-RECEPTOR DENSITY IN RAT CAUDATE

Rat caudate contains a high density of $\beta$-adrenergic receptors (2,7,29) but little (22) or no (23) EPI or NE. The $\beta$-adrenergic receptors in rat caudate are mainly (85%) of the $\beta_1$-subtype, although some $\beta_2$-receptors are also present (18). The possible functional roles of such receptors in a brain region containing no apparent endogenous ligand for the receptors is not understood. Some of the possible explanations for this apparent discrepancy are (a) that these receptors are vestigial and have no function, (b) that they play a developmental role prior to the development of the blood-brain barrier, or (c) that they are located on the peripheral side of the blood-brain barrier and respond to circulating catecholamines.

In order to gain some understanding of the functional role of $\beta_1$- and $\beta_2$-receptors in rat caudate, the effect of various drug treatments and adrenalectomy on the density of $\beta_1$- and $\beta_2$-receptors in rat caudate were examined. Persistent blockade of $\beta$-adrenergic receptors by chronic treatment with propranolol caused a small but significant increase in $\beta_1$-receptor density in rat caudate without affecting $\beta_2$-receptor density (Table 1). Similar effects were observed following adrenalectomy; a small increase in $\beta_1$-receptor density with no change in $\beta_2$-receptor density. Conversely, chronic administration of either pargyline or DMI substantially reduced $\beta_1$-receptor density in rat caudate without affecting $\beta_2$-receptor density (Table 1).

These results demonstrate that the density of $\beta_1$-receptors in rat caudate can be altered by treatments likely to affect the access of adrenergic catecholamines to the receptor. The observation that chronic propranolol administration causes a small increase in $\beta_1$-receptor density in rat caudate raises the possibility that these receptors are normally subject to a tonic activation. Since the removal of circulating catecholamines following bilateral adrenalectomy causes a similar selective increase in $\beta_1$-receptors in rat caudate, it is possible that adrenal catecholamines may contribute a tonic input to $\beta_1$-receptors in rat caudate. Since EPI is generally thought to be unable to permeate the blood-brain barrier, some of these receptors may be located on blood vessels on the peripheral side of the blood-brain barrier. This hypothesis is consistent with the results of Zahniser et al. (34), who showed that destruction of intrinsic striatal neurons with kainic acid did not decrease the density of either $\beta_1$- or $\beta_2$-receptors in rat caudate.

The rather substantial decreases in $\beta_1$-receptor density following chronic administration of pargyline or DMI also suggest that endogenous catecholamines can have access to $\beta_1$-receptors in rat caudate. Wolfe et al. (31) showed that the decrease in $\beta$-adrenergic receptor density in rat cerebral cortex following chronic DMI administration was blocked by pretreatment of the rats with 6-OHDA, suggesting that the effects of DMI on β-adrenergic receptor density in rat cerebral cortex are dependent on the presence of intact noradrenergic nerve terminals and are not a direct effect of the drug. Although this has not yet been demonstrated for the effects of pargyline or DMI on β-adrenergic receptor density in rat caudate, the similar decreases seen with the two different classes of drugs make a direct effect unlikely. It seems more likely that the effects of these two drugs on catecholamine availability are responsible for the observed decreases in $β_1$-receptor density in the caudate. Some reports (10,14) indicate that administration of tricyclic antidepressants or monoamine oxidase inhibitors raise plasma catecholamine levels. It is possible that raised plasma catecholamine levels may be responsible for the observed effects of pargyline and DMI on $β_1$-receptor density in rat caudate, although more definitive experiments will have to be done to be certain of this.

In any case, these experiments show that the $β_1$-receptors in rat caudate can, under certain circumstances, be affected by endogenous catecholamines. In addition, the effects of propranolol and adrenalectomy suggest that some of these receptors may be receiving a tonic input in the normal animal, possibly in the form of catecholamines released from the adrenal medulla. The precise source and identity of the endogenous inputs to rat caudate β-adrenergic receptors remain to be determined.

## ACKNOWLEDGMENT

Portions of this work were supported by USPHS (HL 24353, MH 35043, NS 13289).

## REFERENCES

1. Ahlquist, R. P. (1948): A study of the adrenotropic receptors. *Am. J. Physiol.*, 153:586–600.
2. Alexander, R. W., Davis, J. N., and Lefkowitz, R. J. (1975): Direct identification and characterization of β-adrenergic receptors in rat brain. *Nature (Lond.)*, 258:437–440.
3. Altman, J., and Anderson, W. J. (1973): Experimental reorganization of the cerebellar cortex. II. Effects of elimination of most microneurons with prolonged X-irradiation started at four days. *J. Comp. Neurol.*, 149:123–152.
4. Ariens, E. J., and Simonis, A. M. (1976): Receptors and receptor mechanisms. In: *Beta-Adrenoceptor Blocking Agents*, edited by P. R. Saxena and R. P. Forsyth, pp. 3–27. North Holland, Amsterdam.
5. Berthelsen, S., and Pettinger, W. A. (1977): A functional basis for classification of α-adrenergic receptors. *Life Sci.*, 21:595–606.
6. Bloom, F. E., Hoffer, B. J., and Siggins, G. R. (1972): Norepinephrine mediated cerebellar synapses: A model system for neuropsychopharmacology. *Biol. Psychiatry*, 4:157–177.
7. Bylund, D. B., and Snyder, S. H. (1976): Beta adrenergic receptor binding in membrane preparations from mammalian brain. *Mol. Pharmacol.*, 12:568–580.
8. Carlsson, A. (1959): The occurrence, distribution and physiological role of catecholamines in the nervous system. *Pharmacol. Rev.*, 11:490–493.
9. Carlsson, E., and Hedberg, A. (1977): Are cardiac effects of noradrenaline and adrenaline mediated by different β-adrenoceptors. *Acta Physiol. Scand. (Suppl.)*, 44:47.
10. Chiueh, C. C., and Kopin, I. J. (1978): Centrally mediated release by cocaine of endogenous epinephrine and norepinephrine from the sympathoadrenal medullary system of unanesthetized rats. *J. Pharmacol. Exp. Ther.*, 205:148–154.
11. Hancock, A. A., DeLean, A. L., and Lefkowitz, R. J. (1979): Quantitative resolution of beta-adrenergic receptor subtypes by selective ligand binding: Application of a computerized model fitting technique. *Mol. Pharmacol.*, 16:1–9.

12. Harden, T. K., Mailman, R. B., Mueller, R. A., and Breese, G. R. (1979): Noradrenergic hyperinnervation reduces the density of β-adrenergic receptors in rat cerebellum. *Brain Res.*, 166:194–198.
13. Hoffer, B. J., Siggins, G. R., Oliver, A. P., and Bloom, F. E. (1971): Cyclic AMP mediation of norepinephrine inhibition in rat cerebellar cortex: A unique class of synaptic responses. *Ann. N. Y. Acad. Sci.*, 185:531–549.
14. Kopin, I. J., Lake, R. C., and Ziegler, M. (1978): Plasma levels of norepinephrine. *Ann. Intern. Med.*, 88:671–680.
15. Lands, A. M., Arnold, A., McAuliff, J. P., Luduena, F. P., and Brown, T. G. (1967): Differentiation of receptor systems activated by sympathomimetic amines. *Nature*, 214:597–598.
16. Lands, A. M., Luduena, F. P., and Buzzo, H. J. (1967): Differentiation of receptors responsive to isoproterenol. *Life Sci.*, 6:2241–2249.
17. Minneman, K. P., Dibner, M. D., Wolfe, B. B., and Molinoff, P. B. (1979): $β_1$- and $β_2$-adrenergic receptors in rat cerebral cortex are independently regulated. *Science*, 204:866–868.
18. Minneman, K. P., Hegstrand, L. R., and Molinoff, P. B. (1979): Simultaneous determination of beta-1 and beta-2-adrenergic receptors in tissues containing both receptor subtypes. *Mol. Pharmacol.*, 16:34–46.
19. Minneman, K. P., Hedberg, A., and Molinoff, P. B. (1979): Comparison of beta adrenergic receptor subtypes in mammalian tissues. *J. Pharmacol. Exp. Ther.*, 211:502–508.
20. Minneman, K. P., Pittman, R. N., and Molinoff, P. B. (1981): β-Adrenergic receptor subtypes: Properties, distribution and regulation. *Annu. Rev. Neurosci.*, 4:419–461.
21. Minneman, K. P., Pittman, R. N., Yeh, H. H., Woodward, D. J., Wolfe, B. B., and Molinoff, P. B. (1981): Selective survival of $β_1$-adrenergic receptors in rat cerebellum following neonatal X-irradiation. *Brain Res.*, 209:25–34.
22. O'Donahue, T. L., Crowley, W. R., and Jacobowitz, D. M. (1979): Biochemical mapping of the noradrenergic ventral bundle projection sites: Evidence for a noradrenergic-dopaminergic interaction. *Brain Res.*, 172:87–100.
23. Oke, A., Keller, R., and Adams, R. N. (1978): Dopamine and norepinephrine enhancement in discrete rat brain regions following neonatal 6-hydroxydopamine treatment. *Brain Res.*, 148:245–250.
24. Pittman, R. N., Minneman, K. P., and Molinoff, P. B. (1980): Ontogeny of $β_1$ and $β_2$-adrenergic receptors in rat cerebellum and cerebral cortex. *Brain Res.*, 188:357–368.
25. Pittman, R. N., Minneman, K. P., and Molinoff, P. B. (1980): Alterations in $β_1$ and $β_2$-adrenergic receptor density in the cerebellum of aging rats. *J. Neurochem.*, 35:273–275.
26. Rugg, E. L., Barnett, D. B., and Nahorski, S. R. (1978): Coexistence of beta$_1$ and beta$_2$-adrenoceptors in mammalian lung: Evidence from direct binding studies. *Mol. Pharmacol.*, 14:996–1005.
27. Siggins, G. R., Hoffer, B. J., and Bloom, F. E. (1969): Cyclic adenosine monophosphate: Possible mediator for norepinephrine effects on cerebellar Purkinje cells. *Science*, 165:1018–1020.
28. Sporn, J. R., Harden, T. K., Wolfe, B. B., and Molinoff, P. B. (1976): β-Adrenergic receptor involvement in 6-hydroxydopamine-induced supersensitivity in rat cerebral cortex. *Science*, 194:624–626.
29. Sporn, J. R., and Molinoff, P. B. (1976): β-Adrenergic receptors in rat brain. *J. Cyclic Nucleotide Res.*, 149–161.
30. U'prichard, D. C., Reisine, T. D., Yamamura, S., Mason, S. T., Fibiger, H. C., Ehlert, F., and Yamamura, H. L. (1980): Differential supersensitivity of β-receptor subtypes in rat cortex and cerebellum after central noradrenergic denervation. *Life Sci.*, 26:355–364.
31. Wolfe, B. B., Harden, T. K., Sporn, J. R., and Molinoff, P. B. (1978): Presynaptic modulation of beta adrenergic receptors in cerebral cortex after treatment with antidepressants. *J. Pharmacol. Exp. Ther.*, 207:446–457.
32. Wolfe, B. B., Minneman, K. P., and Molinoff, P. B. (1982): Selective increases in the density of cerebellar $β_1$-adrenergic receptors. *Brain Res.*, 234:474–479.
33. Woodward, D. J., Hoffer, B. J., and Altman, J. (1974): Physiological and pharmacological properties of Purkinje cells in rat cerebellum degranulated by postnatal X-irradiation. *J. Neurobiol.*, 5:283–304.
34. Zahniser, N. R., Minneman, K. P., and Molinoff, P. B. (1979): Persistence of β-adrenergic receptors in rat striatum following kainic acid administration. *Brain Res.*, 178:589–595.

# Possible Influence of Noradrenaline on β-Adrenergic and Muscarinic Cholinergic Receptors in Rat Heart: Effects of 6-Hydroxydopa, Isoproterenol, and Desmethylimipramine

Yasuyuki Nomura, Hiroko Kajiyama, and Tomio Segawa

*Department of Pharmacology, Institute of Pharmaceutical Sciences, Hiroshima University School of Medicine, Hiroshima 734, Japan*

The physiological significance of the interaction between plural neuronal systems is an important subject in neuropharmacological studies. We have reported the interregulation between dopaminergic and cholinergic systems in the striatum (10,14). The close interaction between different types of neurotransmitter receptor systems such as α- and β-adrenoceptors also seems to exist in the brain (6,9). In an earlier study, muscarinic acetylcholine (ACh) receptors involve noradrenaline (NA) release from cardiac sympathetic nerve, suggesting ACh-NA interaction in the heart (7). In contrast, it may be the case in the cardiac tissues that neurons not only excite or inhibit postjunctional cells, but also exert a long-term trophic influence (1,2,4).

To identify whether it is sympathetic neurons or NA secreted from the terminals that affects the receptor systems of postjuncional ACh and β-adrenergic receptor systems in cardiac cells, we examined the influence of neonatal 6-hydroxydopa (6-OHDOPA) treatment, repeated administration of isoproterenol and desmethylimipramine (DMI) on inotropic action of isoproterenol and ACh, isoproterenol-induced stimulation of ornithine decarboxylase (ODC) activity, and specific bindings of [$^3$H]dihydroalprenolol ([$^3$H]DHA) and [$^3$H]quinuclidinyl benzilate ([$^3$H]QNB) in the rat heart.

## MATERIALS AND METHODS

Wistar rats of both sexes were used. 6-OHDOPA (50 or 75 mg/kg) was injected subcutaneously (s.c.) into rats at 0, 2, and 4 days after birth. Treated pups were kept with a mother under normal daylight conditions at 23°C and weaned on day 22. Two- and three-month-old animals were then used for experiments. Isoproterenol (0.1 mg/kg) and DMI (10 mg/kg) were injected subcutaneoulsy into 2-month-old, male rats twice daily (8:00 a.m. and 8:00 p.m.) for 10 days. Animals were sacrificed 19 hr after the last injection of the drugs.

Inotropic action of isoproterenol and ACh in the isolated atria, isoproterenol-induced stimulation of cardiac ODC activity, and specific bindings of [$^3$H]DHA and [$^3$H]QNB to cardiac membranes were examined by the method of Nomura et al. (11,12,14). Protein was determined with the Folin reagent method of Lowry et al. (8). Statistical significance between test and control values was examined by Student's *t*-test.

## RESULTS

### β-Adrenergic Receptors Following Pretreatment with 6-OHDOPA, Isoproterenol, and DMI

#### *Inotropic Action of Isoproterenol*

$EC_{50}$ values of isoproterenol were determined from log concentration-response curves of positive inotropic action of isoproterenol in the isolated atria (Table 1). Neonatal treatment with 6-OHDOPA and repeated administration of isoproterenol did not modify $EC_{50}$ of isoproterenol, but increased significantly ($p < 0.001$) the value in DMI-treated atria.

#### *Isoproterenol-Induced Stimulation of ODC Activity*

Isoproterenol, 0.1 mg/kg s.c., produced 8.3 times elevation of cardiac ODC activity 3 hr after the injection (Table 2). Since a preceding injection of 10 mg/kg propranolol abolished the isoproterenol-induced stimulation (data not shown), the stimulation of ODC activity by isoproterenol appears to be mediated by activating β-adrenergic receptors. In 6-OHDOPA-pretreated animals, isoproterenol markedly

TABLE 1. *$EC_{50}$ of positive inotropic action of isoproterenol in the isolated atria treated with 6-OHDOPA, isoproterenol, and DMI*

| Treatment | $EC_{50}$ (M) | |
|---|---|---|
| Control | $(7.76 \pm 1.94) \times 10^{-10}$ | (6) |
| Neonatal 6-OHDOPA | $(9.04 \pm 2.03) \times 10^{-10}$ | (4) |
| Repeated isoproterenol | $(7.00 \pm 2.62) \times 10^{-9}$ | (11) |
| Repeated DMI | $(5.88 \pm 1.34) \times 10^{-9\,a}$ | (6) |

Neonatal rats were treated with 6-OHDOPA (75 mg/kg s.c.) at 0, 2, and 4 days, and inotropic responses were examined between days 62 and 68. Two-month-old rats were treated with isoproterenol (0.1 mg/kg) and DMI (10 mg/kg) twice a day for 10 days and inotropic responses were examined 19 hr after the last injection. $EC_{50}$ values were determined from the log concentration-response curve. The number of experiments is shown in parenthesis.
[a]Significance: $p < 0.001$ vs control.

TABLE 2. *Isoproterenol-induced stimulation of cardiac ODC activity in rats treated with 6-OHDOPA, isoproterenol, and DMI*

| Treatment | ODC activity (pmol $^{14}CO_2$ formed/mg prot./hr) | |
|---|---|---|
| | Vehicle | Isoproterenol (0.17 mg/kg) |
| Control | 0.75 ± 0.09 (4) | 6.25 ± 0.16$^a$ (7) |
| Neonatal 6-OHDOPA | 0.79 ± 0.15 (6) | 11.14 ± 0.97$^b$ (5) |
| Repeated isoproterenol | 0.76 ± 0.17 (3) | 1.77 ± 0.24$^b$ (8) |
| Repeated DMI | 0.96 ± 0.34 (3) | 0.43 ± 0.28$^b$ (3) |

Treatments with 6-OHDOPA, isoproterenol, and DMI as shown in legend to Table 1. Cardiac ODC activity in rats was examined 3 hr following a s.c. injection of isoproterenol. The number of experiments is shown in parenthesis.
$^a p < 0.001$ vs vehicle.
$^b p < 0.001$ vs controls.

stimulated ODC activity and this stimulation was significantly ($p < 0.001$) higher than that in controls. On the other hand, isoproterenol-induced stimulation of ODC activity was significantly ($p < 0.001$) decreased by repeated isoproterenol and by repeated DMI.

### Specific [³H]DHA Binding

Scatchard analysis of specific [³H]DHA binding to cardiac membranes showed a single component of binding sites with $K_D = 0.67$ nM and $B_{max} = 0.131$ pmol/mg protein (Table 3). 6-OHDOPA treatment resulted in a significant ($p < 0.0001$) increase in $B_{max}$. On the other hand, $B_{max}$ in [³H]DHA binding was significantly ($p < 0.05$, isoproterenol; $p < 0.001$, DMI) reduced by repeated administration of isoproterenol and DMI. $K_D$ values were not changed by any of these treatments.

## Muscarinic ACh Receptors Following Pretreatment with 6-OHDOPA, Isoproterenol, and DMI

### Inotropic Action of ACh

The log ACh concentration-response curve of the 6-OHDOPA-treated atria was shifted to the right of the curve obtained from the control preparations. 6-OHDOPA significantly ($p < 0.05$) increased the $EC_{50}$ value of ACh compared to that in controls (Table 4). $EC_{50}$ of ACh in isoproterenol-treated preparations was lower than that in controls. $EC_{50}$ was increased 4.8 times following repeated DMI.

### Specific [³H]QNB Binding

Table 5 shows saturation parameters in specific [³H]QNB binding in control and treated cardiac membranes. Neonatal 6-OHDOPA and repeated isoproterenol re-

TABLE 3. *Saturation parameters of specific [³H]DHA binding in cardiac membranes of rats treated with 6-OHDOPA, isoproterenol, and DMI*

| Treatment | $K_D$ (nM) | $B_{max}$ (pmol/mg prot.) |
|---|---|---|
| Control | 0.665 ± 0.034 | 0.131 ± 0.003 |
| Neonatal 6-OHDOPA | 0.731 ± 0.030 | 0.166 ± 0.003[a] |
| Repeated isoproterenol | 0.672 ± 0.024 | 0.092 ± 0.010[b] |
| Repeated DMI | 0.600 ± 0.021 | 0.099 ± 0.002[a] |

Procedure of treatments with 6-OHDOPA, isoproterenol, and DMI as shown in legend to Table 1. Cardiac homogenates were incubated with [³H]DHA (final concentration, 0.35–3.7 nM) at 25°C for 20 min. Specific binding was defined as binding displaced by propranolol 5 μM. Saturation parameters were estimated from a Scatchard analysis.
[a] $p < 0.001$ vs controls.
[b] $p < 0.05$ vs controls.

TABLE 4. *$EC_{50}$ of negative inotropic action of ACh in the isolated atria treated with 6-OHDOPA, isoproterenol, and DMI*

| Treatment | $EC_{50}$ (M) | |
|---|---|---|
| Control | $(1.67 \pm 0.34) \times 10^{-8}$ | (6) |
| Neonatal 6-OHDOPA | $(1.51 \pm 0.80) \times 10^{-7}$ [a] | (5) |
| Repeated isoproterenol | $(8.25 \pm 1.46) \times 10^{-7}$ [a] | (12) |
| Repeated DMI | $(7.98 \pm 1.30) \times 10^{-8}$ [b] | (6) |

Neonatal rats were injected with 6-OHDOPA (50 mg/kg s.c.) at 0, 2, and 4 days after birth and inotropic responses to ACh were examined between days 80 and 100. The number of experiments is shown in parenthesis.
[a] $p < 0.05$ vs controls.
[b] $p < 0.001$ vs controls.

sulted in a significant ($p < 0.05$) reduction in $B_{max}$, but repeated DMI significantly ($p < 0.001$) increased $B_{max}$. $K_D$ values were not modified by 6-OHDOPA, isoproterenol, or DMI.

## DISCUSSION

Table 6 shows the outline of the present findings. Biochemical data on ODC activity and [³H]DHA binding suggest 6-OHDOPA-induced β-adrenergic hypersensitivity. This is probably due to compensatory up-regulation of receptor numbers following chemical sympathectomy by 6-OHDOPA, since the neonatal treatment with 6-OHDOPA produced a significant reduction of the cardiac NA content by

TABLE 5. *Saturation parameters of specific [³H]QNB binding in cardiac membranes of rats treated with 6-OHDOPA, isoproterenol, and DMI*

| Treatment | $K_D$ (nM) | $B_{max}$ (pmol/mg prot.) |
|---|---|---|
| Control | 0.291 ± 0.012 | 0.131 ± 0.004 |
| Neonatal 6-OHDOPA | 0.305 ± 0.002 | 0.092 ± 0.003[a] |
| Repeated isoproterenol | 0.296 ± 0.016 | 0.113 ± 0.004[a] |
| Repeated DMI | 0.284 ± 0.017 | 0.163 ± 0.002[b] |

Procedure of treatments with 6-OHDOPA, isoproterenol, and DMI as shown in legend to Table 4. Cardiac homogenates were incubated with [³H]QNB (final concentration, 0.017–0.31 nM) at 25°C for 60 min. Specific binding was defined as binding displaced by atropine 0.1 μM.
[a] $p < 0.05$ vs controls.
[b] $p < 0.001$ vs controls.

TABLE 6. *Outline of the effects of treatments with 6-OHDOPA, isoproterenol, and DMI on cardiac β-adrenergic and muscarinic ACh receptors*

| β-Adrenergic receptors | | | | Muscarinic ACh receptors | |
|---|---|---|---|---|---|
| Inotropism to isoproterenol | [³H]DHA binding | ODC activation | Treatment | Inotropism to ACh | [³H]QNB binding |
| ↑ (tendency) | ↑ | ↑ | Neonatal 6-OHDOPA | ↓ | ↓ |
| ↓ | ↓ | ↓ | Repeated isoproterenol | ↑ | ↑ (tendency) |
| ↓ | ↓ | ↓ | Repeated DMI | ↓ | ↑ |

↑, increase; ↓, decrease; ↑ (tendency), tendency to increase.

32%. In contrast to these biochemical results, inotropic action of isoproterenol was not modified by 6-OHDOPA. Based on the fact that 6-hydroxydopamine (6-OHDA) potentiates inotropic and chronotropic responses to NA but not to isoproterenol, Shibata et al. (17) have explained that 6-OHDA produces the presynaptic type of supersensitivity attributed to a diminished uptake of NA by nerve terminals. The present results may be explained by a presynaptic mechanism and do not suggest an increased number of β-receptors at least in the atrium. Biochemical findings obtained from both atrium and ventricle suggest the involvement of hypersensitivity of postjunctional β-receptors. Thus, both biochemical results seem to be due to hypersensitivity of β-receptors in ventricles. In fact, 6-OHDA evoked potentiation of adenylate cyclase activity in ventricles (3,15).

All results obtained from the experiments concerning repeated isoproterenol administration suggest that repeated isoproterenol results in β-adrenergic hyposensitivity, although repeated isoproterenol did not produce a significant alteration in $EC_{50}$ of isoproterenol in inotropic action compared with controls. The possibility that small amounts of residual isoproterenol interfere with [$^3$H]DHA binding is excluded by a finding that GTP addition did not affect $B_{max}$ in [$^3$H]DHA binding in treated membranes. Repeated isoproterenol markedly increased cardiac weight by 72.8%, suggesting that nonspecific stimulation of isoproterenol on the cardiac metabolism may underlie the reduction of the receptor density. Total binding sites per heart, however, was also decreased by repeated isoproternol. It is likely that repeated isoproternol induces a decrease in the number of the β-receptors. In contrast, repeated DMI produced hyposensitivity to isoproterenol in atrial contraction. Biochemical results suggest a decrease in the number of β-receptors by repeated DMI. One possible explanation for hyposensitivity is that DMI, acting presynaptically, increases the level of NA at NA synapses and induces compensatory decrease in the number of β-receptors (Fig. 1). Long-term DMI treatment induces a decrease

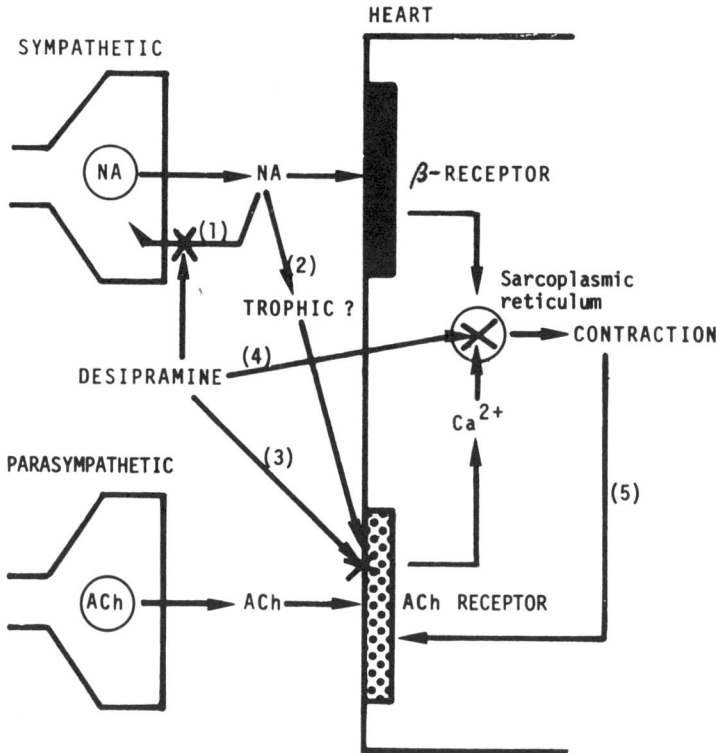

**FIG. 1.** Possible sites of action of repeated DMI on cardiac contraction and on β-adrenergic and muscarinic ACh receptor systems. **(1)** DMI inhibits reuptake of NA, followed by the increase of NA stimulating β-adrenergic receptors. **(2)** NA exerts trophic influence on muscarinic ACh receptors. **(3)** DMI blocks muscarinic ACh receptors. **(4)** DMI injures $Ca^{2+}$ binding sites in sarcoplasmic reticulum. **(5)** Enhanced contraction by increased NA indirectly affects muscarinic ACh receptors.

in the sensitivity of presynaptic receptors, followed by enhanced release of [$^3$H]NA efflux which explains β-adrenergic hyposensitivity in the heart (5). Thus, the long-term exposure of the β-receptors to β-agonists produces down-regulation in the number of β-receptors.

6-OHDOPA reduced the density of [$^3$H]QNB binding sites. $EC_{50}$ for negative inotropic action of ACh was 9.7 times greater for the 6-OHDOPA-treated preparations than for controls. 6-OHDOPA, however, did not modify the maximal response to ACh. Thus, 6-OHDOPA seems to reduce "spare receptors" (18) in postjunctional muscarinic ACh receptors. The mechanism by which 6-OHDOPA produces a decrease in the density of ACh receptors may be the 6-OHDOPA-elicited degeneration of NA nerve terminals, which exert trophic influences on postjunctional muscarinic ACh receptors. However, the following mechanism cannot be ruled out: 6-OHDOPA induces a reduction of presynaptic muscarinic ACh receptors located on NA-ergic nerve terminals, together with degeneration of the terminals, as proposed by Sharma and Banerjee (16).

Repeated isoproterenol decreased the density of [$^3$H]QNB binding sites. Since repeated isoproterenol markedly increased the cardiac weight, isoproterenol-induced stimulation of cellular metabolism may be relevant to the reduction of ACh receptor density. In contrast to the binding results, inotropic action of ACh in the isoproterenol-treated atria shows that the potentiation in inotropic action of isoproterenol following repeated isoproterenol seems to be due to enhanced function at processes between receptor activation and biological responses. Repeated isoproterenol may produce the dramatic change in cardiac physiology and pharmacology as well as in receptor systems.

Repeated DMI administration resulted in the increase of the density of [$^3$H]QNB binding sites. *In vitro* addition of DMI effectively inhibited [$^3$H]QNB binding, indicating that inhibitory influence of DMI produces the compensatory increase in ACh receptors (Fig. 1). Another possible mechanism is that NA increased at synaptic cleft by DMI could produce the increase in the receptor density. This raises the possibility that NA exerts trophic influence on muscarinic ACh receptors, which is supported by the result of 6-OHDOPA induced reduction in the number of ACh receptors (11). The increase in the number of ACh receptors may be due to the antagonistic change in ACh receptors to regulate the muscle contraction accelerated by NA following DMI treatment.

On the other hand, inotropic response to ACh significantly decreased in the DMI-treated atria compared with that in controls. The discrepancy between receptor binding and biological response seems to be solved by the mechanism that repeated DMI injures the excitation-contraction coupling process, since we recently found that repeated DMI significantly reduces $^{45}Ca^{2+}$ binding to sarcoplasmic reticulum fractions from cardiac tissues.

Thus, NA released from sympathetic nerve terminals presumably exerts a long-term trophic influence on the postjunctional muscarinic ACh receptor system in cardiac cells, but the detailed mechanism remains to be explained clearly in future works.

## REFERENCES

1. Black, I. B., and Mytilineou, C. (1976): Transsynaptic regulation of the development of end organ innervation by sympathetic neurons. *Brain Res.*, 101:503–521.
2. Chappineli, V. E., Giacobini, E., Pilar, G., and Uchimura, H. (1976): Induction of cholinergic enzymes in chick ciliary ganglion and iris muscle cells during synapse formation. *J. Physiol.*, 257:749–766.
3. Chiu, T. H. (1978): Chronic effects of 6-hydroxydopamine and reserpine on myocardial adenylate cyclase. *Eur. J. Pharmacol.*, 52:385–388.
4. Costa, E., Guidotti, A., and Hanbauer, I. (1974): Do cyclic nucleotides promote the trans-synaptic induction? *Life Sci.*, 14:1169–1188.
5. Crew, F. T., and Smith, C. B. (1978): Presynaptic alpha-receptor subsensitivity after long-term antidepressant treatment. *Science*, 202:322–324.
6. Johnson, R. W., Reisine, T., Spotnitz, S., Wiech, N., Ursillo, R., and Yamamura, H. I. (1980): Effects of desipramine and yohimbine on $\alpha_2$- and $\beta$-adrenergic sensitivity. *Eur. J. Pharmacol.*, 67:123–127.
7. Lindmar, R., Loffeholz, K., and Muscholl, E. (1968): A muscarinic mechanism inhibiting the release of noradrenaline from peripheral adrenergic nerve fibres by nicotinic agents. *Br. J. Pharmacol.*, 32:289–294.
8. Lowry, O. H., Rosebrough, N. J., Farr, A. L., and Randall, R. J. (1951): Protein measurement with the Folin phenol reagent. *J. Biol. Chem.*, 193:265–275.
9. Maggi, A., U'Prichard, D. C., and Enna, S. J. (1980): $\beta$-Adrenergic regulation of $\alpha_2$-adrenergic receptors in the central nervous system. *Science*, 207:645–647.
10. Nomura, Y., Kajiyama, H., Nakata, Y., and Segawa, T. (1979): Muscarinic cholinergic binding in striatal and mesolimbic areas of the rat: Reduction by 6-hydroxydopa. *Eur. J. Pharmacol.*, 58:125–131.
11. Nomura, Y., Kajiyama, H., and Segawa, T. (1979): Decrease in muscarinic cholinergic response of the rat heart following treatment with 6-hydroxydopa. *Eur. J. Pharmacol.*, 60:323–327.
12. Nomura, Y., Kajiyama, H., and Segawa, T. (1980): Hypersensitivity of cardiac $\beta$-adrenergic receptors after neonatal treatment of rats with 6-hydroxydopa. *Eur. J. Pharmacol.*, 66:225–232.
13. Nomura, Y., Kajiyama, H., and Segawa, T.: Alteration in sensitivity to isoproterenol and acetylcholine following repeated administration of isoproterenol in the rat heart. *J. Pharmacol. Exp. Therap. (in press)*.
14. Nomura, Y., Yotsumoto, I., and Segawa, T. (1981): Ontogenetic development of high potassium- and acetylcholine-induced release of dopamine from striatal slices of the rat. *Dev. Brain Sci.*, 1:171–177.
15. Pick, K., and Wolleman, M. (1977): Catecholamine hypersensitivity of adenylate cyclase after chemical denervation in rat heart. *Biochem. Pharmacol.*, 26:1448–1449.
16. Sharma, V. K., and Banerjee, S. P. (1978): Presynaptic muscarinic cholinergic receptors. *Nature, (Lond.)*, 272:276–278.
17. Shibata, S., Kuchii, M., and Kurahashi, K. (1972): The supersensitivity of isolated rabbit atria and aortic strips produced by 6-hydroxydopamine. *Eur. J. Pharmacol.*, 18:271–280.
18. Stephenson, R. P. (1956): A modification of receptor theory. *Br. J. Pharmacol. Chemother.*, 11:379–386.

# Modulation of *In Vivo* Nigral 5HT Release in the Cat

T. D. Reisine, P. Soubrie, S. Bourgoin, F. Artaud, and J. Glowinski

*INSERM U 114, Groupe NB, College de France, 75231 Paris Cedex 5, France*

Neuroanatomical and biochemical studies indicate that serotonergic (5HT) neurons originating from the raphe nuclei innervate basal ganglionic structures such as the caudate nucleus (CN) and the substantia nigra (SN) (7,8,29). The functional role of such neurons remains unclear. However, electrophysiological evidence has revealed that raphe neurons may exert both a facilitatory and inhibitory action on CN and SN neurons (7,8). Furthermore, 5HT has been implicated in a number of behaviors that have been related to basal ganglia function (8,13).

A number of methodological approaches have been used to study 5HT transmission in the basal ganglia. One such approach which we have utilized extensively is the measurement of the *in vivo* release of $^3$H-5HT continuously formed from $^3$H-tryptophan (16). This release is dependent on 5HT nerve activity and is calcium- and tetrodotoxin-sensitive. Using this technique, it is possible to investigate the various neuronal pathways which influence or regulate 5HT transmission in the brain.

In this review we will focus our discussion on the effect that various transmitters found in the SN have upon *in vivo* nigral $^3$H-5HT release. Furthermore, evidence that the lateral habenula is a link in a possible feedback pathway from the basal ganglia to the raphe nucleus will be presented.

## METHODOLOGY

Experiments were done in cats of either sex, slightly anesthetized (1 to 1.5%) with halothane and stereotaxically implanted with push-pull cannulae, one in each SN (A = +4, L = +4.5, H = −4.5) and one in each CN (A = +14.5, L = +5, H = +5). In some experiments one push-pull cannula was also positioned in the dorsal raphe (A = 1.5, L = 0, H = −2) or in the left lateral habenula (A = +7.5, L = 2, H = +4.5). By means of the push-pull cannula, the brain structures were continuously superfused with an artificial CSF medium containing 40 to 50 Ci/ml of $^3$H-tryptophan and the superfusate containing $^3$H-5HT was collected in serial 12- or 15-min (0.5 ml) fractions. $^3$H-5HT released in the fractions was estimated by liquid scintillation spectrophotometry after its isolation from $^3$H-tryptophan and $^3$H-metabolites using ion-exchange chromatography (16). Under these conditions, the spontaneous release of $^3$H-5HT remains constant for at least 5 hr and represents five to seven times the blank value. Drug applications were generally performed 1.5 hr after the beginning of the superfusion by adding the agent to the artificial CSF, which was delivered by the push-pull cannula to the intended structures. Results were expressed as percent of the mean value of $^3$H-5HT spontaneously released in the four fractions preceding the treatments. Student's $t$-test was then applied to the mean ± SEM of $^3$H-5HT released in corresponding fractions of control and treated cats. (When the $p$ value was ≤ 0.05, a difference was considered to be significant.)

## GAMMA-AMINOBUTYRIC ACID

The SN is known to receive gamma-aminobutyric acid (GABAergic) afferents from the CN and globus pallidus and may also contain intrinsic GABA interneurons (6,7,24). A GABAergic regulation of nigral dopamine (DA) neurons has been described by both release (2) and electrophysiological (31) studies. Our results (25) indicate that GABAergic neurons may also control 5HT transmission in the SN. jWe observed that GABA ($10^{-5}$ M) or muscimol ($10^{-6}$ M), a GABA agonist, when applied into the SN reduced $in$ $vivo$ 5HT release locally (Fig. 1), while the blockade of GABA transmission by the nigral application of picrotoxin ($10^{-5}$ M) facilitated the local $in$ $vivo$ 5HT release (Fig. 2).

This GABAergic control of nigral 5HT transmission may be direct via an action on 5HT nerve terminals. In fact, Gale (11) found a significant population of GABA receptors on nigral 5HT nerve endings. However, GABA may exert an indirect action on $in$ $vivo$ 5HT release by affecting the activity of other nigral transmitter systems. Thus, GABA may influence the release of DA (2) in the SN and we have previously shown that DA released from dendrites has an important influence on the $in$ $vivo$ release of $^3$H-5HT from the SN (17). Furthermore, GABA can modulate the release of substance P in the SN (28). This peptide, as we will show later on in this review also significantly modulates nigral 5HT transmission (21). Thus, the GABAergic control of nigral 5HT transmission could be mediated through several different pathways.

Interestingly, the effects of GABA on nigral $in$ $vivo$ 5HT release were only seen locally. This contrasts with the local and distal (changes in 5HT release in both CN) actions of the nigral application of DA on $in$ $vivo$ 5HT release (17). This may suggest that neurons forming a feedback pathway (7) from the SN to the raphe nucleus are sensitive only to a select group of nigral neurotransmitters. Further studies will thus be necessary to determine which transmitters may affect the activity of such a feedback pathway that regulates 5HT transmission in other brain regions.

## ACETYLCHOLINE

The SN may have a cholinergic innervation since there are detectable levels of choline acetyltransferase activity and muscarinic cholinergic receptors in this structure (7). However, the precise origin of acetylcholine in the SN remains unknown.

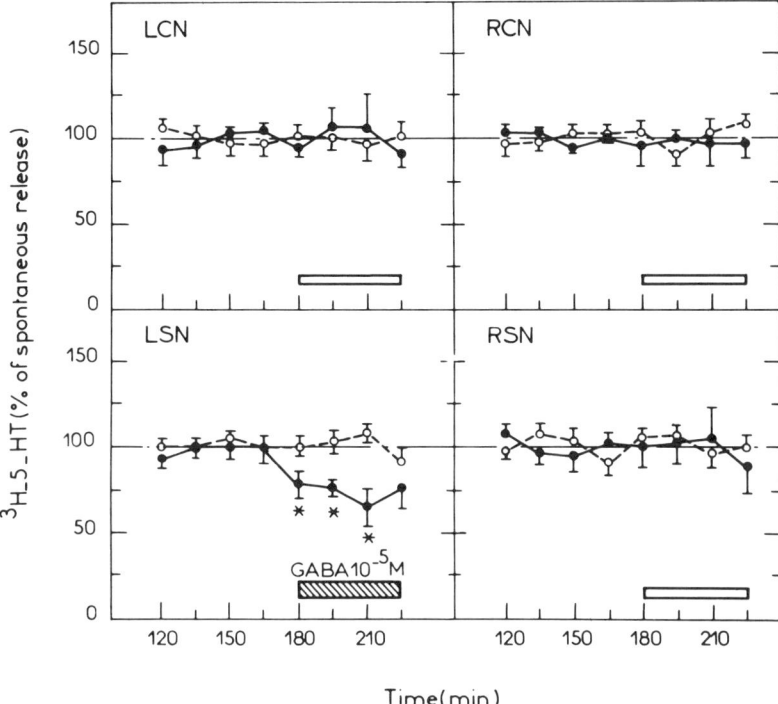

**FIG. 1.** Effects of the unilateral nigral application of GABA on the release of ³H-5HT in the ipsilateral substantia nigra (LSN) and caudate nucleus (LCN) and in the contralateral substantia nigra (RSN) and caudate nucleus (RCN) of the cat. Data are the mean ± SEM (see methodology) of results obtained with groups (*closed circles,* treated cats; *open circles,* control cats) of 4 animals. *$p \leq 0.05$ when compared with corresponding control values.

Acetylcholine may have an important function in regulating neuronal activity in the SN. Recently, Torrens et al. (27) observed that nicotine could inhibit the K⁺-evoked release of substance P from nigral slices and that this effect could be blocked by pempidine, a specific nicotinic receptor antagonist. In contrast, oxotremorine, a muscarinic cholinergic agonist had no effect on the K⁺-evoked release of substance P. These results suggest a cholinergic control of substance P transmission in the SN mediated by nicotinic receptors.

In preliminary studies, we also examined the effect of nigral cholinergic receptor activation on the *in vivo* release of ³H-5HT (Table 1). The application of carbachol ($10^{-5}$ M), a mixed cholinergic agonist, to the SN inhibited the local *in vivo* release of ³H-5HT. No effects in the ipsilateral CN or contralateral CN or SN were observed during or after the drug treatment. These results suggest that acetylcholine may exert a control over 5HT transmission in the SN and support the possibility of a significant cholinergic-serotonergic interaction in the basal ganglia.

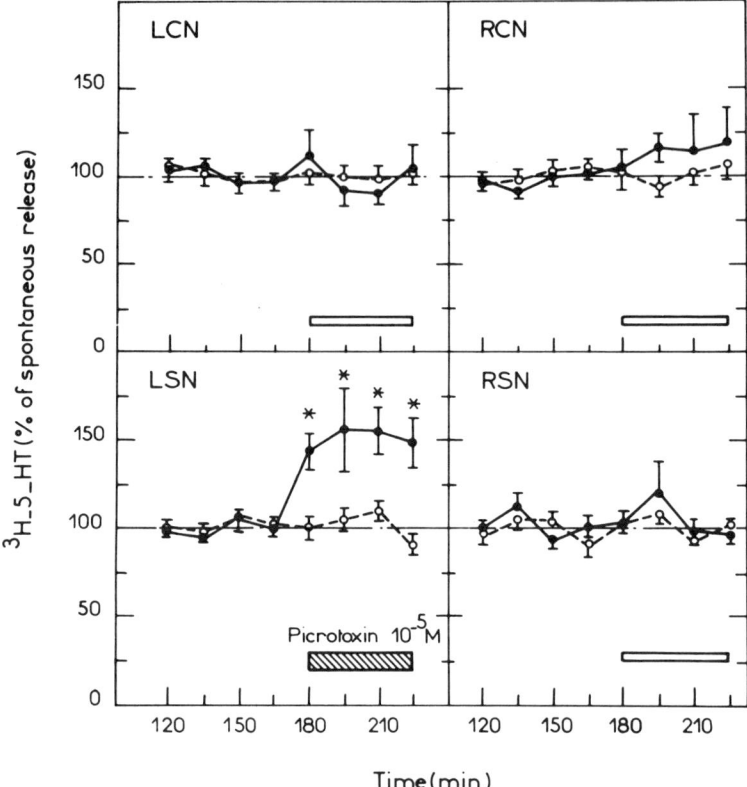

**FIG. 2.** Effects of the application of picrotoxin to the left substantia nigra (LSN) on the release of ³H-5HT in both substantia nigra (LSN and RSN) and both caudate nuclei (LCN and RCN). Data are the mean ± SEM (see methodology) of results obtained with groups (*closed circles*, treated cats; *open circles*, control cats) of 4 animals. *$p \leq 0.05$ when compared with corresponding control values.

## GLUTAMATE

There is substantial evidence for a glutamatergic input to the basal ganglia originating from the cerebral cortex (1,7). Glutamate, released from these neurons, may have an important functional role in the regulation of various neuronal systems in the basal ganglia. This is evident from recent *in vitro* and *in vivo* release experiments (12,19). Our results (21) reveal that glutamate can control 5HT transmission in the SN. Thus, the nigral application of glutamate ($5 \times 10^{-5}$ M) inhibited the local *in vivo* release of ³H-5HT and this effect was blocked by the glutamate receptor antagonist, glutamate diethylester (Fig. 3). Interestingly, the antagonist by itself caused a slight, delayed increase in nigral ³H-5HT release.

The reduction of 5HT release induced by glutamate could result from a direct presynaptic blockade due to excessive depolarization of 5HT nerve terminals. Such a depolarization of nerve terminals by glutamate has been observed in several

TABLE 1. *Effect of the application of carbachol ($10^{-5}$ M) to the left SN on the local release of $^3$H-5HT (N = 4 cats)*

|  | % ± SEM of spontaneous release |
|---|---|
| Baseline release | 99 ± 3.0 |
|  | 104 ± 2.0 |
|  | 96 ± 3.0 |
|  | 102 ± 3.5 |
| Carbachol, $10^{-5}$ M (4 fractions) | 75 ± 3.5[a] |
|  | 69 ± 3.5[a] |
|  | 86 ± 5.0 |
|  | 77 ± 5.5[a] |
| Recovery | 93 ± 4.0 |
|  | 88 ± 5.5 |
|  | 106 ± 7.5 |

[a] $p \leq 0.05$ (Student's *t*-test).

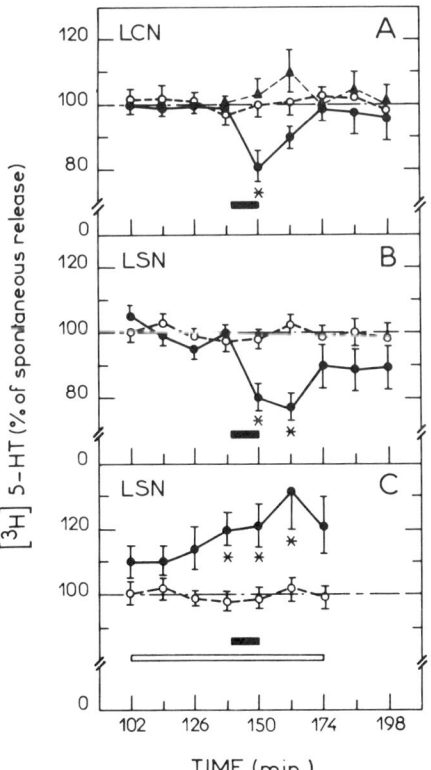

**FIG. 3.** Effect of the application of glutamate in the left caudate or in the left substantia nigra on the local release of $^3$H-5HT in the cat. L-Glutamic acid *(closed bars)* was applied: **(A)** to the left caudate nucleus (LCN) at a concentration of $10^{-7}$ M *(triangles, N = 5 cats)* or $5 \times 10^{-5}$ M *(closed circles, N = 7 cats)*; **(B)** to the left substantia nigra (LSN) at a concentration of $5 \times 10^{-6}$ M *(closed circles, N = 7 cats)*; **(C)** to the left substantia nigra (LSN) at a concentration of $5 \times 10^{-5}$ M *(closed circles, N = 5 cats)* in the presence of L-glutamic acid diethylester ($10^{-4}$ M; *open bars*). *$p \leq 0.05$ when compared with corresponding values of control cats *(open circles)*.

invertebrate species (10). Yet an indirect action upon GABA, substance P, or DA transmission within the nigra cannot be excluded in explaining glutamate's regulation of nigral 5HT release.

An action of glutamate on nigral *in vivo* 5HT release may indicate a role for cortical glutamatergic inputs in the regulation of nigral 5HT transmission. In fact, a cerebral cortical control of striatal and nigral DA release (19) has been observed and studies are now in progress to determine whether stimulation of the cerebral cortex may also influence 5HT transmission in the basal ganglia.

## SUBSTANCE P

The excititory neuropeptide, substance P, is found in high amounts in the SN and is believed to be contained within neurons of striatal origin (5,7). Its central physiological role remains unclear. However, recently it was shown to inhibit the *in vivo* release of DA from dendrites in the SN (3). This supports its role in the control of nigral-striatal dopaminergic neuronal activity. We have found that substance P (21), when applied into the SN, also affects the *in vivo* release of $^3$H-5HT (Fig. 4). Substance P ($10^{-7}$ M) induced an increase of $^3$H-5HT release, locally, that was slow in onset. The delayed appearance of substance P's effect is rather unusual. However, electrophysiological studies conducted in the rat SN have shown that the iontophoretic application of substance P elicits a facilitation of nigral cell firing that is also slow in onset (4,5). An explanation for the delayed action of substance P on neuronal firing and *in vivo* 5HT release is unknown. Yet it may suggest a rather unique mechanism of action of this peptide on neuronal activity.

Substance P's actions on *in vivo* 5HT release may be direct upon 5HT nerve terminals. However, as suggested by Reubi et al. (23), substance P's enhancement of nigral *in vitro* 5HT release may also be mediated via DA neurons. In fact, substance P inhibits *in vivo* nigral DA release and as mentioned previously, DA reduces *in vivo* $^3$H-5HT release (17). Furthermore, the time of application required for substance P to induce its maximal effects on nigral *in vivo* DA and 5HT release corresponds very closely. Also, the facilitation of *in vitro* $^3$H-5HT release from nigral slices by substance P is blocked by the DA receptor antagonist, fluphenazine (23). Thus, by modulating nigral dopaminergic transmission, substance P may indirectly control nigral 5HT release.

In addition to its local effects, substance P induced an immediate increase in $^3$H-5HT release in the contralateral CN. This rapid increase is in contrast with the delayed onset of action seen locally for substance P. This may suggest that substance P acts upon a different population of cells in the SN to produce its local versus its distal effects. Support for this proposal comes from studies by Collingridge and Davies (4) who showed that substance P, when iontophoretically applied to the SN, facilitated nigral firing with a slow onset in some cells but with an immediate onset in other neurons. The neuronal pathways mediating this effect on *in vivo* 5HT release in the contralateral CN are not known. However, recent anatomical evidence indicates that a crossed nigral-contralateral striatal neuronal pathway exists (9). This

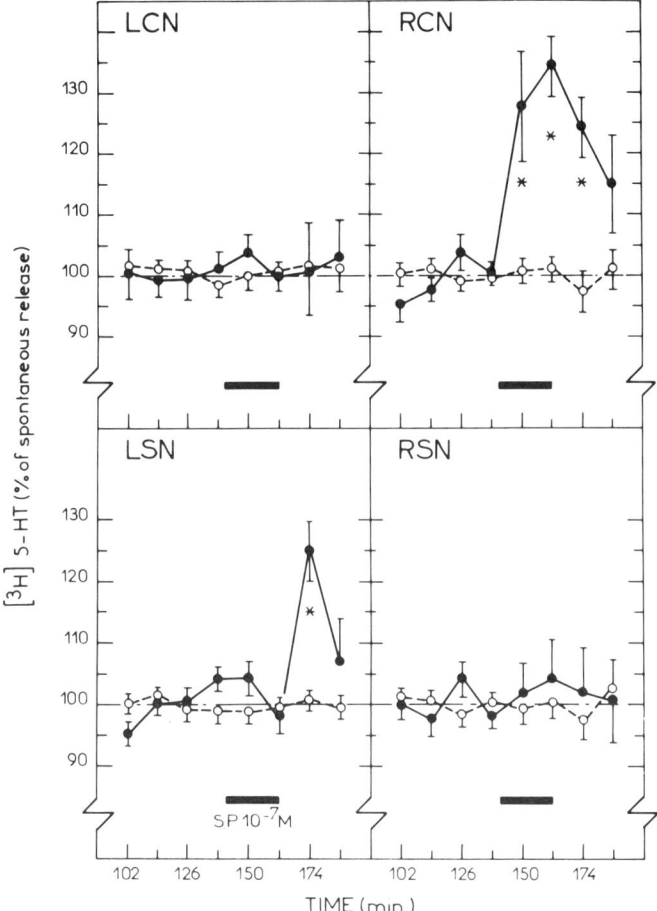

**FIG. 1.** Effect of the application of substance P to the left substantia nigra (LSN) on the release of ³H-5HT in both substantia nigra (LSN and RSN) and both caudate nuclei (LCN and RCN). Data are the mean ± SEM (see methodology) of results obtained with groups of 7 treated cats *(closed circles)* and 4 control cats *(open circles)*. *$p \leq 0.05$ when compared with corresponding control values.

pathway may be important in mediating the contralateral effects of substance P on *in vivo* ³H-5HT release.

## FEEDBACK PATHWAY AND LATERAL HABENULA

The distal effects on ³H-5HT release induced by the nigral application of DA and substance P have led us to identify feedback pathways from the basal ganglia to the raphe that may act to regulate 5HT neurons projecting to the CN or SN. An important link in one such putative feedback pathway is the lateral habenula. This nuclei receives inputs from the basal ganglia and sends a massive projection to the dorsal and median raphe (14,15,18,20). In a preliminary study (26), we observed that the application of KCl (60 mM) to the lateral habenula could simultaneously facilitate the *in vivo* release of $^3$H-5HT release in both CN and both SN. These results suggested to us that lateral habenular-raphe neurons may control the activity of raphe 5HT cells.

These initial studies inspired us to try to dissect out the various components of this feedback pathway.

Recent biochemical studies have shown that the globus pallidus sends GABAergic neurons to the lateral habenula (18). To test whether this pathway is important in regulating 5HT release in the basal ganglia, we interrupted GABA transmission in the lateral habenula by applying picrotoxin ($10^{-5}$ M) and measured the effect of this manipulation on *in vivo* 5HT release in both CN and both SN. As revealed in Table 2, picrotoxin applied into one lateral habenula reduced $^3$H-5HT release in both SN. However, 5HT release was not altered in either CN during or after this treatment (data not shown). This finding suggests that 5HT neurons innervating the SN may be differentially regulated from those 5HT neurons projecting to the CN. Support for this proposal comes from experiments on the effect of auditory and visual stimuli on the release of $^3$H-5HT in both CN and both SN of awake, encephale isole cats (22). In these studies, we found that light flashes and click noises could

TABLE 2. $^3$H-5HT release in the SN (% ± SEM of spontaneous release)

| A. Effect of unilateral application of picrotoxin ($10^{-5}$ M) into the lateral habenula ($N = 6$ cats) | Left SN | Right SN |
|---|---|---|
| Baseline release | 102 ± 1.5 | 100 ± 2.0 |
| | 98 ± 2.0 | 97 ± 2.0 |
| | 97 ± 1.5 | 103 ± 3.0 |
| | 103 ± 1.5 | 99 ± 1.5 |
| Picrotoxin, $10^{-5}$ M (4 fractions) | 86 ± 3.0[a] | 84 ± 4.0[a] |
| | 76 ± 3.5[a] | 82 ± 3.5[a] |
| | 82 ± 4.0[a] | 81 ± 3.0[a] |
| | 75 ± 4.5[a] | 80 ± 4.0[a] |
| B. Effect of the application of substance P ($10^{-7}$ M) into the dorsal raphe ($N = 7$ cats) | Left SN | Right SN |
| Baseline release | 100 ± 2.0 | 101 ± 2.0 |
| | 99 ± 2.0 | 103 ± 2.5 |
| | 104 ± 1.5 | 100 ± 0.5 |
| | 97 ± 2.5 | 97 ± 2.5 |
| Substance P, $10^{-7}$ M (2 fractions) | 82 ± 4.5[a] | 82 ± 2.5[a] |
| | 80 ± 5.0[a] | 81 ± 4.0[a] |
| Recovery | 78 ± 4.0[a] | 87 ± 10.0 |
| | 76 ± 3.0[a] | 83 ± 8.0 |

[a] $p \leq 0.05$ (Student's *t*-test).

facilitate $^3$H-5HT release in both SN without affecting $^3$H-5HT release in either CN.

As mentioned previously, the lateral habenula sends an important input to the dorsal raphe nucleus (15,25). The transmitters associated with this projection have not been clearly identified. However, there is some evidence to suggest that substance P is contained within some of those neurons (30). Thus, we have applied substance P into the dorsal raphe and found a significant inhibition of 5HT release in both SN (Table 2). In this study we also saw a slight inhibition of 5HT release in both CN. However, this effect was very small compared with the decrease in nigral $^3$H-5HT release. These results must be viewed in light of the finding of Van der Kooy and Hattori (29) who showed that in the rat the dorsal raphe innervation to the SN exists as a branched collateral of neurons projecting to the CN. Further anatomical studies will therefore be necessary to determine whether in the cat distinct dorsal raphe 5HT neurons innervate the SN and not the CN.

The inhibition of nigral 5HT release found after picrotoxin application to the lateral habenula or substance P addition to the dorsal raphe supports the existence of a feedback pathway from the basal ganglia to the raphe with the lateral habenula as a relay nuclei. The different effects on nigral versus striatal 5HT release seen in these experiments indictes that this putative pathway may selectively control 5HT neurons projecting to the SN as compared with 5HT neurons innervating the CN.

## CONCLUSION

We have observed that several neurotransmitters in the SN can significantly modulate $^3$H-5HT release locally. Some of these transmitters affect 5HT release only locally, whereas others can alter 5HT transmission in the contralateral basal ganglia. The local effects on $^3$H-5HT release may be due to a direct action of the transmitter on 5HT terminals or indirectly via other nigral elements. The distal effects on $^3$H-5HT release could be mediated by feedback pathways that may control the activity of raphe 5HT neurons. One such pathway may have the lateral habenula as an integral component. Further studies will be necessary to clearly identify the neuronal systems responsible for controlling 5HT transmission in the basal ganglia. However, our results suggest that in some cases 5HT transmission in the SN and CN are differentially regulated.

## ACKNOWLEDGMENTS

This research was supported by grants from INSERM, DRET (79/077), and Rhône Poulenc S.A. Dr. T. D. Reisine is a post-doctoral fellow of the NINCDS (F 32-N.S. 0646-01).

## REFERENCES

1. Carter, C. J. (1980): Evidence for glutamatergic projections from the prefrontal cortex to the striatum, nucleus accumbens, amygdaloid complex and substantia nigra in the rat. *Neurosci. Lett (suppl.)*, 5:580.

2. Chéramy, A., Nieoullon, A., and Glowinski, J. (1978): Gabaergic processes involved in the control of dopamine release from nigrostriatal dopaminergic neurons in the cat. *Eur. J. Pharmacol.*, 48:281–290.
3. Chéramy, A., Nieoullon, A., Michelot, R., and Glowinski, J. (1977): Effects of the intranigral application of dopamine and substance P in the *in vivo* release of newly synthetized ³H-dopamine in the ipsilateral caudate nucleus of the cat. *Neurosci. Lett.*, 4:105–109.
4. Collingridge, C., and Davies, J. (1980): Effect of substance P (SP) and morphine on substantia nigra neurones. *Neurosci. Lett. (Suppl.)*, 5:557.
5. Davies, J., and Dray, A. (1976): Substance P in the substantia nigra. *Brain Res.*, 107:623–627.
6. Di Chiara, G., Morelli, M., Porceddu, M., Mulas, M., and Del Fiacco, M. (1980): Effect of discrete kainic acid-induced lesions of corpus caudatus and globus pallidus on glutamic acid decarboxylase of rat substantia nigra. *Brain Res.*, 189:193–199.
7. Dray, A. (1977): The striatum and substantia nigra. A commentary of their relationships. *Neuroscience*, 4:1407–1439.
8. Dray, A., Davies, J., Oakley, N. R., Tomgroach, P., and Veelucci, S. (1978): The dorsal and medial raphe projections to the substantia nigra in the rat: electrophysiological, biochemical and behavioral observations. *Brain Res.*, 151:431–442.
9. Fass, B., and Butcher, L. (1981): Evidence for a crossed nigrostriatal pathway in rats. *Neurosci. Lett.*, 22:109–113.
10. Florey, E., and Woodcock, B. (1968): Presynaptic excitatory action of glutamate applied to crab nerve-muscle preparation. *Comp. Biochem. Physiol.*, 26:651–661.
11. Gale, K. (1979): GABA receptors in rat substantia nigra: changes in response to lesions and chronic drug treatment. *Neurosci. Abstr.*, 9:71.
12. Giorguieff, M. F., Kemel, M. L., and Glowinski, J. (1977): Presynaptic effect of L-glutamic acid on the release of dopamine in rat striatal slices. *Neurosci. Lett.*, 6:73–77.
13. Giambalvo, C., and Snodgrass, S. (1978): Biochemical and behavioral effects of serotonin neurotoxine on the nigrostriatal dopamine system: comparison of injection sites. *Brain Res.*, 152: 555–566.
14. Herkenham, M., and Nauta, W. (1977): Afferent connections of the habenular nuclei in the rat. A horseradish peroxidase study, with a note on the fiber-of-passage problem. *J. Comp. Neurol.*, 173:123–146.
15. Herkenham, M., and Nauta, W. (1979): Efferent connections of the habenular nuclei in the rat. *J. Comp. Neurol.*, 187:19–48.
16. Hery, F., Simonnet, G., Bourgoin, S., Soubrie, P., Artaud, F., Hamon, M., and Glowinski, J. (1979): Effect of nerve activity on the *in vivo* release of ³H-serotonin continuously formed from L-³H-tryptophan in the caudate nucleus of the cat. *Brain Res.*, 169:317–334.
17. Hery, F., Soubrie, P., Borugoin, S., Montastruc, J., Artaud, F., and Glowinksi, J. (1980): Dopamine released from dendrites in the substantia nigra control the nigral and striatal release of serotonin. *Brain Res.*, 193:143–151.
18. Nagy, J. I., Carter, D., Lehmann, J., and Fibiger, H. C. (1978): Evidence for a GABA containing projection from the entopeduncular nucleus to the lateral habenula in the rat. *Brain Res.*, 145: 360–364.
19. Nieoullon, A., Cheramy, A., and Glowinski, J. (1978): Release of dopamine evoked by electrical stimulation of the motor and visual areas of the cerebral cortex in both caudate nuclei and in the substantia nigra in the cat. *Brain Res.*, 145:69–84.
20. Phillipson, O., and Griffith, A. (1980): The neurones of origin for the mesohabenular dopamine pathway. *Brain Res.*, 197:213–218.
21. Reisine, T. D., Soubrie, P., Artaud, F., and Glowinksi, J. (1982): Application of glutamate and substance P into the substantia nigra modulate *in vivo* ³H-serotonin release in the basal ganglia of the cat. *Brain Res.*, 236:317–327.
22. Reisine, T. D., Soubrie, P., Artaud, F., and Glowinksi, J. (1982): Sensory stimuli differentially affect *in vivo* nigral and striatal ³H-serotonin release in the cat. *Brain Res.*, 232:77–87.
23. Reubi, J., Emson, P., Jessell, T., and Iversen, L. L. (1978): Effects of GABA, dopamine and substance P on the release of newly synthetized ³H-5-hydroxytryptamine from rat substantia nigra *in vitro*. *Naunyn Schmiedebergs Arch. Pharmacol.*, 304:271–275.
24. Ribak, C., Vaughn, J., and Roberts, E. (1980): GABAergic nerve terminals decrease in the substantia nigra following hemitransections of the striatonigral and pallidonigral pathways. *Brain Res.*, 192:413–423.

25. Soubrie, P., Montastruc, J., Bourgoin, S., Reisine, T., Artaud, F., and Glowinski, J. (1981): *In vivo* evidence for GABAergic control of serotonin release in the cat substantia nigra. *Eur. J. Pharmacol.*, 69:483–488.
26. Soubrie, P., Reisine, T., Artaud, F., and Glowinski, J. (1981): Role of the lateral habenula in modulating nigral and striatal *in vivo* ³H-serotonin release in the cat. *Brain Res.*, 225.
27. Speciale, S., Neckers, L., and Wyatt, J. (1980): Habenular modulation of raphe indolamine metabolism. *Life Sci.*, 27:2367–2372.
28. Torrens, Y., Beaujouan, J., Besson, M. J., Michelot, R., and Glowinski, J. (1981): Inhibitory effects of GABA, L-glutamic acid and nicotine on the potassium-evoked release of substance P in substantia nigra slices of the rat. *Eur. J. Pharmacol.*, 71:383–392.
29. Van der Kooy, D., and Hattori, T. (1980): Dorsal raphe cells with collateral projections to the caudate-putamen and substantia nigra: A fluorescent retrograde double labeling study in the rat. *Brain Res.*, 186:1–7.
30. Vincent, S., Staines, W., McGeer, E., and Fibiger, H. (1980): Transmitters contained in the efferents of the habenula. *Brain Res.*, 195:479–484.
31. Waszcak, B., Eng, N., and Walters, J. (1980): Effects of muscimol and picrotoxin on single unit activity of substantia nigra neurons. *Brain Res.*, 188:185–197.

# $^3$H-Serotonin Binding Sites: Pharmacological and Species Differences

*David L. Nelson, *†Rick Schnellmann, and *†Mark Smit

*Department of Pharmacology and Toxicology, College of Pharmacy; and †Department of Pharmacology, College of Medicine, University of Arizona, Tucson, Arizona 85721

Serotoneric neurons form a very complex system within the central nervous system (CNS). Anatomical studies have demonstrated that these neurons arise from at least nine separate cell groups in the brainstem and project to practically all areas of the CNS (3,10). Biochemical findings have been consistent with this and have shown relatively high concentrations of serotonin (5-hydroxytryptamine, 5-HT) in most areas of the brain and spinal cord (24). The existence of such a broadly distributed system is also reflected in behavioral and physiological findings. Thus, the involvement of 5-HT has been implicated in a broad range of behaviors and disease states including the perception of pain, release of pituitary hormones, eating, sleeping, depression, and schizophrenia to name just a few (5,7,13). The complexity of its distribution and actions has made it difficult to study the specific effects of 5-HT on discrete systems, a problem that has been compounded by the lack of specificity of the drugs which have been used to study serotonergic systems. Unfortunately, most of these compounds, particularly the antagonists, have significant interactions with other neurotransmitter receptors (19). In order to better understand the actions of 5-HT and to try and develop more selective pharmacological agents, many studies have turned to the examination of 5-HT receptors. Such investigations have demonstrated that there are multiple types of 5-HT receptors, that they mediate different types of cellular responses, that they have different regional distributions, and that they have different pharmacological profiles.

The first results suggesting multiple types of 5-HT receptors came from studies of smooth muscle in the periphery. As early as 1954, Gaddum and Hameed (15) had suggested the existence of two different types of peripheral 5-HT receptors, and this has been confirmed by a number of subsequent works (4,9,30). Later, with the development of electrophysiological techniques the concept of multiple 5-HT receptors was extended to neural tissue. For example, Gerschenfeld and Paupardin-Tritsch (16,17) characterized 5-HT responses in the ganglia of *Aplysia*. On the basis of the ionic changes and the pharmacological properties of the receptors that mediated these changes, they postulated the existence of as many as six different 5-HT receptors in the ganglia of this invertebrate. Electrophysiological studies in the mammalian CNS also suggested a heterogeneity of 5-HT receptors. Thus, 5-HT was found to produce either excitation or inhibition postsynaptically (2). The excitatory effect of 5-HT could also be blocked by "classical" 5-HT antagonists, such as LSD, methysergide, and cinanserin (6,28), whereas the inhibitory action could not (18). Thus, the 5-HT receptors linked to these two responses appeared to be pharmacologically distinct. In addition to the postsynaptic receptors there also appeared to be a presynaptic autoreceptor. Stimulation of this receptor caused decreased firing of serotonergic neurons (18), and the pharmacological profile of this receptor appeared different from the postsynaptic receptors. Thus, it was found that hallucinogens such as LSD, psilocin, and $N,N$-dimethyltryptamine were more potent at the autoreceptors than at postsynaptic sites (1). *In vitro* studies have confirmed the existence of presynaptic 5-HT receptors which can regulate the release of serotonin and have demonstrated the ability of these sites to discriminate between different 5-HT antagonists. Cerrito and Raiteri (8) found that methiothepin blocked the 5-HT-induced inhibition of $^3$H-5-HT release from synaptosomes while other 5-HT antagonists (cyproheptadine, methysergide, and mianserin) were inactive.

Biochemical measures of 5-HT receptor activity have also suggested the possibility of multiple types of 5-HT receptors. For example, two different 5-HT-stimulated adenylate cyclase systems have been described in the mammalian CNS. In one of these (low-sensitivity type) half-maximal stimulation of adenylate cyclase occurs at 0.5 to 1.0 μM 5-HT (12,31), whereas in the other (high-sensitivity type) half-maximal stimulation occurs with 1 to 4 nM 5-HT (14). In addition, in cultured neuroblastoma brain cell hybrids it has been shown that the 5-HT receptors that stimulate adenylate cyclase activity are distinct from the 5-HT receptors that mediate depolarization and acetylcholine release in these cells (20).

The results of ligand-binding studies are also consistent with the concept of multiple 5-HT receptors. Peroutka and Snyder (27) have suggested the classification of central 5-HT receptors into two groups based on the results of ligand-binding studies. One of these, the 5-HT$_1$ receptor, is defined by the high-affinity binding of $^3$H-5-HT, and the other, the 5-HT$_2$ receptor, is defined by the binding of $^3$H-spiperone in the rat frontal cortex. The comparison of the pharmacological profiles of these two sites with those of 5-HT receptors that have been identified electrophysiologically led Peroutka et al. (26) to postulate that the 5-HT$_1$ receptors represent the sites which mediate the inhibitory effects of 5-HT in the CNS, whereas the 5-HT$_2$ receptors represent those sites which mediate the excitatory effects of 5-HT. The 5-HT$_2$ sites also appear to represent the receptors involved in both tryptamine-induced seizures in the rat (19) and 5-hydroxytryptophan-induced head twitches in the mouse (26).

The 5-HT$_1$ receptors themselves appear to be heterogeneous. It has been shown, for example, that a number of compounds produce logit-log inhibition curves of $^3$H-5-HT binding that have slopes that are less than unity, suggesting the possibility of multiple binding sites (22). The neuroleptic spiperone actually gives biphasic inhibtion curves of $^3$H-5-HT binding in membranes from rat brain and shows regional differences in its potency. Analysis of these inhibition curves shows that they are consistent with at least two populations of binding sites (25). One of these

(5-HT$_{1-A}$) has relatively high affinity for spiperone ($K_D$ = 2–13 nM) while the other (5-HT$_{1-B}$) has low affinity ($K_D \simeq$ 35,000 nM).

The work described below deals with one aspect of multiple 5-HT receptors, i.e., the heterogeneity of 5-HT$_1$ sites. It is an extension of our earlier studies with spiperone in the rat, and it demonstrates that multiple $^3$H-5-HT binding sites exist in other species and that compounds other than the neuroleptics discriminate between different types of $^3$H-5-HT binding sites.

## MUTLIPLE $^3$H-5-HT BINDING SITES

### METHODS

The binding assays for $^3$H-5-HT were carried out as previously described (22,25). Male Sprague-Dawley rats were killed by decapitation, and cats were killed by pentobarbital overdose. The brains were rapidly removed and placed on ice for dissection. The tissues were homogenized in 40 volumes of Tris-HCl buffer (50 mM, pH 7.4) using a Brinkmann Polytron (setting 5 for 15 sec). The homogenates were centrifuged (48,000 × g for 10 min), the pellets were washed by resuspension in buffer, and the process was repeated three more times. Between the second and third washes the resuspended homogenates were incubated for 10 min at 37°C. The final pellet was resuspended in 50–100 volumes of the Tris buffer for use in the binding assay. The assay tubes (final volume, 2 ml) contained the following: 0.5 ml of the tissue homogenate, 5.7 mM ascorbate, 10 μM pargyline, 4 mM CaCl$_2$, 50 mM Tris, $^3$H-5-HT, and added drugs for a final pH of 7.4. The samples were incubated for 7 min at 37°C, and then the incubation was terminated by vacuum filtration through Whatman GF/B filters. This was followed by three, 5-ml washes with cold buffer. Radioactivity in the filters was measured by liquid scintillation spectrometry. Specific $^3$H-5-HT binding was defined as the difference between total binding and that occurring in the presence of either 0.3 μM unlabeled 5-HT or 1 μM metergoline and represented 50–80% of the total bound radioactivity trapped by the filters.

Nonlinear regression analysis of the inhibition of $^3$H-5-HT binding by the various drugs was accomplished by the computer program NONLIN (21) as previously described (11,25). Using this procedure it was determined if the inhibition curves were consistent with interactions at a single population of binding sites or whether they indicated more than a single type of site. When more than one site was suggested, the data were analysed according to a two-site model. The finding that data fit a two-site better than a one-site model only indicates that there are at least two populations of sites and does not preclude the possibility that the two groups of sites themselves might be heterogeneous.

### RESULTS

#### Spiperone Inhibition of $^3$H-5-HT Binding in the Cat

As was described at the opening of this chapter, previous studies of spiperone inhibition of $^3$H-5-HT binding in the rat had demonstrated the presence of at least two different high-affinity $^3$H-5-HT binding sites (25). In the present work, similar studies were carried out in the cat to determine if this heterogeneity of binding sites occurred in other species. Analysis of saturation curves for the binding of $^3$H-5-HT using Scatchard plots revealed a single high-affinity binding site in tissues from the cat. As seen in Table 1, there were no significant differences between the $K_D$ values in tissues from the cat compared with the rat. However, the brain areas of the cat did appear to have slightly higher concentrations of receptors than the corresponding areas of the rat brain.

Examination of the inhibition of $^3$H-5-HT binding by spiperone revealed differences between different brain areas of the cat. An example of this is shown in Fig. 1 which contrasts the spiperone inhibition curve found in the corpus striatum (CS) with that found for the dorsal half of the hippocampus (DH). Table 2 shows the IC$_{50}$ values (concentrations causing 50% inhibition of specific $^3$H-5-HT binding) for the spiperone inhibition curves in these two tissues as well as for ventral hippocampus (VH) and frontal cortex (FC). As can be seen, these values were spread over a 30-fold range of concentrations. It can also be seen in this figure that the slopes derived from logit-log plots of the inhibition curves were less than unity.

Analysis of the inhibition curves by nonlinear regression and computer curve fitting showed that they fit a two-site model significantly better than a one-site model, and the results of the analysis according to a two site-model are shown in Table 3. It was seen that the site having high affinity for spiperone ($K_H$) had similar affinities for this compound in all four structures. However, there were large regional differences in the sites having low affinity ($K_L$) for spiperone. Thus, FC and CS exhibited $K_L$ sites which had very low affinity for spiperone and which resembled those previously described in the rat (25). However, VH and DH exhibited $K_L$ values which were much less than those in FC or CS.

## Discrimination of Multiple $^3$H-5-HT Binding Sites by Tryptamine Analogues

Since previous work had shown that certain neuroleptics could discriminate between different types of $^3$H-5-HT binding sites, the possibility that other types of

TABLE 1. *Kinetic analysis of $^3$H-5-HT binding in regions of the rat and cat brain*

| Species | Area | $K_D$ (nM) | $B_{max}$ (fmol/mg tiss.) |
|---|---|---|---|
| Rat | Hippo. | 2.85 ± 0.65 | 16.3 ± 1.4 |
|  | FC | 2.71 ± 0.55 | 9.6 ± 0.8 |
| Cat | Hippo. | 2.94 ± 0.58 | 23.7 ± 0.1[a] |
|  | FC | 2.41 ± 0.34 | 12.9 ± 0.7 |

$K_D$ and $B_{max}$ represent, respectively, the dissociation constant and the total number of specific binding sites determined by Scatchard analysis in the hippocampus (Hippo.) and frontal cortex (FC). Each point represents the mean ± SEM of six separate experiments for the tissues from the rat and two separate experiments for those from the cat.
[a] Significantly different from rat hippocampus, $p < 0.05$.

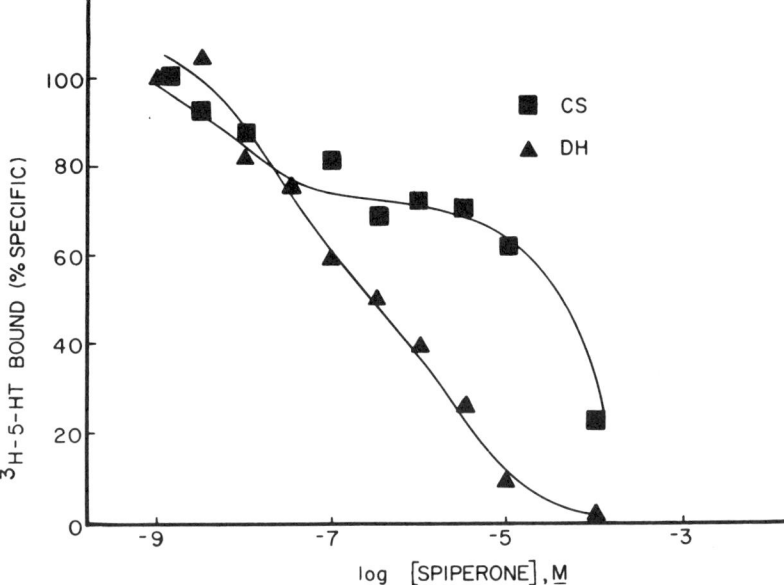

**FIG. 1.** Inhibition of ³H-5-HT binding in cat corpus striatum (CS) and dorsal hippocampus (DH) by spiperone. ³H-5-HT (1.8 nM) binding was measured as described in Methods. Each point is the mean from three separate experiments and the curves represent the best fit for a two-site model determined by nonlinear regression analysis. The data are expressed as percent of the specific ³H-5-HT binding which occurred in the absence of added drugs.

TABLE 2. *Regional differences in cat brain for the potency of spiperone in inhibiting $^3$H-5-HT binding*

| Area | $IC_{50}$ (nM) | Slope |
|---|---|---|
| CS | 8900 ± 874[a] | 0.29 ± 0.07 |
| FC | 1197 ± 449 | 0.28 ± 0.06 |
| VH | 344 ± 85 | 0.64 ± 0.12 |
| DH | 286 ± 93 | 0.56 ± 0.07 |

$IC_{50}$ values (concentration in nM causing 50% inhibition of specific ³H-5-HT binding) and slope values were derived from Hill or logit-log plots of the inhibition of ³H-5-HT binding by spiperone. Each value represents the mean ± SEM of values from three separate experiments. CS, corpus striatum; FC, frontal cortex; VH, ventral hippocampus; DH, dorsal hippocampus.

[a] Significantly different from the $IC_{50}$ values in the other tissues at $p < 0.005$.

TABLE 3. *Kinetic properties of spiperone's inhibition of $^3$H-5-HT binding in the cat brain*

| Area | $K_H$ (nM) | $B_H$ | $K_L$ (nM) | $B_L$ |
|------|-----------|-------|-----------|-------|
| CS | 5.1 | 0.29 | 51,600 | 0.71 |
| FC | 20.5 | 0.60 | 52,800 | 0.40 |
| VH | 5.7 | 0.50 | 823 | 0.50 |
| DH | 13.1 | 0.53 | 1,400 | 0.47 |

Data from curves of the inhibition of specific $^3$H-5-HT binding by spiperone were analyzed by nonlinear regression as described in Methods. $K_H$ and $K_L$ are the dissociation constants of spiperone for the high- and low-affinity sites, respectively. $B_H$ and $B_L$ are the proportions of high- and low-affinity sites measured at 1.8 nM $^3$H-5-HT. The abbreviations for the tissue areas are the same as in Table 2. The inhibition curves for all brainareas fit a two-site model significantly better than a one-site model (FC, $p < 0.001$; CS, $p < 0.001$; DH, $p < 0.001$; VH, $p < 0.05$).

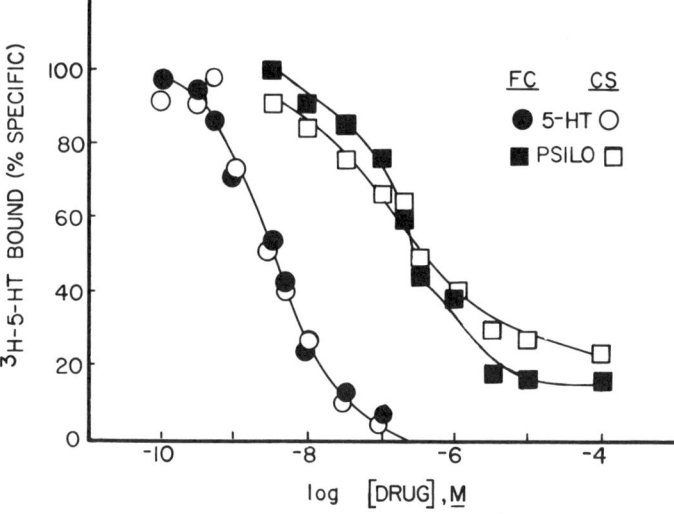

**FIG. 2.** Inhibition of $^3$H-5-HT binding in rat corpus striatum (CS) and frontal cortex (FC) by psilocybin (PSILO) and 5-HT. Each point represents the mean of five separate experiments for 5-HT, four experiments with psilocybin in FC, and three experiments using psilocybin in CS. Data are expressed as in Fig. 1.

compounds might also distinguish between these sites was examined. In the present study two tryptamine analogs were found to be particularly interesting. One of these, psilocybin (*O*-phosphoryl-4-hydroxy-*N,N*-dimethyltryptamine), produced somewhat unique inhibition curves. As can be seen in Fig. 2, the inhibition curves in both rat FC and CS began to plateau at a concentration of about 3 μM. There was little additional change with concentrations of psilocybin as high as 100 μM. In FC 10 to 20% of the specific $^3$H-5-HT binding sites appeared resistant to inhibition by psilocybin, whereas in CS these made up about 15 to 30% of the sites. Nonlinear regression analysis showed that the inhibition curves generated by psilocybin fit a two-site model better than a one-site model, and the results of this analysis are shown in Table 4. Because of the shape of the curves it was not possible to accurately estimate the affinity (if any) of psilocybin for the low-affinity sites.

5-Methoxy-$N,N$-dimethyltryptamine [5(OMe)DMT] was another tryptamine derivative which appeared to distinguish between different types of $^3$H-5-HT binding sites (Fig. 3; Table 4). Like psilocybin, its inhibition curve fits a two-site model significantly better than a one-site model. However, unlike psilocybin, it was possible to obtain complete inhibition of specific $^3$H-5-HT binding.

One of the questions raised by the inhibition curves produced with the tryptamines was whether the two groups of sites which they could discriminate were identical to the sites discriminated by spiperone. The results with psilocybin suggested that they were probably different (see Discussion below). To test the correlations between the sites differentiated by 5(OMe)DMT and spiperone, the inhibition of $^3$H-5-HT binding by 5(OMe)DMT was measured in both the presence and absence of 1 μM spiperone (Fig. 3). It had previously been shown that 1 μM spiperone completely inhibits $^3$H-5-HT binding to the 5-HT$_{1-A}$ site while hardly affecting its binding to the 5-HT$_{1-B}$ site (25). If the two populations of sites found with 5(OMe)DMT corresponded to the sites seen with spiperone, the presence of 1 μM spiperone should convert the 5(OMe)DMT inhibition curve to one having a Hill coefficient of 1.0, and the $K_D$ of 5(OMe)DMT for the remaining sites should be equal to that of one of the populations of sites identified in the absence of spiperone. As can be seen in Fig. 3, the presence of 1 μM spiperone produced an increase in the slope of the inhibition curve. This can also be seen in Table 4 where the Hill coefficient changed from 0.52 in the absence of spiperone to 0.92 in the presence of spiperone. Nonlinear regression analysis showed that in the presence of spiperone the curve was consistent with a single population of sites. The $K_D$ of 5(OMe)DMT, which

TABLE 4. *Binding parameters for the inhibition of $^3$H-5-HT binding in the rat brain by tryptamine derivatives*

| Drug | Area | $K_H$ (nM) | $K_L$ (nM) | $B_H$ | $B_L$ | $S$ |
|---|---|---|---|---|---|---|
| Psilocybin | FC | 177.3 | >100,000 | 0.78 | 0.15 | — |
|  | CS | 94.1 | >100,000 | 0.58 | 0.32 | — |
| 5(OMe)DMT | CTX | 19.2 | 2996 | 0.69 | 0.24 | 0.52 |
| 5(OMe)DMT + 1 μM spiperone | CTX | 145.9 | — | 0.90 | — | 0.92 |

These values were derived from the data shown in Fig. 2 (psilocybin) and Fig. 3 [5(OMe)DMT] using nonlinear regression analysis as described under Methods. $K_H$, $K_L$, $B_H$, and $B_L$ are defined in Table 3. FC, frontal cortex; CS, corpus striatum; CTX, cortex dorsal to the rhinal sulcus. $S$ is the slope or Hill coefficient determined by nonlinear regression analysis. The curves for which $K_H$ and $K_L$ are shown fit two-site models better than one-site models ($p < 0.01$). The curve for 5(OMe)DMT + 1 μM spiperone did not fit the two-site model better and was therefore analyzed according to a one-site model.

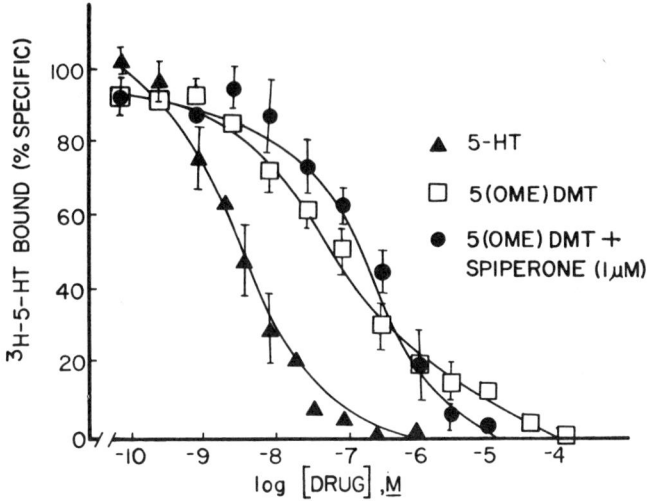

**FIG. 3.** Effect of spiperone on the inhibition of $^3$H-5-HT binding by 5(OMe)DMT. Each point is the mean of five separate experiments for the 5-HT curve, nine experiments for the 5(OMe)DMT curve, and five experiments for 5(OME)DMT + spiperone. The tissue used in these experiments was rat cortex dorsal to the rhinal sulcus. Data are expressed as in Fig. 1. In the case of 5(OME)DMT + spiperone, the control value (100%) was taken as that which occurred in the presence of 1 μM spiperone without any added 5(OME)DMT. This concentration of spiperone inhibited specific $^3$H-5-HT binding by 50 to 60%.

was calculated for these sites, fell in between the $K_D$ values for the high- and low-affinity sites which were calculated in the absence of spiperone (Table 4).

## DISCUSSION

The data presented here confirm and extend the previous findings which suggested the existence of multiple high-affinity binding sites for $^3$H-5-HT in the mammalian brain. In the cat, as in the rat, it appeared that $^3$H-5-HT has high affinity for a population of sites which it recognized as a homogeneous group, but which could be divided into subgroups according to their differential affinities for various drugs. The findings in the cat suggest that the subdivision of $^3$H-5-HT binding sites into only two groups, as was done based on data from the rat CS and FC (25), may be an over-simplification. In the four brain areas of the cat that were examined the $^3$H-5-HT binding sites having high affinity for spiperone gave $K_D$ values that were all within the same range ($K_D$ = 5–21 nM), and these agreed well with the values reported by Pedigo et al. (25) in the rat. However, the low affinity sites appeared to exist as two separate groups. In the cat FC and CS, these sites had very low affinity for spiperone ($K_D \simeq 50$ μM; Table 4), which agreed with that found in the rat brain, where the $K_D$ values were about 35 μM. The low-affinity sites in the two areas of the hippocampus had $K_D$ values that were about 50 times lower than the values in CS and FC, suggesting the possibility of a third type of $^3$H-5-HT binding site. In preliminary studies using tissues from rabbit and guinea pig, all of the brain areas that have been examined, including FC and CS, showed low-affinity sites ($K_D$ values ranging from 0.4 to 3.0 μM) which resembled those found in the cat DH and VH.

The studies of the inhibition of $^3$H-5-HT binding by the tryptamine analogs also suggested that in the rat brain the two populations of sites that can be discriminated by the use of spiperone, may themselves actually be heterogeneous. For example, there appeared to be sites in both the rat CS and FC that were resistant to inhibition by psilocybin. In the CS these comprised about 30% of the specific $^3$H-5-HT binding sites and in the FC they made up about 15% of the sites. However, in studies with spiperone it was found that the proportion of 5-HT$_{1-A}$ to 5-HT$_{1-B}$ sites was 18:82 in the CS and 59:41 in the FC (24). Thus, the two sites discriminated by psilocybin in CS and FC did not correspond to the sites discriminated by spiperone. The results with 5(OMe)DMT also suggested that the two populations of sites differentiated by this compound were not the same as those found with spiperone. As discussed under Results, the inhibition curve generated by 5(OMe)DMT was consistent with the existence of at least two different populations of $^3$H-5-HT binding sites. If these sites were identical to the two types of sites discriminated by spiperone, then the addition of 1 μM spiperone (a concentration that blocks $^3$H-5-HT binding to 5-HT$_{1-A}$ sites but not 5-HT$_{1-B}$ sites) to the assays should convert the 5(OMe)DMT inhibition curve to one which would be consistent with a single population of sites. In addition, the $K_D$ of 5(OMe)DMT for the sites not blocked by spiperone should represent either the high- or the low-affinity sites identified in the absence of spiperone. As seen under Results (Fig. 3; Table 4), the addition of spiperone did convert the 5(OMe)DMT inhibition curve to one which was consistent with a single population of sites. However, the curve was not clearly shifted either to the right or the left as would have been expected if spiperone was blocking only one group of sites. Rather, at low concentrations of 5(OMe)DMT it appeared that the curve was shifted to the right, whereas at higher concentrations it was shifted to the left. Thus, the $K_D$ value calculated for 5(OMe)DMT in the presence of spiperone fell in between the values calculated for the high- and low-affinity sites in the absence of spiperone. This suggested then that the two populations of sites which could be discriminated by the use of 5(OMe)DMT were not identical to the two groups of sites found with spiperone.

The data discussed above raise a number of questions. One of the most obvious concerns the identity of these sites. It has often been suggested that the high-affinity binding sites for $^3$H-5-HT represent a physiologically relevant receptor, although the evidence suggesting this is somewhat minimal. The most compelling data are probably those which show that the numbers of these binding sites can be regulated either upwards or downwards in response to conditions which either decrease or increase the access of 5-HT to its receptors (23). In addition, Fillion et al. (14) have suggested that the high-affinity 5-HT binding sites may represent the receptors that are linked to the high-sensitivity 5-HT-stimulated adenylate cyclase, and Peroutka et al. (26) have suggested that these may represent the 5-HT receptors which mediate inhibitory events in the CNS. If $^3$H-5-HT binding sites do in fact represent receptors, then the question must be posed as to whether all of the subpopulations of these sites represent subpopulations of serotonergic receptors. If they do correspond to different types of 5-HT receptors, then the current data which shows that they have different pharmacological profiles would suggest that it may eventually be possible to develop compounds that could act selectively at certain types of these receptors.

Another question raised by the finding that there may be more than two types of $^3$H-5-HT binding sites concerns the usefulness of $^3$H-5-HT as a ligand to study the properties of these sites. Certainly, if the radioactive ligand in a binding assay binds with approximately the same affinity to more than two populations of sites, then the accurate analysis of the individual sites becomes very difficult. These findings point to the need to develop ligands that are selective for specific types of 5-HT$_1$ sites. Currently, the investigation of analogs of tryptamine would seem a potentially profitable direction to take. From the studies described above, it can be seen that certain indoleamines can discriminate between different types of $^3$H-5-HT binding sites. In addition, the tryptamines have the advantage that they seem to have very low affinity for the 5-HT$_2$ receptors (29) and, in general, have relatively low affinity for the receptors for other monoaminergic neurotransmitters.

Not only is there a need to develop new ligands for specific subtypes of 5-HT$_1$ sites, but there is a general need for compounds, either agonists or antagonists, that act specifically at 5-HT$_1$ receptors. Most of the so-called 5-HT antagonists that are currently available are much more potent at 5-HT$_2$ sites than at 5-HT$_1$ sites, and in addition practically all of these compounds have significant interactions with other neurotransmitter receptors (19). Thus, the development of specific 5-HT$_1$ agonists and antagonists would significantly aid the biochemical, physiological, and behavioral studies attempting to characterize the roles and actions of 5-HT in the CNS.

## ACKNOWLEDGMENTS

The authors wish to thank Michelle Soble and Laura Weber for their excellent technical assistance and Alice Hazard for her preparation of this manuscript. This work was supported by a Biomedical Research Development Grant (ISO-RR09094-01) and a grant from the Pharmaceutical Manufacturers Association Foundation.

## REFERENCES

1. Aghajanian, G. K., and Haigler, H. J. (1975): Hallucinogenic indoleamines: preferential action upon presynaptic serotonin receptors. *Psychopharmacol. Commun.*, 1:619–629.
2. Aghajanian, G. K., and Wang, R. Y. (1978): Physiology and pharmacology of central serotonergic neurons. In: *Psychopharmacology: A Generation of Progress*, edited by M. A. Lipton, A. DiMascio, and K. F. Killam, pp. 171–183. Raven Press, New York.
3. Anden, N.-E., Dahlstrom, A., Fuxe, K., Larson, K., Olson, L., and Ungerstedt, U. (1966): Ascending monoamine neurons to the telencephalon and diencephalon. *Acta Physiol. Scand.*, 67:313–326.
4. Apperley, E., Feniuk, W., Humphrey, P. P. A., and Levy, G. P. (1980): Evidence for two types of excitatory receptor for 5-hydroxytryptamine in dog isolated vasculature. *Br. J. Pharmacol.*, 68:215–224.

5. Barchas, J., and Usdin, E., editors (1973): *Serotonin and Behavior.* Academic Press, New York.
6. Boakes, R. J., Bradley, P. B., Briggs, I., and Dray, A. (1970): Antagonism of 5-hydroxytryptamine by LSD 25 in the central nervous system: a possible neuronal basis for the actions of LSD 25. *Br. J. Pharmacol.*, 40:202–218.
7. Boullin, D. J., editor (1978): *Serotonin in Mental Abnormalities.* Wiley, New York.
8. Cerrito, F., and Raiteri, M. (1979): Serotonin release is modulated by presynaptic autoreceptors. *Eur. J. Pharmacol.*, 57:427–430.
9. Costa, M., and Furness, J. B. (1979): The sites of action of 5-hydroxytryptamine in nerve-muscle preparations from the guinea-pig small intestine and colon. *Br. J. Pharmacol.*, 65:237–248.
10. Dahlstrom, A., and Fuxe, K. (1965): Evidence for the existence of monoamine neurons in the cell bodies of brain stem neurons. *Acta Physiol. Scand.*, 62(Suppl. 232):1–55.
11. Ehlert, F. J., Roeske, W. R., Rosenberger, L. B., and Yamamura, H. I. (1980): The influence of guanyl-5′- yl imidodiphosphate and sodium on muscarinic receptor binding in the rat brain and longitudinal muscle of the rat ileum. *Life Sci.*, 26:245–252.
12. Enjalbert, A., Hamon, M., Bourgoin, S., and Bockaert, J. (1978): Postsynaptic serotonin-sensitive adenylate cyclase in the central nervous system. II. Comparison with dopamine- and isoproterenol-sensitive adenylate cyclases in rat brain. *Mol. Pharmacol.*, 14:11–23.
13. Essman, W. B., editor (1978): *Serotonin in Health and Disease*, Vols. I–V. S.P. Medical and Scientific Books, New York.
14. Fillion, G., Beaudoin, D., Rousselle, J. C., Deniau, J. M., Fillion, M. P., Dray, F., and Jacob, J. (1979): Decrease of [$^3$H]5-HT high affinity binding and 5-HT adenylate cyclase activation after kainic acid lesion in rat brain striatum. *J. Neurochem.*, 33:567–570.
15. Gaddum, J. H., and Hameed, K. A. (1954): Drugs which antagonize 5-hydroxytryptamine. *Br. J. Pharmacol.*, 9:240–248.
16. Gerschenfeld, H. M., and Paupardin-Tritsch, D. (1974): Ionic mechanisms and receptor properties underlying the responses of molluscan neurones to 5-hydroxytryptamine. *J. Physiol. (Lond.),* 243:427–456.
17. Gerschenfeld, H. M., and Paupardin-Tritsch, D. (1974): On the transmitter function of 5-hydroxytryptamine at excitatory and inhibitory monosynaptic junctions. *J. Physiol. (Lond.),* 243:457–481.
18. Haigler, H. J., and Aghajanian, G. K. (1974): Peripheral serotonin antagonists: failure to antagonize serotonin in brain areas receiving a prominent serotonergic input. *J. Neural Transm.*, 35:257–273.
19. Leysen, J. E., Awouters, F., Kennis, L., Laduron, P. M., Vandenberk, J., and Janssen, P. A. J. (1981): Receptor binding profile of R 41 468, a novel antagonist at 5-HT$_2$ receptors. *Life Sci.*, 28:1015–1022.
20. MacDermot, J., Higashida, H., Wilson, S. P., Matsuzawa, H., Minna, J., and Nirenberg, M. (1979): Adenylate cyclase and acetylcholine release regulated by separate serotonin receptors of somatic hybrid cells. *Proc. Natl. Acad. Sci. USA*, 76:1135–1139.
21. Metzler, C. M., Elfring, G. L., and McEwan, A. J. (1974): *A Users Manual for NONLIN.* The Upjohn Company, Michigan.
22. Nelson, D. L., Herbet, A., Bourgoin, S., Glowinski, J., and Hamon, M. (1978): Characteristics of central 5-HT receptors and their adaptive changes following intracerebral 5,7-dihydroxytryptamine administration in the rat. *Mol. Pharmacol.*, 14:983–995.
23. Nelson, D. L., Pedigo, N. W., and Yamamura, H. I. (1980): Multiple types of serotonin receptors. In: *Psychopharmacology and Biochemistry of Neurotransmitter Receptors*, edited by H. I. Yamamura, R. W. Olsen, and E. Usdin, pp. 325–338. Elsevier North Holland, New York.
24. O'Brien, R. A. (1978): Cerebral distribution of serotonin. In: *Serotonin in Mental Abnormalities*, edited by D. J. Boullin, pp. 41–70. John Wiley, New York.
25. Pedigo, N. W., Yamamura, H. I., and Nelson, D. L. (1981): Discrimination of multiple $^3$H-5-hydroxytryptamine binding sites in rat brain by neuroleptics. *J. Neurochem.*, 36:220–226.
26. Peroutka, S. J., Lebovitz, R. M., and Snyder, S. H. (1981): Two distinct central serotonin receptors with different physiological functions. *Science*, 212:827–829.
27. Peroutka, S. J., and Snyder, S. H. (1979): Multiple serotonin receptors: Differential binding of [$^3$H]5-hydroxytryptamine, [$^3$H]lysergic acid diethylamide and [$^3$H]spiroperidol. *Mol. Pharmacol.*, 16:687–699.
28. Roberts, M. H. T., and Straughan, D. W. (1967): Excitation and depression of cortical neurones by 5-hydroxytryptamine. *J. Physiol. (Lond.),* 193:269–294.
29. Seeman, P., Westman, K., Coscina, D., and Warsh, J. J. (1980): Serotonin receptors in hippocampus and frontal cortex. *Eur. J. Pharmacol.*, 66:179–191.

30. Shaw, E., and Woolley, D. W. (1954): Pharmacological properties of some antimetabolites of serotonin having unusually high activity on isolated tissues. *J. Pharmacol. Exp. Ther.*, 111:43–53.
31. Von Hungen, K., Roberts, S., and Hill, D. F. (1975): Serotonin-sensitive adenylate cyclase activity in immature rat brain. *Brain Res.*, 84:257–267.

*Molecular Pharmacology of Neurotransmitter Receptors*, edited by T. Segawa et al.
Raven Press, New York © 1983.

# Central Serotonin Receptors: Regulation Mechanism at the Molecular Level

## Gilles Fillion

*Laboratory of Pharmacology, Pasteur Institute,
Paris Cédex 15, France*

Studies of the receptors to 5-hydroxytryptamine (5-HT or serotonin) were initiated by Gaddum and Picarelli (20) and suggested the existence of two types of receptors to 5-HT in the peripheral tissue. The first attempt to determine directly the binding of 5-HT to specific sites was done by Marchbanks (28), and later Farrow and van Vunakis (11) studied the binding of $^3$H-LSD used as a serotoninergic ligand. Since these early studies, other works have been devoted to the 5-HT receptors, studying either the binding of serotonergic ligands or the activation of an adenylate cyclase system in various preparations. Among the ligands that have been used are: $^3$H-5-HT (4,16,19,29,30,31,33,36,39,41,42,44,45), $^3$H-LSD (2,3,19,26,27), $^3$H-spiperone (26,40), $^3$H-metergoline (21), and $^3$H-methiothepine (32).

The activation of an adenylate cyclase induced by 5-HT has been studied in cerebral tissues: von Hungen et al. (25) were the first to describe an activation with an apparent affinity corresponding to a $K_D$ close to 1 μM. Enjalbert et al. (9,10) confirmed and extended these results. Fillion et al. (17,18) also observed this low-affinity adenylate cyclase, but in addition, they reported a second type of activation corresponding to a high-affinity constant (apparent $K_D$ = 1 nM).

The first part of this chapter presents data related to the binding of $^3$H-5-HT to cerebral preparations, and the second part presents those related to the activation of an adenylate cyclase by 5-HT. The results indicate the existence of two different types of 5-HT receptors and justify the hypothesis of a mechanism of function of the 5-HT postsynaptic receptor.

The material used in these experiments is either prepared from rat or horse brains or is constituted from cultured cells (cultured glial cell lines $C_6$, primary cultured glial or neuronal cells).

Brain tissue preparations obtained as described by Fillion et al. (19) were as follows: homogenates of various brain areas (cerebral cortex, hippocampus, striatum), crude mitochondrial fractions, synaptosomal membrane fractions prepared according to Cotman and Matthews (8) and glial membrane fractions prepared from glial cell fractions obtained as described by Blomstrand and Hamberger (6).

$^3$H-5-HT binding was assayed in various experimental conditions (19). After incubation of the tissue in the presence of $^3$H-5-HT at a given concentration for a given time, the incubate was filtered through glass fiber filter and the radioactivity bound measured by liquid scintillation spectrometry. The activation of the adenylate cyclase was measured by determining the cyclic adenosine monophosphate (cAMP) production induced by 5-HT using a radioimmunoassay (17,18).

## NEURONAL AND GLIAL RECEPTORS FOR 5-HT

It has been shown previously that in enriched synaptic membrane preparations from various brain areas $^3$H-5-HT bound specifically to recognition sites with a high-affinity constant (16). Using crude membrane preparations, Peroutka and Snyder (36), and Nelson et al. (31) also observed this high-affinity binding for $^3$H-5-HT; however, other observers (19,43,44) found, in addition to this first type of high-affinity binding, a second one corresponding to a lower affinity ($K_D$ close to 12 nM). Fillion et al. (12) showed that the high-affinity binding corresponded to neuronal and, more precisely, postsynaptosomal sites. The nature of the lower affinity binding sites was unknown. The same authors presented experimental arguments which strongly suggested a correspondence to a glial component (13).

A similar situation was observed for the activation of the adenylate cyclase induced by 5-HT. Von Hungen et al. (25) and Enjalbert et al. (9,10) observed, in homogenates of newborn rat cerebral tissue, a serotonin-activated adenylate cyclase which corresponded to a low apparent affinity constant ($K_D$ close to 1 µM); they were unable to observe a significant increase in cAMP production using adult rat brain homogenates.

Fillion et al. (17,18) using horse, bovine, or rat brain observed two types of adenylate cyclase sensitive to 5-HT: One, corresponding to an apparent $K_D = 1$ µM, and a second to 1 nM; the two activations were present in homogenates of various brain areas. In addition, it was shown that purified synaptic membranes contained only the high-affinity type of adenylate cyclase activation (apparent $K_D = 1$ nM). This latter activation corresponded to a neuronal and, more precisely, postsynaptosomal localization (12). The nature of the low-affinity activation was not known, although Enjalbert et al. (9,10) postulated its postsynaptosomal localization. Fillion et al. (13) presented several arguments in favor of the glial nature of this adenylate cyclase; in particular, it was present in glial cell membrane preparation isolated from brain striatum.

Because glial cell fractions prepared from cerebral tissue are contaminated to a certain extent with neuronal elements (16), it was interesting to measure the adenylate cyclase activation induced by 5-HT in preparations devoid of neuronal contamination. Glial cell lines ($C_6$) have been tested for their capacity to produce cAMP after incubation in the presence of various concentrations of 5-HT. The observed activation corresponded clearly to a low apparent affinity constant (apparent $K_D$ close to 1 µM) (Fig. 1). It was antagonized preferentially by 5-HT antagonists, whereas nonserotoninergic drugs were less efficient (Beaudoin et al., *in preparation*). A similar activation curve has been obtained (Beaudoin et al., *in preparation*) on primary cultured glial cells obtained according to Berwald-Netter and co-workers

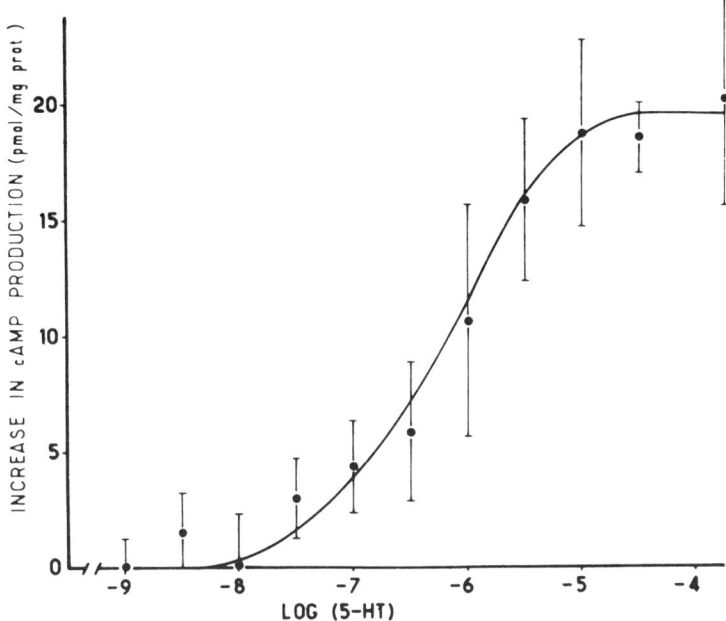

**FIG. 1.** Increase in adenylate cyclase activity induced by 5-HT in $C_6$ glial cell line preparation. Aliquots of cells suspension were incubated for 8 min at 37°C in the presence of various concentrations of 5-HT. The cAMP production was measured by radioimmunoassay. The basal level was 62.9 ± 1.7 pmole/mg protein. The values represent the mean of three experiments.

(5) (Fig. 2). These cells were not sensitive to 5-HT at low-concentration ranges (concentration < .5 μM), whereas a clear activation was observed for higher concentration ($K_D$ close to 2 μM). It is interesting to note that neuronal primary cultured cells prepared according to Berwald-Netter et al. (5) were sensitive to 5-HT with an apparent affinity constant corresponding to a high affinity ($K_D$ close to 1 nM) as shown in Fig. 2.

These results strongly suggest that the low-affinity adenylate cyclase activity is not neuronal, but glial. It might be related to the 5-HT recognition sites found in the same preparation and binding the amine with a low-affinity constant.

Thus, it appears that at least two distinct types of 5-HT units are located on neuronal cells and on glial cells. A neuronal postsynaptic recognition site is able to bind $^3$H-5-HT with a high affinity, whereas the glial cells bind $^3$H-5-HT with a lower affinity. In parallel, neuronal membranes contain an adenylate cyclase sensitive to 5-HT with a high affinity, and glial membranes are sensitive to 5-HT with a low affinity.

These results are in agreement with those of Bockaert et al. (7), indicating that the sites binding 5-HT with a high affinity are not identical to those involved in the activation of the adenylate cyclase of low affinity. Indeed, these two serotoninergic units are located in two different preparations. Our results, on the contrary, suggest that the adenylate cyclase activated by 5-HT with a low affinity is not

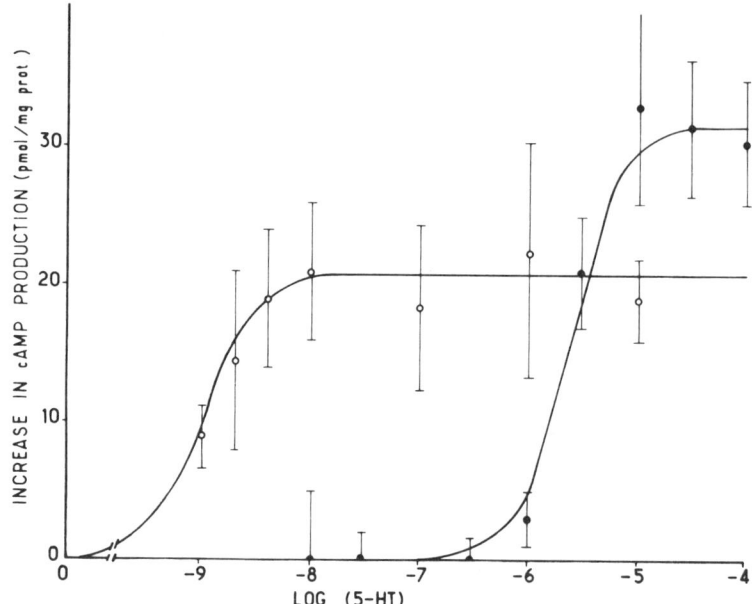

**FIG. 2.** Increase in cAMP production measured in primary cultured cells: neuronal cells *(open circles)* and glial cells *(closed circles)*. The cells were incubated at 37°C for 8 min in the presence of various concentrations of 5-HT. The basal levels were 128.7 ± 6 and 127.5 ± 8 pmole/mg protein, respectively.

postsynaptically located, as has been reported previously (31), but is very likely glial.

Below are some experimental arguments indicating that, in neuronal membranes, the recognition sites might be directly related to the activation of the adenylate cyclase; however, this conclusion will be certain only when solubilization and reconstitution of the receptor is achieved. Similarly, the relationship between the glial recognition site and the glial adenylate cyclase is not yet directly evidenced, although it is indicated by several arguments.

## REGULATION MECHANISM OF THE POSTSYNAPTIC RECEPTOR

The 5-HT receptor located on postsynaptic membranes consists, presumably, of a recognition site able to bind $^3$H-5-HT with a high affinity ($K_D$ = 2–3 nM), coupled to an adenylate cyclase activated by 5-HT with a high affinity (apparent $K_D$ = 1 nM). Binding experiments and adenylate cyclase assays have been performed in order to approach the mechanism involved in the transfer of the physiological signal corresponding to the binding of the ligand to its site.

The experiments have been realized using purified synaptic membranes which, in previously used experimental conditions, contained only a single population of binding sites and a single type of adenylate cyclase activation. The incubation of the membranes in the presence of $^3$H-5-HT (0.5–4.0 nM) at 22°C for a relatively long duration period (30 to 45 min) corresponds to the existence of a high-affinity binding population ($K_D$ = 2–3 nM).

However, when the membranes are incubated in parallel for a shorter time (8–10 min at 22°C), the observed binding corresponds to a lower affinity constant ($K_D$ = 12–15 nM); the maximal number of sites is constant. Intermediate incubation durations correspond to biphasic binding curves resulting in the same total number of sites, partly of a high-affinity type, partly of a low-affinity type; the ratio high/low affinity increases with the incubation time.

Preexposure of the membranes to 10 nM 5-HT for 5 min at 37°C or 10 to 15 min at 22°C followed by a wash (dilution and centrifugation) induces a modification of the $^3$H-5-HT binding, that is, a binding of $^3$H-5-HT with a high-affinity constant, even after a short incubation time. These results suggest that the binding site for 5-HT might exist under two different structural conformations corresponding to different affinities for the ligand; the binding of the agonist itself would induce a structural conformation change of the receptor protein. We previously presented experimental evidence which indicated that these structural changes were blocked by sulfhydryl-group reagents and that the structure corresponding to a low affinity appeared stabilized by guanosine 5'-triphosphate (GTP).

In a like manner, the adenylate cyclase activation induced by 5-HT and corresponding to a high affinity constant ($K_D$ = 1 nM) has been observed in purified synaptosomal membranes to study the effect of the preexposure to 5-HT. Non-preexposed or buffer preexposed membranes were activated by 5-HT and produced cAMP. The same membranes preexposed to 10 nM for 10 min at 22°C and then incubated for 2 min in the control conditions were not any more sensitive to 5-HT. The presence of GTP ($10^{-4}$ M) during the induction procedure resulted in the suppression of the inhibiting effect of the 5-HT preexposure (Fig. 3).

The hypothesis of a regulation mechanism of the postsynaptic receptor for 5-HT might be based on the fact that modifications of the structural conformation of the

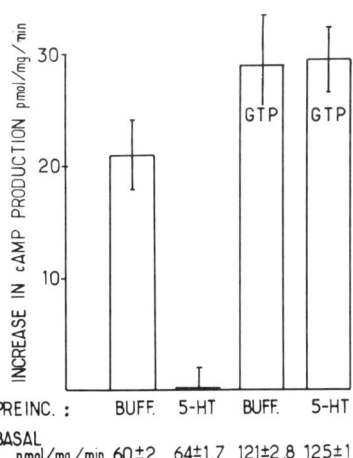

**FIG. 3.** Increase in cAMP production induced by 10 nM 5-HT in enriched synaptic membrane fraction. Membranes were preexposed in buffer (buff) or in 10 nM serotonin (5-HT) for 10 min in the presence or absence of GTP.

binding site for 5-HT appear to correspond to changes in the reactivity of the adenylate cyclase to the amine. In experimental conditions inducing a structural change of the recognition site binding 5-HT toward a state of low affinity, a serotoninergic activation of the adenylate cyclase is observed. On the contrary, in conditions that induce the binding of 5-HT with a high affinity, no enzymatic activation is observed; the affinity change of the binding appears related to the activity of the enzymatic system.

A three-state model has been proposed for the cholinergic nicotinic receptor (22,23); a similar hypothetical model might be suggested for the postsynaptic 5-HT receptor. This assumption would indicate that the recognition site involved in the opening of an ionophore as well as that involved in an enzymatic activation behave according to the same basic princeps. Little is known about the role of GTP in the phenomenon. Presumably, a nucleotide binding protein analogous to that originally described by Pfeuffer (37) for the β-adrenergic receptor also exists for the 5-HT receptor; it probably plays an important role in its mechanism of regulation. Although some analogies might be shown with the β-adrenergic receptor, it seems that the two systems might not be identical.

## INTERRELATION OF TRICYCLIC ANTIDEPRESSANTS WITH THE POSTSYNAPTIC 5-HT RECEPTOR

The pharmacology of the 5-HT receptor has been widely studied (4,9,10,18,26,29,30,33,34,36,39,41,43–45). It has to be noted that in many works being performed using homogenates of cerebral tissue, the binding studied generally referred not only to postsynaptosomal sites but, also, to a significant part to glial sites. Thus, the determination of $IC_{50}$ for various drugs might reflect an effect on a complex system.

Two types of drugs interacting with the receptors may be observed: first, those that act through a direct binding to the 5-HT site, and thus compete with the amine to occupy the receptor site; and second, those that act through an indirect mechanism. In this latter class, the antidepressant drugs constitute an interesting group.

It was generally considered that antidepressants acted on the serotoninergic system by increasing the amount of 5-HT available at the receptor level (38); they would either inhibit the monoaminoxydase responsible for the degradative process of 5-HT, or they would inhibit the reuptake of 5-HT. However, some recent antidepressant drugs are devoid of monoaminoxydase-inhibiting properties and do not modify the uptake of 5-HT. Therefore, the possibility that they act at the postsynaptic level has to be considered. Such an hypothesis has been proposed already on a pharmacological basis (1,46).

Our experiments consisted in preexposure of synaptosomal membranes to various drugs (generally 10 nM), namely serotonin agonists and antagonists, neuroleptics, and antidepressants of various nature; the preparations were then simply diluted 20 times and the binding of $^3H$-5-HT tested as usual. It was shown that tricyclic antidepressants, including those unable to inhibit the uptake of 5-HT, had in common

TABLE 1.

| Preexposure | Affinity constant for $^3$H-5-HT ($K_D$ nM) |
|---|---|
| Buffer | 15.3 ± 1.26 |
| 5-HT | 1.8 ± 0.4 |
| Imipramine | 2.42 ± 0.22 |
| Chlorimipramine | 1.72 ± 0.99 |
| Amitryptiline | 4.2 ± 0.35 |
| Trimeprine | 4.0 ± 0.3 |
| Iprindole | 3.9 ± 1.02 |
| Mianserine | 2.9 ± 0.88 |
| Chlorpromazine | 14.24 ± 1.95 |
| Fluphenazine | 10.7 ± 1.9 |

The affinity constant for $^3$H-5-HT was measured using fractions enriched in synaptosomal membranes. Membranes were pre-exposed for 10 min at 37°C with 10 nM of the drug and usually diluted twenty times in buffer. Binding curves for $^3$H-5-HT were determined in a concentration range from 2 to 30 nM. The affinity constants are the means of three to six individual assays.

the property of increasing the affinity of the 5-HT binding site for $^3$H-5-HT. It was shown that the high-affinity binding corresponded to a state of the receptor incapable of activating the adenylate cyclase. This property was not shared by neuroleptics (haloperidol) or nonantidepressant drugs (chlorpromazine, fluphenazine) (14), (Table 1).

The antidepressant drugs may act on the serotoninergic system through a mechanism corresponding to the inactivation of the receptor. It is obviously too early to directly relate this effect of the antidepressants to their clinical properties; however, these findings might constitute a novel approach in the search for their mechanism of action.

## CONCLUSION

The existence of multiple receptors for 5-HT has been suggested by Nelson et al. *(this volume)* who presented experimental evidence supporting this hypothesis. We have presented here additional results that introduce another level of complexity in the serotoninergic receptor system, since postsynaptosomal receptors have to be distinguished from glial ones. The study of the mechanism of function of these types of "regulating systems" introduces new information and may explain some effects of drugs acting at this level.

## ACKNOWLEDGMENT

This study was supported by Grant ATP No. 4173 from the CNRS.

## REFERENCES

1. Aprison, M. H., Takahashi, R., and Tachiki, K. (1978): Hypersensitive serotoninergic receptors involved in clinical depression—a theory. In: *Neuropharmacology and Behavior*, edited by B. Haber and M. M. Aprison, pp. 23–53. Plenum Press, New York.
2. Bennett, J. L., and Aghajanian, G. K. (1974): Stereospecific binding of d-LSD on physiological response of serotoninergic neurones. *Fed. Proc.*, 33:256.
3. Bennett, J. P., and Snyder, S. (1975): Stereospecific binding of d-lysergic acid diethylamide (LSD) to brain membranes: relationship to serotonin receptors. *Brain Res.*, 94:523–544.
4. Bennett, J. P., and Snyder, S. H. (1976): Serotonin and lysergic acid diethylamide binding in rat brain membranes: relationship to postsynaptic serotonin receptors. *Mol. Pharmacol.*, 12:373–389.
5. Berwald-Netter, Y., Martin-Moutot, N., Koulakoff, A., and Courand, F. (1981): $Na^+$ channel associated scorpion toxin receptor sites as probe for neuronal evolution *in vivo* and *in vitro*. *Proc. Natl. Acad. Sci. USA*, 78:1245–1249.
6. Blomstrand, C., and Hamberger, A. (1970): Amino acid incorporation *in vitro* in proteins of neuronal and glial cell enriched fractions. *J. Neurochem.*, 17:1187–1195.
7. Bockaert, J., Nelson, J. L., Herbert, A., Adrien, J., Enjalbert, A., and Hamon, M.: Serotonin-receptors coupled with an adenylate cyclase in the rat brain. Non identity with $^3$H-5-HT binding sites. In: *Serotonin—Current Aspects of Neurochemistry and Function*, edited by B. Haber. Plenum Press, New York *(in press)*.
8. Cotman, C. W., and Matthews, D. A. (1971): Synaptic plasma membranes from rat brain synaptosomes: isolation and partial characterization. *Biochim. Biophys. Acta*, 249:380–394.
9. Enjalbert, A., Bourgoin, S., Hamon, M., Adrien, J., and Bockaert, J. (1978): Postsynaptic serotonin-sensitive adenylate cyclase in the central nervous system. I. Development and distribution of serotonin and dopamine sensitive adenylate cyclase in rat and guinea pig brain. *Mol. Pharmacol.*, 14:2–10.
10. Enjalbert, A., Hamon, M., Bourgoin, S., and Bockaert, J. (1978): Postsynaptic serotonin sensitive adenylate cyclase in the central nervous system. II. Comparison with dopamine and isoproterenol sensitive adenylate cyclase in rat brain. *Mol. Pharmacol.*, 14:11–23.
11. Farrow, J. T., and van Vunakis, H. (1972): Binding of d-lysergic acid diethylamide to subcellular fractions from rat brain. *Nature*, 237:164–166.
12. Fillion, G., Beaudoin, D., Rousselle, J. C., Deniau, J. M., Fillion, M. P., Dray, F., and Jacob, J. (1979): Decrease of $^3$H 5-HT high affinity binding and 5-HT adenylate cyclase activation after kainic acid lesion in rat brain striatum. *J. Neurochem.*, 33:567–570.
13. Fillion, G. M. B., Beaudoin, D., Rousselle, J. C., and Jacob, J. (1980): $^3$H 5-HT binding sites and 5-HT sensitive adenylate cyclase in glial cell membrane fraction. *Brain Res.*, 198:361–375.
14. Fillion, G., and Fillion, M. P. (1980): Transitional states of the neuronal serotoninergic site. *Eur. J. Pharmacol.*, 65:109–112.
15. Fillion, G., and Fillion, M. P.: Modulation of affinity of postsynaptic serotonin receptors by antidepressant drugs. *Nature (in press)*.
16. Fillion, G., Fillion, M. P., Spirakis, C., Bahers, J. M., and Jacob, J. (1976): 5-hydroxytryptamine binding to synaptic membranes from rat brain. *Life Sci.*, 18:65–74.
17. Fillion, G., Rousselle, J. C., Beaudoin, D., Pradelles, P., Goiny, M., Dray, F., and Jacob, J. (1979): Serotonin sensitive adenylate cyclase in horse brain synaptosomal membranes. *Life Sci.*, 24:1813–1822.
18. Fillion, G., Rousselle, J. C., Goiny, M., Pradelles, Ph., Dray, F., and Jacob, J. (1977): Activation adényl cyclasique sensible à la 5-hydroxytryptamine sur des préparations membranaires synaptosomales de cerveau. *C.R. Acad. Sci. Paris*, 295:265–268.
19. Fillion, G., Rousselle, J. C., Fillion, M. P., Beaudoin, D., Goiny, M., Deniau, J. M., and Jacob, J. (1978): High affinity binding of $^3$H 5-hydroxytryptamine to brain synaptosomal membranes: Comparison with $^3$H lysergic acid diethylamide binding. *Mol. Pharmacol.*, 14:50–59.
20. Gaddum, J. H., and Picarelli, Z. P. (1957): Two kinds of tryptamine receptor. *Br. J. Pharmacol.*, 12:323–328.
21. Hamon, M., Mallet, M., Herbet, A., Nelson, D., Audinot, M., Pichat, L., and Glowinski, J. (1980): $^3$H metergoline: a new ligand of 5-HT receptors in the rat brain. *J. Neurochem.*, 1981.
22. Heidmann, T., and Changeux, J. P. (1979): Fast kinetic studies on the interaction of fluorescent agonist with the membrane bound acetylcholine receptor from *Torpedo marmorata*. *Eur. J. Biochem.*, 91:255–279.
23. Heidmann, T., and Changeux, J. P. (1979): Fast kinetic studies on the allosteric interactions between acetylcholine receptor and local anesthetic binding sites. *Eur. J. Biochem.*, 94:281–296.
24. Heltzel, J. A., Boehme, D. H., and Vogel, W. (1981): Serotonin binding to different regions of human brain. *Brain Res.*, 204:451–454.

25. von Hungen, K., Roberts, S., and Hill, D. F. (1974): Developmental and regional variations in neurotransmitter sensitive adenylate cyclase systems in cell free preparations from rat brain. *J. Neurochem.*, 22:811–817.
26. Leysen, J. E., and Laduron, P. M. (1977): A serotonergic component of neuroleptic receptors. *Arch. Int. Pharmacodyn.*, 230:337–339.
27. Lovell, R. A., and Freedman, D. X. (1976): Stereospecific receptor sites for d-lysergic acid diethylamide in rat brain: effects of neurotransmitters, amines antagonists and other psychotropic drugs. *Mol. Pharmacol.*, 12:620–630.
28. Marchbanks, R. M. (1966): Serotonin binding to nerve ending particles and other preparations from rat brain. *J. Neurochem.*, 13:1481–1493.
29. Middlemiss, D., Blakeborough, L., and Leather, S. R. (1977): Direct evidence for an interaction of β adrenergic blockers with the 5-HT receptor. *Nature*, 267:289–290.
30. Nelson, D. L., Herbet, A., Bourgoin, S., Glowinski, J., and Hamon, M. (1978): Characteristics of central 5-HT receptors and their adaptive changes following intracerebral 5-7-dihydroxytryptamine administration in the rat. *Mol. Pharmacol.*, 14:983–995.
31. Nelson, D., Herbet, A., Enjalbert, A., Bockaert, J., and Hamon, M. (1980): Serotonin-sensitive adenylate cyclase and $^3$H serotonin binding sites in the CNS of the rat. I and II. *Biochem. Pharmacol.*, 29:2445–2453.
32. Nelson, D., Herbet, A., Pichat, L., and Glowinski, J. (1979): *In vitro* and *in vivo* disposition of $^3$H methiothepin in brain tissue. *Arch. Pharmacol.*, 310:25–33.
33. Ögren, S. O., Fuxe, K., Agnati, L. F., Gustafsson, J. A., Jönsson, G., and Holm, A. C. (1979): Reevaluation of the indoleamine hypothesis of depression. Evidence for a reduction of functional activity of central 5-HT systems by antidepressant drugs. *J. Neurol. Transm.*, 46:85–103.
34. Pedigo, N. W., Yamamura, H. I., and Nelson, D. L. (1981): Discrimination of multiple [$^3$H]5-hydroxytryptamine binding sites by the neuroleptic spiperone in rat brain. *J. Neurochem.*, 36: 220–226.
35. Peroutka, S. J., Lebovitz, R. M., and Snyder, S. H. (1979): Serotonin receptor binding sites affected differentially by guanine nucleotides. *Mol. Pharmacol.*, 16:700–708.
36. Peroutka, S., and Snyder, S. (1979): Multiple serotonin receptors: differential binding of $^3$H 5-hydroxytryptamine, $^3$H lysergic acid diethylamide and $^3$H spiroperidol. *Mol. Pharmacol.*, 16: 687–699.
37. Pfeuffer, T. (1977): GTP binding proteins in membranes and the control and adenylate cyclase activity. *J. Biol. Chem.*, 252:7224–7234.
38. van Praag, H. M. (1974): *Pharmacopsychiatry*, 7:281–292.
39. Quayle, E. S., Pagel, J., Monti, S. A., and Christian, S. (1977): Specific serotonin binding and adenylate cyclase stimulation: a correlative study using isolated synaptosomal membranes from mature rat brain. *Ala. J. Med. Sci.*, 14:259–263.
40. Quick, M., and Iversen, L. L. (1979): Regional study of $^3$H spiperone binding and the dopamine sensitive adenylate cyclase in rat brain. *Eur. J. Pharmacol.*, 56:323–330.
41. Samanin, R., Mennine, T., Ferraris, A., Bendotti, C., and Borsini, F. (1980): Hyper and hyposensitivity of central serotonin receptors: [$^3$] serotonin binding and functional studies in the rat. *Brain Res.*, 189:449–457.
42. Segal, M. (1981): The action of serotonin in the rat hippocampus. In: *Serotonin: Current Aspects of Neurochemistry and Function. Symposium INS, Athens*, edited by B. Haber. Plenum Press, New York *(in press)*.
43. Segawa, T., Midzuta, T., and Nomura, Y. (1979): Modifications of central 5-hydroxytryptamine binding sites in synaptic membranes from rat brain after long-term administration of tricyclic antidepressants. *Eur. J. Pharmacol.*, 58:75–83.
44. Shih, J. C., and Young, H. (1978): The alteration of serotonin binding sites in aged human brain. *Life Sci.*, 23:1441–1448.
45. Snyder, S. H., and Bennett, J. (1975): Biochemical identification of the postsynaptic serotonin receptor in mammalian brain. *Pre- and Postsynaptic Receptors*, 3:191–206.
46. Sulser, F. (1979): New perspective on the mode of action of antidepressant drugs. *Trends Pharmacol. Sci. Rev.*, 1:92–94.

*Molecular Pharmacology of Neurotransmitter Receptors*, edited by T. Segawa et al.
Raven Press, New York © 1983.

# Dopamine Receptors in the Central Nervous System

Ian Creese, David R. Sibley, Mark W. Hamblin, and Stuart E. Leff

*Department of Neurosciences, University of California, San Diego, School of Medicine, La Jolla, California 92093*

## PHARMACOLOGICAL CHARACTERIZATION OF DOPAMINE RECEPTORS

Kebabian and Calne (13) in a seminal review have divided dopamine (DA) receptors into two general categories, D-1 and D-2. D-1 receptors are responsible for DA stimulation of adenylate cyclase activity. The location for the prototype D-1 receptor is the parathyroid gland where DA agonists stimulate cyclic adenosine monophosphate (cAMP) synthesis concomitantly with parathyroid hormone release (1). D-2 receptors, whose prototype is found in the pituitary, inhibit hormone-stimulated adenylate cyclase activity (18a,2) and regulate prolactin and alpha-MSH release from the anterior and intermediate pituitary glands respectively.

The pharmacological profiles of D-1 and D-2 receptors are clearly distinct. Agonists consistently demonstrate higher affinities in eliciting a biochemical or physiological response at D-2 receptors than at D-1 receptors. Apomorphine (APO) is a potent agonist with full intrinsic activity at D-2 receptors in contrast to its partial agonist activity at D-1 receptors. Similarly, various dopaminergic ergots (such as bromocryptine) are full, potent (nM) agonists at D-2 receptors but only weak, partial agonists or antagonists at D-1 receptors. With respect to antagonists, phenothiazines and thioxanthenes are potent antagonists of D-2 receptors; however, they also exhibit high affinity for D-1 receptors. In contrast, butyrophenones (BUTYs) and related drugs (e.g., domperidone) are very potent antagonists of D-2 receptors but exhibit only low affinity for D-1 receptors. Similarly, substituted benzamides such as sulpiride which are inactive at D-1 receptors exhibit potent behavioral DA antagonism and moderate affinity at D-2 receptors.

This review addresses the question: Can these pharmacologically identified receptors be studied by radioligand binding techniques?

## RADIOLIGAND BINDING TO DOPAMINE RECEPTORS IN THE PITUITARY

Our binding studies have indicated that bovine anterior pituitary (BAP) cells possess a homogeneous population of D-2 receptors through which DA inhibits prolactin release (22–25). These studies provide a good starting point to discuss radioligand DA receptor identification. The binding of the radiolabeled DA butyrophenone antagonist, [$^3$H]spiroperidol or spiperone (SP), to BAP membranes is homogeneous, saturable, and of high affinity with a dissociation constant ($K_D$) of 0.3 nM. Whereas all antagonist competition curves exhibit monophasic, mass-action characteristics with pseudo-Hill coefficients ($n_H$) equal to 1, agonist/[$^3$H]SP competition curves exhibit heterogenous characteristics with pseudo-Hill coefficients less than unity. For example, in the absence of guanine nucleotides (GN), the APO/[$^3$H]SP curve is shallow ($n_H = 0.58$) with computer analysis indicating that the data are best explained by a two site/state binding model (Table 1). The two sites/states are present in approximately equal proportions in the membranes. In the presence of GTP or its nonmetabolizable analog Gpp(NH)p, the APO curve is shifted to the right and steepened ($n_H = 0.94$). Moreover, computer analysis of the data now indicates a single homogeneous population of binding sites whose affinity for APO is not significantly different from the $K_L$ value of the control curve. Other agonists give qualitatively identical results.

The radiolabeled agonist [$^3$H]N-propylnorapomorphine (NPA) labels DA receptors in BAP membranes (22,23), a tissue with no direct dopaminergic innervation, reinforcing our hypothesis that under our assay conditions [$^3$H]agonists can label postsynaptic receptors (3). Its $B_{max}$ is approximately 50% of that of [$^3$H]SP's, suggesting that it labels only the high affinity agonist site/state ($R_H$) seen in agonist/[$^3$H]SP curves. This is confirmed by the finding that agonist/[$^3$H]NPA competition curves are homogeneous with single affinities that are not significantly different from the $K_H$ values obtained from the corresponding agonist/[$^3$H]SP curve. Furthermore, saturating concentrations of GNs completely abolish specific [$^3$H]NPA binding to pituitary membranes. We suggest that the $R_H$ and $R_L$ sites represent high and low affinity agonist binding states of a single D-2 receptor molecule with GNs regulating an interconversion between the high and the low affinity states (Table 1). Supporting evidence was obtained using BAP cells, dispersed via collagenase treatment and then used in the binding experiment. Strikingly, the (−)APO/[$^3$H]SP curve is now steep ($n_H = 0.86$) and comparable to the (−)APO/[$^3$H]SP + Gpp(NH)p

TABLE 1. *Model of anterior pituitary D-2 receptor*

| High antagonist affinity | | High antagonist affinity |
|---|---|---|
| $R_H$ | GTP ⇌ | $R_L$ |
| High agonist affinity ($K_H$) | | Low agonist affinity ($K_L$) |

curve in membranes. Additionally, exogenously added GNs no longer affect the (−)APO/[$^3$H]SP curve. Thus, in whole cells endogenous GTP regulates agonist binding in a fashion identical to that of exogenously added GTP in membrane preparations. Importantly, specific [$^3$H]NPA binding is not detectable in intact cells, directly confirming the absence of a detectable $R_H$ state in these cells. However, membranes prepared from these cells exhibit identical binding properties as membranes directly prepared from the whole gland, indicating that the lack of high affinity agonist binding is not the result of receptor degradation occurring during the dispersion. Thus, the $R_H$ and $R_L$ sites are presumably not functionally discrete receptor molecules, since if they were they would *both* be demonstrable in whole cells as well as in membranes.

## DA RECEPTORS IN THE STRIATUM

The very first CNS DA receptor binding studies utilized the agonist [$^3$H]DA and the antagonist [$^3$H]haloperidol (HAL) as ligands (3,20). [$^3$H]HAL bound to a site with high affinity very much like the D-2 receptor since described in anterior pituitary. Bovine striatum also possessed high affinity sites for [$^3$H]DA and other agonist ligands that, unlike the $R_H$ state of the pituitary D-2 receptor, had very low (approximately μM) affinity for BUTYs (Table 2). Much of the controversy over the last few years within this area of research has centered around the neuronal localization of these two sites, whether, in fact, they could represent distinct receptors, and their possible relationship to the DA-sensitive adenylate cyclase. Further disputes have involved whether or not these binding sites can be further subdivided, and whether or not there exists yet more DA receptor subtypes detectable under different assay conditions.

### [$^3$H]Butyrophenone Binding Sites

The majority of high affinity binding sites for [$^3$H]BUTYs in the striatum are identical to the D-2 pituitary receptor. As in pituitary, [$^3$H]agonist ligands can, under appropriate conditions, label these same sites with high affinity (*vida infra*); and the affinity of agonists is reduced by GNs with a specificity similar to that of pituitary (10,32).

Biochemically, the function of the striatal D-2 receptor is not yet known. However, they may mediate the inhibition of adenylate cyclase activity as they do in the pituitary. On the behavioral level, by contrast, the functional relevance of the striatal D-2 receptors is extremely well documented. The affinities of a number of structurally diverse DA antagonists for BUTY binding sites correlate highly with their molar potencies in antagonism of DA-mediated behaviors. Of greatest clinical importance is the correlation between the potencies of these drugs as antipsychotic agents in man, and their potency in competition for [$^3$H]BUTY binding (4,21). The affinity of an antagonist for [$^3$H]BUTY binding is thus a powerful predictor of *in vivo* DA receptor antagonism and antipsychotic activity.

Recently, Sokoloff and co-workers (26) have proposed the existence of another BUTY binding site ("D-4" receptor) in striatum, characterized by high affinity for

TABLE 2. *Characteristics of dopaminergic binding sites in membrane preparations*

| | D-1 | D-2 $R_H \rightleftharpoons R_L$ | | D-3 |
|---|---|---|---|---|
| Usable radioligands | | | | |
| [$^3$H]thioxanthenes | + | + | + | ?[a] |
| [$^3$H]BUTY | − | + | + | − |
| [$^3$H]agonists | ?[b] | + | − | + |
| Agonist affinity | μM | nM | μM | nM |
| BUTY affinity | μM | nM | nM | μM |
| Adenylate cyclase association | Stimulatory | Inhibitory or unassociated | | ?[c] |
| GN Sensitivity | + | + | − | + |
| Function | (a) Parathyroid hormone release (b) In striatum: unknown | (a) Regulation of pituitary hormone release (b) DA-mediated behavioral responses and their antagonism by neuroleptics | | Autoregulation of DA neurones? |
| Striatal location | Intrinsic neurons | (a) Intrinsic neurons (b) Corticostriate afferents?[d] | | Nigrostriatal terminals[e] |
| Pituitary location | − | + | | − |

[a] [$^3$H]flupentixol binding to D-3 receptors has yet to be investigated.
[b] [$^3$H]agonists may label a high affinity state of D-1 receptors.
[c] Autoreceptors are definitely not linked to stimulation of cAMP levels; however, their association with inhibition of adenylate cyclase has not been studied. Postsynaptic D-3 binding sites may be a high agonist-affinity state of D-1 receptors.
[d] [$^3$H]BUTY binding sites on corticostriate terminals may be a distinct D-2 receptor subtype as they have low agonist affinity and no GN sensitivity.
[e] D-3 binding sites appear to be found both on, and postsynaptic to, DA terminals in the striatum.

BUTYs and other DA antagonists but with low affinity for DA agonists. As these authors note, however, D-2 receptors appear to convert to the D-4 type with the addition of GTP. This strongly suggests that, rather than being a separate receptor subtype, the "D-4" site is merely the $R_L$ state of the D-2 receptor. The use of the term "D-4" receptor should therefore be abandoned in the interest of clarity and consistency with the nomenclature of other receptor systems.

Some evidence exists, however, that [$^3$H]BUTY binding sites in pituitary and striatum do differ. As noted above, GNs shift the pseudo-Hill coefficient of agonist/[$^3$H]BUTY competition curves in pituitary membranes to approximately 1, indicating the existence of only one [$^3$H]BUTY binding site in this tissue. This GN change in pseudo-Hill slope, however, is incomplete for some agonists in the striatum (32), despite the fact that these agonist displacement curves are shifted to the right and steepened by GNs. Furthermore, the GN shift is of a lower magnitude in the striatum compared with the pituitary. Thus, in striatum there may well be more than one [$^3$H]BUTY binding site. One of these D-2 subtypes may be identical to that found in pituitary, itself interconverting between two agonist affinity states under the influence of GNs; a separate D-2 receptor subtype may be present which is insensitive to GNs. Kainic acid lesion studies have lent some support for this suggestion *(vide infra)*—it has proved possible to selectively remove GN sensitive [$^3$H]BUTY binding sites, found on intrinsic striatal neurons, leaving a population of nucleotide-insensitive sites intact on the terminals of the corticostriate pathway (9). Thus there is evidence, albeit incomplete at this time, for two distinct subtypes of BUTY binding D-2 receptors in both rat and bovine brain.

### [$^3$H]Agonist Binding Sites

Putative DA receptors in striatum have also been identified by the binding of a number of tritiated DA agonists. Unlike the binding of the [$^3$H]BUTY ligands, that of the [$^3$H]agonist ligands is markedly dependent upon assay conditions. Under some conditions [$^3$H]agonist ligands can bind to D-2 receptors with high affinity, as they do in anterior pituitary. A subset of the [$^3$H]agonist binding sites, however, differ from the BUTY labeled D-2 binding sites in that BUTYs have micromolar affinities for these sites. Thus, it has been proposed that these [$^3$H]agonist binding sites represent yet another distinct DA receptor, the "D-3" receptor (28). It should be noted that it remains a possibility that this D-3 agonist binding is actually to a high affinity agonist binding state of the D-1 receptor. For the purposes of this review, we will, for now, continue to use the D-3 nomenclature.

The D-3 receptors are operationally defined as binding sites with high affinity for [$^3$H]DA, [$^3$H]APO, [$^3$H]NPA or [$^3$H]ADTN and low affinity for BUTYs. They are apparently absent in pituitary which lacks a DA innervation. In bovine striatal membranes at 37°C in the presence of "physiological" (extracellular) concentrations of ions, [$^3$H]DA specifically labels only D-3 sites, with a $K_D$ of about 10–20 nM (3). Such sites have also been labeled in both calf and rat striatum under various conditions with [$^3$H]APO, [$^3$H]NPA, and [$^3$H]ADTN with affinities ($K_D$) in the nanomolar range. Oddly, under roughly these same physiological conditions, high affinity [$^3$H]DA binding to rat striatal membranes is not reproduceably found, although Seeman and co-workers have been able to obtain such binding under other conditions (16,28). We have recently explained these divergent results by characterizing the effects of temperature and ionic conditions on [$^3$H]DA binding in rat caudate membranes. In the absence of metal cations and chelating agents, following a preincubation in buffer at 37°C, specific [$^3$H]DA binding is entirely to D-3 sites. Addition of millimolar $Ca^{2+}$, $Mg^{2+}$, $Mn^{2+}$, or $Co^{2+}$ allows increased D-3 [$^3$H]DA binding and also allows labeling of D-2 and D-3 sites with nearly equal affinity. This reflects prevention by these cations of an irreversible degradation of D-2 sites, as previously described using [$^3$H]SP to define D-2 receptors (31). EDTA and EGTA (0.1 μM–10 mM) paradoxically have a similar effect, although the maximal enhancement in [$^3$H]agonist D-2 binding seen with chelators is less than that seen with divalent cations. Chelators and divalent cations have a further effect in greatly decreasing nonspecific binding of [$^3$H]DA. $Na^+$ (10–150 mM) on the other hand, decreases [$^3$H]DA binding to both D-2 and D-3 sites by decreasing agonist, but not antagonist affinity. This $Na^+$-mediated decrease in agonist but not antagonist affinity is similar to that observed for the opiate receptor, the alpha-1 and the alpha-2 adrenergic receptors, and the histamine-1 receptor. [$^3$H]DA binding to both D-2 and D-3 sites is also reduced by increasing incubation temperature, although [$^3$H]BUTY binding to D-2 sites is not. The combined effect of sodium and temperature are sufficient to place [$^3$H]DA affinity for D-3 sites in rat membranes when assayed at 37°C in the presence of Na$^+$ outside the range detectable in filtration assays. At 22–25°C in the absence of sodium, however, [$^3$H]DA displays a $K_D$ of about 2 nM for D-3 sites. [$^3$H]NPA (30) and [$^3$H]APO (6) also label D-2 receptors with high affinity, as they do in anterior pituitary, as well as D-3 sites. This dual labeling of D-2 and D-3 receptors by these agonists leads to their biphasic displacement by BUTY antagonists with both high (nM) and low (μM) affinity components. Thus depending on tissue preparation and incubation conditions DA [$^3$H]agonists can label either D-2 or D-3 receptors selectively, or both.

The function of the D-3 sites is unclear. Antagonist affinities at these sites do not correlate with their antipsychotic (4) or anti-Parkinsonian (29) potencies nor do they correspond well with their ability to block stimulation of DA-sensitive adenylate cyclase. Lesion studies suggest that the D-3 site may represent autoreceptors on nigrostriatal terminals *(vide infra)*.

## IRREVERSIBLE MODIFICATION OF DA RECEPTORS

### Phenoxybenzamine-Selective Alkylation of [$^3$H]BUTY Binding Sites

Recently, we have shown that phenoxybenzamine selectively and irreversibly eliminates [$^3$H]BUTY labeled D-2 binding sites while producing little effect on [$^3$H]DA labeled D-3 binding sites in bovine striatum (12). Thus, as suggested earlier by displacement studies, binding sites for [$^3$H]DA and [$^3$H]BUTYs appear to be physically distinct and do not interconvert under the conditions of the assay. This decrease in [$^3$H]SP binding is mediated by a decline in the number of binding sites with little change in their affinity, consistent with a covalent attachment of phenoxybenzamine at this site, as suggested for its action at the alpha-adrenergic receptor. This is further supported by the resistance of this inhibition to reversal by repeated washings. [$^3$H]SP binding sites are protected from phenoxybenzamine attack by occupancy, both by agonists and antagonists, indicating that the phenoxybenzamine effect is mediated through site-directed attack and not merely through a nonspecific membrane effect.

Binding of the agonist ligand [$^3$H]APO assayed under identical conditions is affected to a degree intermediate to that of [$^3$H]SP and [$^3$H]DA. The decrease in [$^3$H]APO binding that is seen, as with that for [$^3$H]SP binding, occurs in a site-directed manner, with a decrease in $B_{max}$ unaccompanied by a major change in $K_D$. The increased sensitivity of [$^3$H]APO high affinity binding sites in comparison with those for [$^3$H]DA suggested that even under conditions where [$^3$H]DA binding is D-3 selective, [$^3$H]APO labels *both* the relatively phenoxybenzamine-resistant D-3 site and the relatively phenoxybenzamine-sensitive D-2 site. Displacement of total [$^3$H]APO specific binding from control membranes by SP (6) is clearly biphasic with an overall pseudo-Hill slope of about 0.5, consistent with the presence of more than one type of [³H]APO binding site.

As anterior pituitary is believed to contain D-2 but not D-3 binding sites, it would be anticipated that [³H]APO binding would show identical phenoxybenzamine sensitivity to [³H]SP binding in this tissue. This is indeed the case reinforcing the hypothesis that both agonist and antagonist [³H]ligands label the same singular D-2 receptor in the anterior pituitary.

### Heat Treatment-Multiple Effects Mimicking GTP

Lew and Goldstein (15) first reported that briefly raising the temperature of striatal homogenates to 53°C results in a large decrease in [³H]DA binding, while leaving [³H]SP binding largely unchanged. This was interpreted as a heat-induced denaturation of [³H]DA binding sites, but not the separate [³H]SP binding site. Additional evidence now suggests that it is not the D-3 [³H]DA binding site itself which is denatured. Exposure of caudate homogenates to 53°C causes a rapid decrease in specific binding of *both* agonist ligands [³H]APO and [³H]DA with more than one-half eliminated within 30 sec. The binding of [³H]SP is unaffected. Unlike treatment with phenoxybenzamine, heat treatment equally affects the binding of [³H]DA, which under the conditions employed here labels only the D-3 site, and that of [³H]APO, which labels both D-2 and D-3 sites. Thus, heat treatment not only eliminates [³H]DA and [³H]APO binding to the D-3 site, but also the binding of [³H]APO to the D-2 site, despite a lack of any alteration in [³H]SP binding to the D-2 site. Thus this effect cannot be explained merely as a loss of the D-2 binding sites *per se*, and is highly reminiscent of the effects of GNs on agonist binding. In addition to causing an apparent reduction in the number of high affinity [³H]agonist binding sites, heat treatment has a second effect in causing a reduction in potency of unlabeled agonists in displacement of [³H]SP—the $IC_{50}$'s for DA and APO are shifted 10–15-fold higher after exposure of homogenates to 53°C for 4 min. Micromolar concentrations of GDP, GTP, or Gpp(NH)p also cause a similar decrease in agonist potency. The effects of 4 min heat treatment and maximal GTP included in the assay are not additive, consistent with a common site of action. Finally, heat treatment has a third effect, it causes an increase in the pseudo-Hill slope of DA/[³H]SP displacements from 0.4 for control homogenates to 0.8 in those exposed to 53°C for 4 min. This steepening of the displacement curve is once again an effect on D-2 binding also seen with addition of GNs (7,32).

A single explanation of these three common, nonadditive effects of heat treatment and GNs is suggested by the characterization of a GTP-binding regulatory protein ("N") that modulates beta-adrenergic receptor function (18). This protein, when coupled with the beta-receptor—and possibly many other neurotransmitter and hormones receptors—enables high affinity binding of [³H]agonist ligands and potent displacement of [³H]antagonists by agonists. When N/receptor association is prevented, either by the addition of GTP or manipulations eliminating N directly, high affinity [³H]agonist binding is lost, and agonist/[³H]antagonist displacements are right-shifted and steepened. Antagonist binding remains unaffected. Thus, heat denaturation of such a regulatory moiety, rather than the D-2 and D-3 receptors themselves, would explain the observed selective decreases in the binding of [³H]agonists to both D-2 and D-3 sites.

## NEUROANATOMICAL LOCALIZATION OF DA RECEPTORS IN THE CNS

Studies in rat striatum have provided evidence for a differential localization of D-1, D-2, and D-3 receptor subtypes. Kainic acid-induced lesions of intrinsic striatal neurons almost completely eliminates striatal DA-sensitive adenylate cyclase activity, indicating that almost all of this enzyme (and thus presumably D-1 receptors) is present on these cells (11,19). Seventy-five percent of the binding of [³H]flupentixol, which labels D-1 receptors, is also eliminated after kainic acid lesion. Striatal kainate lesions also indicate that about 50% of [³H]BUTY binding sites are localized on intrinsic neurons. These [³H]BUTY binding sites exhibit GN-sensitive agonist binding. Most of the remaining BUTY binding sites in the striatum appear to be localized on corticostriate terminals and are removable by cortical ablation (19). In contrast, these latter sites appear to have low affinity for agonists and are GN-insensitive (9). In the absence of additional supporting data, however, the presence of a separate non-GN-sensitive D-2 receptor on cortical afferents must remain tentative. It remains a possibility, for example, that kainic acid removes GTP regulation of cortical afferent D-2 receptors by reducing the level of active N protein.

Studies comparing striatal kainate lesion-induced losses in the binding of [³H]BUTYs and [³H]agonists (9,14) reported that high affinity [³H]agonist sites were decreased to a greater extent than [³H]BUTY binding. Since this greater loss of agonist binding (70% or greater) correlated more closely with the loss seen in DA-sensitive adenylate cyclase activity, and since both measures show GN sensitivity, it was hypothesized that [³H]agonists may label a high affinity agonist binding state of the D-1 receptor in striatal membrane preparations. This conjecture has yet to be disproved.

The localization of D-3 sites identified with [³H]agonists under different assay conditions has been elusive leading to a lack of consensus concerning the pharmacological specificity, neuronal localizations and functional roles of these sites (7). 6-Hydroxydopamine (6-OHDA) lesions of the nigrostriatal pathway have been used to remove presynaptic DA terminals in the striatum to determine if D-3 sites are presynaptic autoreceptors. However, since denervation hypersensitivity of striatal DA receptors results from these lesions, they could result in an elimination of the binding to presynaptic receptors masked by a concomitant increase in binding to postsynaptic receptors. Indeed, increased numbers of putative DA receptors in striatum were identified by both [³H]BUTY binding (5,17) and with [³H]APO (8). Contrary to Creese's finding, Nagy et al. (17), using different assay conditions, reported a decrease in [³H]APO binding in striata ipsilateral to the 6-OHDA lesion, which led them to hypothesize that [³H]APO specifically labels presynaptic autoreceptors. A recent study by Sokoloff et al. (27) found a change in the distribution of pharmacologically differentiable [³H]APO sites in striatum after 6-OHDA lesions of the nigrostriatal tract. [$^3$H]APO sites having nM affinity for BUTYs and domperidone (D-2 sites—termed by them as class I) increased 25–30% in density whereas sites having lower or μM affinity for BUTYs and domperidone (D-3 sites—termed by them as class II) showed 30–50% decreases in density. In this same study, striatal kainate lesions produced a 57% decrease in class I sites and no change in class II sites. However, we have recently shown that reserpine mimics the 6-OHDA reduction in "D-3" binding, suggesting that DA depletion, rather than terminal degeneration is responsible for the loss in D-3 sites. While the above studies are consistent with the hypothesis that [$^3$H]agonists can label both pre- and postsynaptic receptor sites, they are only correlative. Future studies will be required to pursue the pharmacological and morphological identity of these putative subclasses of DA receptors in order to further comprehend their role in the physiological and behavioral function of the neostriatum.

## CONCLUDING COMMENTS

Table 2 summarizes our present understanding of DA receptor classification. The advantage to the terminology used over other classification schemes is that it (a) takes into account the historical development of the field and (b) attempts to encompass the pharmacological classification of DA receptors, association of receptors with adenylate cyclase, and identification of binding sites within a common nomenclature. Noted in the table are some points of contention for which there is insufficient data at present to draw firm conclusions. The availability of selective agonists and antagonists is central to receptor classification. The advent of selective D-1, D-2, and D-3 agents in the future may not only allow the resolution of the above questions, but also lead to better pharmacological treatment of disorders such as schizophrenia, tardive dyskinesia, Parkinson's disease, Huntingtons chorea, galactorrhea, and hyperprolactinemia, which certainly involve these receptor subtypes and their regulation.

## ACKNOWLEDGMENTS

The authors wish to thank Dolores Taitano for manuscript typing and Andre De Lean, M.D., for computer analysis. This research was supported by PHSMH 32990. I. C. is a recipient of a RSDA PHSMH00316.

## REFERENCES

1. Attie, M. F., Brown, E. M., Gardner, D. G., Spiegel, A. M., and Aurbach, G. D. (1980): Characterization of dopamine-responsive adenylate cyclase of bovine parathyroid cells and its relationship to parathyroid hormone secretion. *Endocrinology*, 107:1776–1781.
2. Cote, T. E., Grewe, C. W., and Kebabian, J. W. (1981): Stimulation of the D-2 dopamine receptor in the intermediate lobe of the rat pituitary gland decreases the responsiveness of the beta-adrenoceptor: Biochemical mechanism. *Endocrinology*, 108:420–426.
3. Creese, I., Burt, D. R., and Snyder, S. H. (1975): Dopamine receptor binding: Differentiation of agonist and antagonist states with $^3$H-dopamine and $^3$H-haloperidol. *Life Sci.*, 17:993–1002.
4. Creese, I., Burt, D. R., and Snyder, S. H. (1976): Dopamine receptor binding predicts clinical and pharmacological potencies of antischizophrenic drugs. *Science*, 192:481–483.
5. Creese, I., Burt, D. R., and Snyder, S. H. (1977): Dopamine receptor binding enhancement accompanies lesion-induced behavioral supersensitivity. *Science*, 197:596–598.

6. Creese, I., Prosser, T., and Snyder, S. H. (1978): Dopamine receptor binding: Specificity, localization and regulation by ions and guanyl nucleotides. *Life Sci.*, 23:495–500.
7. Creese, I., and Sibley, D. R. (1979): Radioligand binding studies: Evidence for multiple dopamine receptors. *Commun. Psychopharmacol.*, 3:385–395.
8. Creese, I., and Snyder, S. H. (1979): Nigrostriatal lesions enhance striatal $^3$H-apomorphine and $^3$H-spiroperidol binding. *Eur. J. Pharmacol.*, 56:277–281.
9. Creese, I., Usdin, T., and Snyder, S. H. (1979): Guanine nucleotides distinguish between two dopamine receptors. *Nature*, 278:577–578.
10. Creese, I., Usdin, T. B., and Snyder, S. H. (1979): Dopamine receptor binding regulated by guanine nucleotides. *Mol. Pharmacol.*, 16:69–75.
11. Govoni, S., Olgiati, V. R., Trabucchi, M., Garau, L., Stefanini, E., and Spano, P. F. (1978): [$^3$H]Haloperidol and [$^3$H]spiroperidol receptor binding after striatal injection of kainic acid. *Neurosci. Lett.*, 8:207–210.
12. Hamblin, M., and Creese, I. (1980): Phenoxybenzamine discriminates multiple dopamine receptors. *Eur. J. Pharmacol.*, 65:119–121.
13. Kebabian, J. W., and Calne, D. B. (1979): Multiple receptors for dopamine. *Nature*, 277:93–96.
14. Leff, S., Adams, L., Hyttel, J., and Creese, I. (1981): Kainate lesion dissociates striatal dopamine receptor radioligand binding sites. *Eur. J. Pharmacol.*, 70:71–75.
15. Lew, J. Y., and Goldstein, M. (1979): Dopamine receptor binding for agonists and antagonists in thermal exposed membranes. *Eur. J. Pharmacol.*, 55:429–430.
16. List, S., Titeler, M., and Seeman, P. (1980): High-affinity $^3$H-dopamine receptors ($D_3$ sites) in human and rat brain. *Biochem. Pharmacol.*, 29:1621–1622.
17. Nagy, J. I., Lee, T., Seeman, P., and Fibiger, H. C. (1978): Direct evidence for presynaptic and postsynaptic dopamine receptors in brain. *Nature*, 274:278–281.
18. Ross, E. M., and Gilman, A. G. (1980): Biochemical properties of hormone-sensitive adenylate cyclase. *Annu. Rev. Biochem.*, 49:533–564.
18a. Onali, P., Schwartz, J. P., and Costa, E. (1981): Dopaminergic modulation of adenylate cyclase stimulation of vasoactive intestinal peptide (VIP) in anterior pituitary. *Proc. Natl. Acad. Sci. USA*, 78:6531–6534.
19. Schwarcz, R., Creese, I., Coyle, J. T., and Snyder, S. H. (1978): Dopamine receptors localised on cerebral cortical afferents to rat corpus striatum. *Nature*, 271:766–768.
20. Seeman, P., Chau-Wong, M., Tedesco, J., and Wong, K. (1975): Brain receptors for antipsychotic drugs and dopamine: Direct binding assays. *Proc. Natl. Acad. Sci. USA*, 72:4376–4380.
21. Seeman, P., Lee, T., Chau-Wong, M., and Wong, K. (1976): Antipsychotic drug doses and neuroleptic/dopamine receptors. *Nature*, 261:717–719.
22. Sibley, D. R., and Creese, I. (1979): Multiple pituitary dopamine receptors: Effects of guanine nucleotides. *Soc. Neurosci. Abstr.*, 5:352.
23. Sibley, D. R., and Creese, I. (1980): Anterior pituitary dopamine receptors: Heterogeneity of agonist binding. *Fed. Proc.*, 39:1098.
24. Sibley, D. R., De Lean, A., and Creese, I. (1982): Anterior pituitary dopamine receptors: I. Demonstration of high and low affinity states of the incontravertible D-2 dopamine receptor. *J. Biol. Chem. (in press).*
25. Sibley, D. R., and Creese, I. (1982): Anterior pituitary dopamine receptors: II. Guanine nucleotides mediate state interconversions of the D-2 dopamine receptor. *J. Biol. Chem.*, 257:6351–6361.
26. Sokoloff, P., Martres, M. P., and Schwartz, J. C. (1980): Three classes of dopamine receptor (D-2, D-3, D-4) identified by binding studies with $^3$H-apomorphine and $^3$H-domperidone. *Naunyn Schmiedebergs Arch. Pharmacol.*, 315:89–102.
27. Sokoloff, P., Martres, M.-P., and Schwartz, J.-C. (1980): $^3$H-Apomorphine labels both dopamine postsynaptic receptors and autoreceptors, *Nature*, 288:283–286.
28. Titeler, M., List, S., and Seeman, P. (1979): High affinity dopamine receptors ($D_3$) in rat brain. *Commun. Psychopharmacol.*, 3:411–420.
29. Titeler, M., and Seeman, P. (1978): Antiparkinsonian drug doses and neuroleptic receptors. *Experientia*, 34:1490–1492.
30. Titeler, M., and Seeman, P. (1979): Selective labeling of different dopamine receptors by a new agonist $^3$H-ligand: $^3$H-N-propylnorapomorphine. *Eur. J. Pharmacol.*, 56:291–292.
31. Usdin, T. B., Creese, I., and Snyder, S. H. (1980): Regulation by cations of $^3$H-spiroperidol binding associated with dopamine receptors of rat brain. *J. Neurochem.*, 34:669–676.
32. Zahniser, N. R., and Molinoff, P. B. (1978): Effect of guanine nucleotides on striatal dopamine receptors. *Nature*, 275:453–455.

*Molecular Pharmacology of Neurotransmitter Receptors*, edited by T. Segawa et al.
Raven Press, New York © 1983.

# Identification and Localization of the Recognition Binding Subunit of the $D_1$ Dopamine Receptor

## C. Tanaka, T. Kuno, T. Mita, and T. Ishibe

*Department of Pharmacology, Kobe University School of Medicine, Kobe 650, Japan*

The dopamine receptors have been well characterized in binding assays and pharmacological experiments, and these receptors have been classified into distinct sets of two or more subtypes. Kebabian and Calne (5) have proposed to distinguish the $D_1$ receptor, affected by dopamine at micromolar concentrations and linked to adenylate cyclase from other dopamine receptors not associated with adenylate cyclase. Nishikori et al. (9) reported the solubilization and separation of two distinct dopamine receptors, using canine striatal membranes photolabeled with [$^3$H]dopamine. However, molecular characterization of the recognition site of the dopamine receptor has heretofore not been fully determined. We report here identification of the binding subunit of the $D_1$ receptor from rat striatal synaptic membranes and autoradiographic localization of the $D_1$ receptor after photoaffinity labeling.

## METHODS

Male Wistar rats weighing about 200 g were decapitated and the striatum, frontal cortex, hypothalamus, and cerebellum were rapidly removed. A fraction enriched in synaptic membranes, designated $M_1$, was prepared from four brain areas by the method of DeRobertis et al. (4). All procedures were conducted at 0 to 4°C.

### Determination of Dopamine-Sensitive Adenylate Cyclase

Dopamine-sensitive adenylate cyclase activity was determined by measuring the amount of cyclic adenosine monophosphate (cAMP) formed during incubation in the absence and presence of dopamine, by the method of Nishikori et al. (9).

### Photoaffinity Labeling of the Dopamine Receptor

The technique of photoaffinity labeling of the dopamine receptor with [$^3$H]dopamine described by Nishikori et al. (9) was used—but with slight modification. The $M_1$ membranes were preincubated with a micromolar concentration of [$^3$H]dopamine (ethyl-$^3$H-dopamine, 21.53 Ci/m mol, New England Nuclear) in the assay mixture for dopamine sensitive adenylate cyclase, as described above except for omission of GTP, at 0 or 30°C for 10 min. Thereafter, photolysis was performed for various times at 0 or 30°C. The photolabeled membranes were washed repeatedly with a cold 50-mM Tris/maleate buffer to remove free [$^3$H]dopamine.

## SDS-Polyacrylamide Gel Electrophoresis

The $M_1$ membranes recovered from the photolysis were solubilized and reduced with 2% sodium dodecylsulfate (SDS) and 5% β-mercaptoethanol in 0.0625 M Tris/HCl buffer, pH 6.8 containing 10% glycerol and 0.001% bromophenol blue by boiling for 5 min. These treated $M_1$ membranes were analyzed using SDS-10% polyacrylamide slab gel electrophoresis, by the method of Ames (1). After protein staining, the gel slab was dried for the fluorography on Kodak X-Omat R film at −70°C by the method of Chamberlain (2). Intensity of the darkness of bands on the film was measured quantitatively by scanning with a dual-wavelength TCL scanner CS-910 (Shimadzu). The molecular weights of bands on the gels were estimated by comparing their mobility with that of marker proteins, bovine serum albumin, ovalbumin, and α-chymotrypsinogen-A (Sigma), by the method of Weber and Osborn (12).

## Kainic Acid-Induced Lesions

Kainic acid, 3 μg dissolved in 1 μl of phosphate buffered saline, was stereotaxically injected at a rate of 0.2 μl/30 sec into the right caudate nucleus. Three unilateral injections of 1 μg each were used to maximize the amount of striatal tissue lesioned, and the lesions were verified by histological changes in the striatum and by ipsilateral turning behavior which followed intraperitoneal administration of apomorphine 3 weeks after the kainic acid injection.

## Microscopic Autoradiography of the $D_1$ Receptor

The brain perfused with 0.03% paraformaldehyde in 0.01 M phosphate buffered saline was rapidly frozen. The 10-μm thick coronal frozen sections were thaw-mounted onto precleaned gelatin-coated slides and air dried. Before beginning autoradiographic experiments, we carried out biochemical experiments to determine the optimal conditions for photoaffinity labeling of the dopamine receptor in the slide mount tissue with [$^3$H]dopamine. The sections were incubated with [$^3$H]dopamine at various micromolar concentrations in the standard incubation mixture as used for photoaffinity labeling of the membrane fraction, under UV illumination. After various rinsings, the sections were scraped from the slides and the incorporated radioactivity was measured. Under the optimal condition for maximal specific to nonspecific ratios, photoaffinity labeling of the slide mount brain sections with [$^3$H]dopamine was performed. After extensive washing with phosphate buffered saline and water at 25°C, slides were air dried and dipped into Kodak NTB-2 emulsion. After coated slides were stored at 4°C for 2–3 weeks, they were developed and counter-stained with toluidine blue. The localization of silver grains was microscopically examined under dark-field and bright-field illumination.

## Chemical Assay for Dopamine

Five milliliters of 0.4 N perchloric acid containing 5 mg $Na_2S_2O_5$ and 20 mg EDTA was added to the incubation mixture and the preparation was centrifuged for 10 min at 10,000 rpm. The supernatants were assayed for dopamine using high-performance liquid chromatography with electrochemical detection, by the method of Keller et al. (6).

## RESULTS

### Photoaffinity Labeling of the $D_1$ Receptor with Micromolar [$^3$H]Dopamine

When the striatal membranes were incubated with 5 μM of [$^3$H]dopamine at 0°C, specific incorporation of [$^3$H]dopamine into the $M_1$ membranes gradually increased with increase in the illumination time and reached a plateau after 60 min (Fig. 1A). We defined nonspecific incorporation as that in the presence of 1 mM nonradioactive dopamine, and specific incorporation as the difference between total and nonspecific incorporation. Photolabeling of the membranes with increasing concentrations of [$^3$H]dopamine showed a saturable specific incorporation. On the other hand, when photolysis was performed at 30°C, [$^3$H]dopamine was rapidly incorporated into the striatal membranes and the amount of [$^3$H]dopamine incorporated was double that when photolysis was performed for 120 min at 0°C (Fig. 1A). To determine whether dopamine in the incubation medium is degraded during photolysis, dopamine contents in the incubation medium were measured. When incubation was carried out in the absence of the membranes, the concentration of dopamine did not change with UV illumination both at 0 and 30°C. However, when dopamine was incubated with the striatal membranes, photolysis at 30°C resulted in a loss of 70% of initial dopamine content during 60 min. When photolysis was carried out at 0°C for 120 min the loss of dopamine in the incubation medium was about 20% of that prior to photolysis. To determine whether [$^3$H]dopamine would label the dopamine receptor upon photolysis, effects of dopamine agonists and antagonists on photoaffinity labeling were examined. Incorporation was reduced by the addition of nonradioactive dopamine when the concentrations were increased from 10 μM to 1 mM, in a concentration-dependent manner.

Specific incorporation of [$^3$H]dopamine was inhibited slightly by the addition of norepinephrine but not by L-DOPA or isoproterenol. Apomorphine, bromocriptine, and haloperidol at micromolar concentrations markedly inhibited specific incorporation which was not significantly changed by sulpiride, a $D_2$ receptor blocker (11) and benztropine, a blocker of the reuptake of dopamine (3) (Fig. 2).

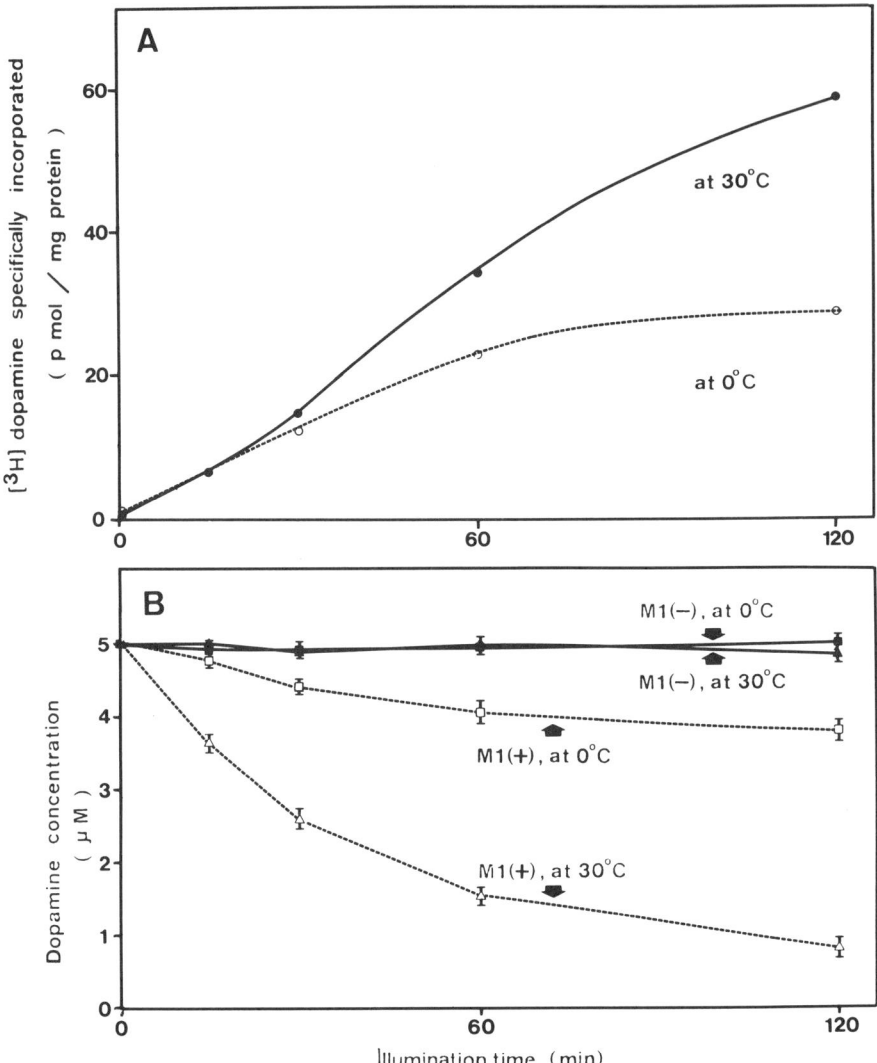

**FIG. 1. A:** Time dependency of specific [$^3$H]dopamine incorporation into rat striatal membranes at 0°C *(open circles)* and 30°C *(closed circles)*. Membrane fraction from rat striatum ($M_1$:1 mg protein/ml) was preincubated with 5 μM [$^3$H]dopamine in 0.5 ml of 80 mM Tris/maleate buffer, pH 7.4, containing 8 mM MgSO$_4$, 2 mM ATP, 0.5 mM 3-isobutyl-1-methylxanthine, 0.6 mM EGTA, 0.02% ascorbic acid, in the presence and absence of 1 mM nonradioactive dopamine, for 10 min at 0°C. The samples were then illuminated by UV light at 0°C or 30°C. $M_1$ was washed repeatedly in cold 50 mM Tris/maleate buffer, pH 7.4, and the radioactivity was measured. Specific [$^3$H]dopamine incorporation into rat striatal membrane was determined as the difference between the incorporation in the absence (total) and presence (nonspecific) of 1 mM nonradioactive dopamine. The results are means of duplicate determinations. **B:** Dopamine degradation during the photolysis. Dopamine concentration in the incubation mixture was determined using high-performance liquid chromatography with electrochemical detection in the absence of $M_1$ at 0°C *(closed squares)*, or 30°C *(closed triangles)*, and the presence of $M_1$ at 0°C *(open squares)*, or 30°C *(open triangles)*, under the same preincubation and incubation as **A**. The results are means and standard errors of triplicate determinations.

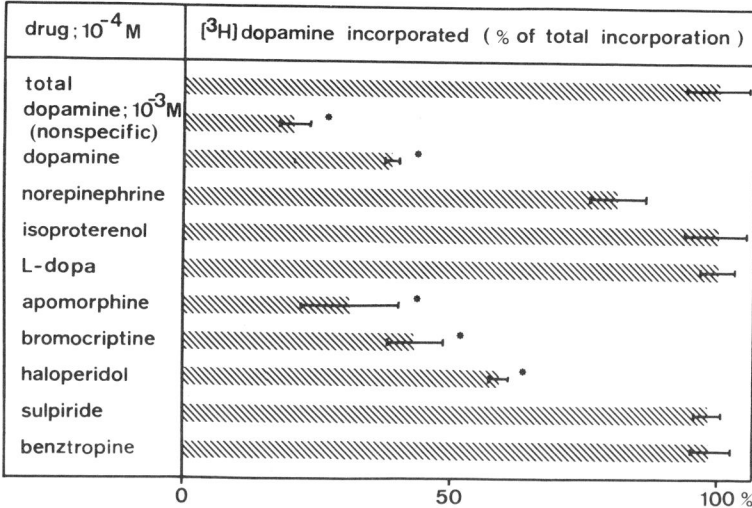

**FIG. 2.** Drug inhibition of [³H]dopamine incorporation into rat striatal membranes. $M_1$ was preincubated with 5μM [³H]dopamine in the same assay mixture in the absence (total) and presence of various indicated drugs for 10 min at 0°C and then illuminated by UV light for 120 min at 0°C. The results are means and standard errors of triplicate determinations. The *closed circles* indicate significant difference from total; $p < 0.001$.

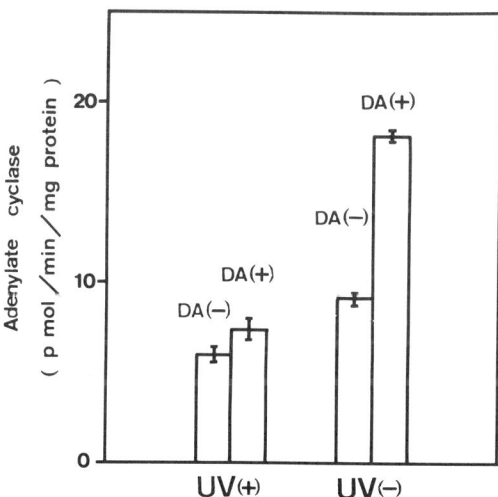

**FIG. 3.** Inactivation of dopamine-stimulated activity of adenylate cyclase in rat striatal membranes by photoaffinity labeling. Dopamine-sensitive adenylate cyclase activity was determined by measuring the amount of cyclic AMP formed during a 5-min incubation in the presence and absence of 100 μM dopamine under the standard conditions at 30°C with the samples ($M_1$: 0.5 mg/ml) which were or were not preilluminated by UV light, in the presence of 1 mM nonradioactive dopamine, for 120 min at 0°C and followed by five washings. Each column represents the mean of five replicate samples with standard error indicated by vertical bands.

## Inactivation of Dopamine-Sensitive Adenylate Cyclase

To determine if dopamine would covalently label the $D_1$ receptor upon photolysis, causing irreversible inactivation of the dopamine-stimulated adenylate cyclase, this enzyme activity was assayed in the prephotolyzed striatal membrane. Photolysis in the presence of 1 mM dopamine resulted in an approximately 80% loss in dopamine-stimulated adenylate cyclase activity, as compared with findings in nonilluminated control membranes (Fig. 3). There was some loss of the basal activity of adenylate cyclase by UV illumination; however, the dopamine-stimulated response remained intact and this inactivation of dopamine-stimulated adenylate cyclase activity by photoaffinity labeling was prevented by the presence of haloperidol but not by sulpiride in the assay mixture (data not shown).

## SDS Polyacrylamide Slab Gel Electrophoresis

The photolabeled mmbranes were solubilized with SDS and reduced by β-mercaptoethanol, after which the solubilized membranes were analyzed by electrophoresis on 10% polyacrylamide slab gels. When the striatal membranes were photolabeled at 30°C for 60 min, several labeled bands appeared on the fluorograph (Fig. 4F). When photolabeling was carried out at 0°C for 120 min, a strongly labeled band appeared among several weakly labeled bands (Fig. 4A, Fig. 5D). Molecular weight of the labeled band was estimated to be about 57,000 daltons by comparing its mobility with those of the proteins with known molecular weights. The labeling of 57,000-dalton protein was inhibited in a concentration-dependent manner by the addition of nonradioactive dopamine to the incubation medium during photolysis, and was abolished in the presence of 1 mM dopamine (Fig. 4B and C). Haloperidol also reduced the labeling (Fig. 4D) but sulpiride, a specific $D_2$ receptor blocker, had no effect on the labeling of this band, even at 100 μM (Fig. 4E).

## Effect of Kainic Acid Lesion

Three weeks after unilateral intrastriatal injection of kainic acid, specific incorporation of [$^3$H]dopamine radioactivity in the lesion side was 53% of that in the contralateral striatum. Labeled $M_1$ membranes were then analyzed by SDS polyacrylamide slab gel electrophoresis after solubilization and reduction. The 57,000-dalton band was very weakly labeled on the lesioned side as compared with that in the intact side (Fig. 4G and H), suggesting that this protein localized on the neural elements which had degenerated after kainic acid treatment.

## Regional Distribution of [$^3$H]Dopamine Binding Subunit

As shown in Fig. 5, the 57,000-dalton band was intensely labeled in tissue from the frontal cortex and the striatum and the weakest labeling occurred in the cerebellum.

When coronal sections of rat forebrain were incubated with [$^3$H]dopamine upon photolysis, high densities of grains were observed in dopaminergic brain areas such as the caudoputamen and the nucleus accumbens. In the caudoputamen, grains were seen to surround the striatal neurons (Fig. 6A). White matter areas such as corpus callosum and capsula interna and fiber bundles in the caudoputamen had negligible specific binding. When sections were photolabeled in the presence of 1 mM nonradioactive dopamine, the densities of grains were markedly decreased, as shown in Fig. 6B.

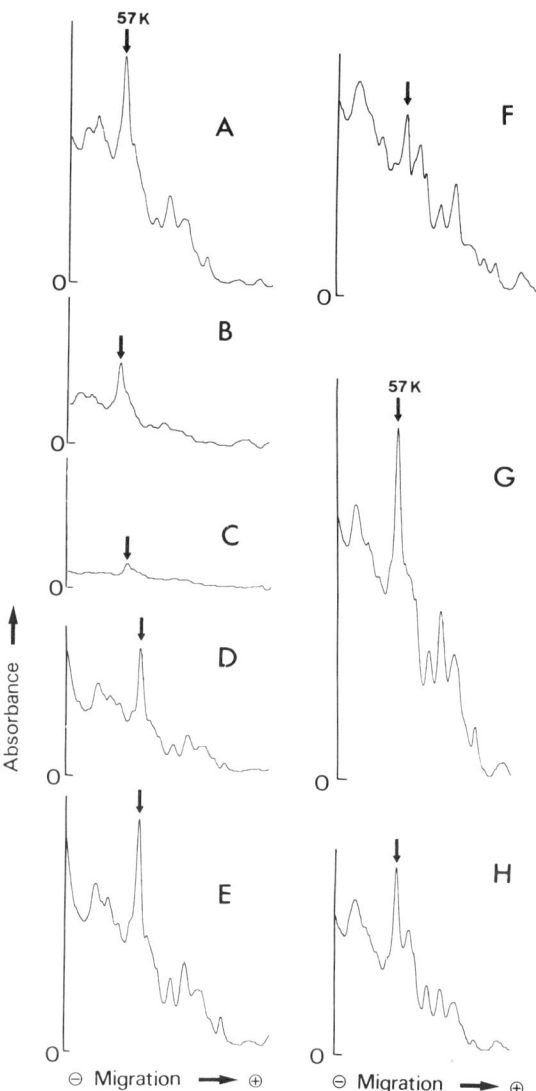

**FIG. 4.** Densitogram obtained from fluorograph of rat striatal membranes labeled with [$^3$H]dopamine. $M_1$ was labeled with 5 μM [$^3$H]dopamine at 0°C for 120 min in the absence **(A)** and presence of $10^{-4}$ M dopamine **(B)**, $10^{-3}$ M dopamine **(C)**, $10^{-4}$ M haloperidol **(D)**, $10^{-4}$ M sulpiride **(E)**, and at 30°C for 60 min **(F)**. $M_1$ fractions from intact **(G)** and kainic acid lesioned **(H)** side were also labeled with 5 μM [$^3$H]dopamine at 0°C for 120 min. The *arrows* indicate the 57,000-dalton bands.

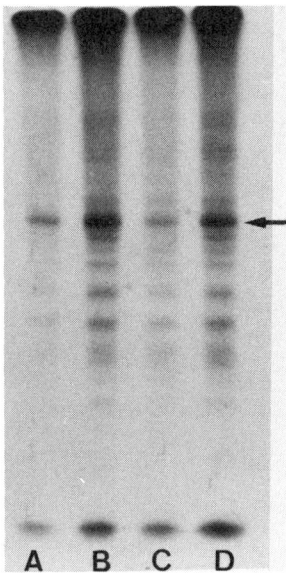

FIG. 5. Regional distribution of 57,000-dalton proteins. Fluorographs of rat brain membranes from hypothalamus **(A)**, frontal cortex **(B)**, cerebellum **(C)**, and striatum **(D)** photolabeled with 5μM [$^3$H]dopamine for 120 min at 0°C.

## DISCUSSION

Photoaffinity labeling of the $D_1$ receptor was initiated by Nishikori et al. (9). As the $D_1$ receptor subunit on SDS polyacrylamide slab gels could not be visualized by fluorography, under the condition used in their experiment for photolabeling of canine striatal membranes with 0.5 μM [$^3$H]dopamine carried out at 30°C for 40 min, the optimal condition was determined in our first experiment. When the striatal membranes were photolabeled with 5 μM [$^3$H]dopamine at 30°C for 60 min, several bands on the gels were labeled and 120-min photolysis induced the labeling of multiple protein bands. As a loss of 70% of initial dopamine was found 60 min after photolyzing at 30°C, enzymatic degradation may occur during photolysis and result in labeling of multiple bands, because photodecomposition and thermal degradation of dopamine itself were negligible. Therefore, photolysis was carried out at 0°C in this experiment.

Micromolar dopamine was irreversibly linked to the rat striatal $M_1$ membranes upon ultraviolet (UV) illumination. This labeling was inhibited markedly by dopamine, apomorphine, bromocriptine, and haloperidol, slightly by norepinephrine, but not by L-DOPA, isoproterenol, benztropine, and sulpiride. These findings indicate that specific incorporation of [$^3$H]dopamine probably represents its covalent attachment to the $D_1$ receptor. If so, dopamine-sensitive adenylate cyclase should be affected by photoaffinity labeling of the $D_1$ receptor with dopamine. In fact, dopamine-stimulated adenylate cyclase activity in the $M_1$ prephotolysed with 1 mM dopamine was markedly lower as compared with the nonilluminated control. These findings suggest that the receptor photolabeled with [$^3$H]dopamine linked to dopamine-sensitive adenylate cyclase.

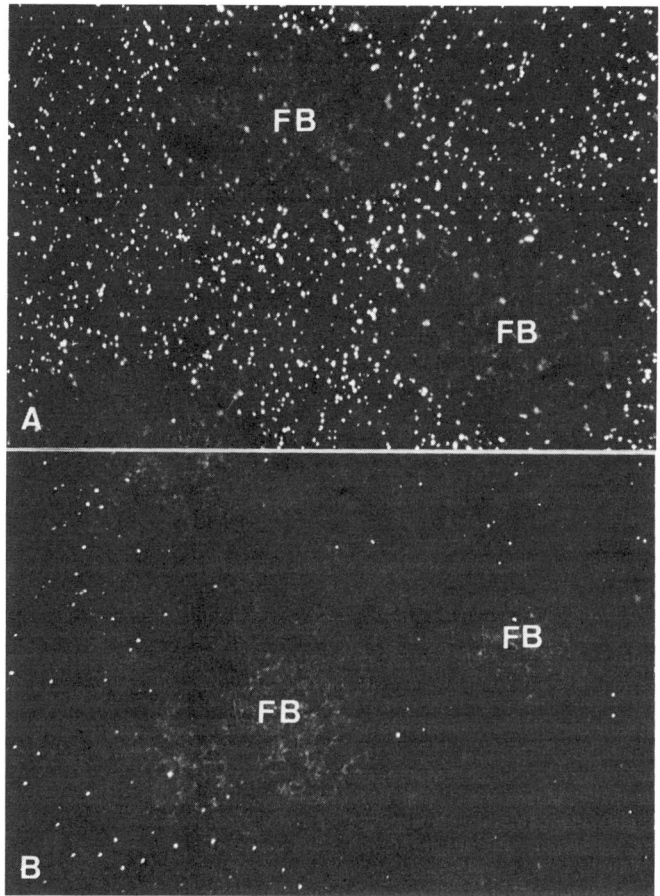

**FIG. 6.** Dark-field photomicrograph of autoradiograms of photolabeled [³H]dopamine in rat caudoputamen section (×64). Formaldehyde-treated (10 μm) sections were preincubated in 5 μM [³H]dopamino for 30 min at 0°C in the absence **(A)** and presence **(B)** of 1 mM nonradioactive dopamine, thereafter photolysed for 120 min at 0°C. Note high density grains in the tissue, except for nerve fiber bundles of the dark-field photographs. Nonradioactive dopamine, 1 mM, eliminated most specific labels, as demonstrated in **B**.

To identify the $D_1$ receptor binding subunit, the $M_1$ membrane photolabeled with [³H]dopamine was analyzed by electrophoresis on SDS polyacrylamide slab gels. When photolysis was carried out at 0°C, a strongly labeled band appeared among several weakly labeled bands on the fluorograph. Molecular weight of this main band was estimated to be about 57,000. This band was hardly detected by protein staining, indicating that it constitutes only a minute fraction of the total protein. The labeling of 57,000-dalton protein was inhibited by dopamine and haloperidol but not by sulpiride, a specific $D_2$ receptor blocker. These findings suggest that 57,000-dalton polypeptide is the recognition subunit of the dopamine receptor linked to adenylate cyclase, the $D_1$ receptor.

Dopamine-sensitive adenylate cyclase has been shown to exist in the postsynaptic membranes of rat striatum by means of kainate lesions (8).

We have demonstrated that the $D_1$ receptor binding subunit with an apparent molecular weight of 57,000 is also located on the neural elements which degenerated after kainic acid treatment. The 57,000-dalton subunit is located preferentially in dopaminergic areas, highest in the frontal cortex, followed by the striatum and the hypothalamus and lowest in nondopaminergic areas.

We developed a new method for dopamine receptor autoradiography using photo-affinity labeling by which [$^3$H]dopamine binding sites of a micromolar order were visualized in the rat striatum. The dopamine receptor in our slide-mounted tissue sections fixed by formaldehyde had all of the characteristics found in biochemical studies with the $M_1$ fraction (data not shown). As shown in the autoradiograms, high densities of the dopamine receptor photolabeled with [$^3$H]dopamine were found in the dopaminergic areas such as the caudoputamen and the nucleus accumbens. In the caudoputamen specific labels were seen to surround the striatal neurons but such labels were not evident within nerve cell bodies and nerve fiber bundles. The intrastriatal distribution of [$^3$H]dopamine binding sites is generally in agreement with previously reported distributions of dopaminergic nerve terminals (7), and of [$^3$H]spiperone binding sites (10).

## CONCLUSIONS

It was demonstrated that 57,000-dalton polypeptide is the recognition subunit of the dopamine receptor linked to adenylate cyclase, the $D_1$ receptor, and is located preferentially in postsynaptic neuronal membranes in dopaminergic areas, the frontal cortex, and the striatum.

## ACKNOWLEDGMENTS

This work was supported by grants from the Ministry of Education, Science and Culture and the Ministry of Health and Welfare, Japan. We thank Dr. H. Maeno and Dr. K. Nishikori, Department of Pharmacology and Biochemistry, Central Research Laboratories, Yamanouchi Pharmaceutical Co., Ltd., and Dr. M. Yoshioka, Department of Analytical Chemistry, Faculty of Pharmaceutical Sciences, University of Tokyo, for pertinent advice on photoaffinity labeling of dopamine receptor and M. Ohara of Kyushu University for critical reading of the manuscript.

## REFERENCES

1. Ames, G. F.-L. (1974): Resolution of bacterial proteins by polyacrylamide gel electrophoresis on slab. *J. Biol. Chem.*, 249:634–644.
2. Chamberlain, J. P. (1979): Fluorographic detection of radioactivity in polyacrylamide gels with the water-soluble fluor, sodium salicylate. *Anal. Biochem.*, 98:132–135.
3. Coyle, J. T., and Snyder, S. H. (1969): Antiparkinsonian drugs: Inhibition of dopamine uptake in the corpus striatum as a possible mechanism of action. *Science*, 166:899–901.
4. DeRobertis, E., Rodriguez De Lores Arnaiz, G., and Alberici, M. (1967): Subcellular distribution of adenyl cyclase and cyclic phosphodiesterase in rat brain cortex. *J. Biol. Chem.*, 242:3487–3497.

5. Kebabian, J. W., and Calne, D. B. (1979): Multiple receptors for dopamine. *Nature*, 277:92–96.
6. Keller, R., Oke, A., Mefford, I., and Adams, R. N. (1976): Liquid chromatographic analysis of catecholamines—routine assay for regional brain mapping. *Life Sci.*, 19:995–1004.
7. Lindvall, O., and Björklund, A. (1974): The organization of the ascending catecholamine neuron systems in the rat brain as revealed by the glyoxylic acid fluorescence method. *Acta Physiol. Scand. (Suppl.)*, 412:1–48.
8. McGeer, E. G., Innanen, V. T., and McGeer, P. L. (1976): Evidence on the cellular localization of adenyl cyclase in the neostriatum. *Brain Res.*, 118:356–358.
9. Nishikori, K., Noshiro, O., Sano, K., and Maeno, H. (1980): Characterization, solubilization, and separation of two distinct dopamine receptors in canine caudate nucleus. *J. Biol. Chem.*, 255:10909–10915.
10. Palacios, J. M., Niehoff, D. L., and Kuhar, M. J. (1981): [$^3$H]spiperone binding sites in brain: Autoradiographic localization of multiple receptors. *Brain Res.*, 213:277–289.
11. Trabucchi, M., Longoni, R., Fresia, P., and Spano, P. F. (1975): Sulpiride: A study of the effects on dopamine receptors in rat neostriatum and limbic forebrain. *Life Sci.*, 17:1551–1556.
12. Weber, K., and Osborn, M. (1969): The reliability of molecular weight determinations by dodecyl sulfate-polyacrylamide gel electrophoresis. *J. Biol. Chem.*, 244:4406–4412.

*Molecular Pharmacology of Neurotransmitter Receptors*, edited by T. Segawa et al.
Raven Press, New York © 1983.

# Demonstration of a Complex Subunit Composition of a Unitary Dopamine Receptor: Effects of Lesions and Proteolytic Enzymes on Stereospecific Binding

J. E. Leysen, W. Gommeren, and P. Van Gompel

*Department of Biochemical Pharmacology, Janssen Pharmaceutica Research Laboratories, B-2340 Beerse, Belgium*

Many different hypotheses regarding the multiplicity of dopamine receptors have been put forward from *in vitro* binding studies with different labeled dopamine agonists and antagonists (2,13). In contrast to the hypothesis that $^3$H-dopamine antagonists and $^3$H-dopamine agonists would label distinct dopamine receptors, called $D_2$- and $D_3$-receptors (13), we proposed a concept of a unitary dopamine receptor, which probably contains different subunit sites, and which is localized on different types of membranes and cells (8). Our hypothesis is based on the finding of an obvious relationship between the binding affinities of a wide variety of drugs for $^3$H-agonist and $^3$H-antagonist labeled sites in the striatum and limbic areas of rat brain and on the concomitant distribution of the stereospecific binding sites at regional, cellular, and subcellular level. Nevertheless, competition in binding between agonists and antagonists revealed irregular binding equilibrium patterns, and optimal assay conditions for measuring $^3$H-agonist and $^3$H-antagonist binding appeared to be different (10).

In the described study, the concomitant distribution of $^3$H-agonist and $^3$H-antagonist binding sites is further scrutinized and the neuronal localization of stereospecific binding sites recovered in different subcellular fractions is investigated. To that purpose, unilateral striatal kainic acid lesions and cortical ablations were performed in rats, and the effects on binding parameters of $^3$H-apomorphine and $^3$H-spiperone were examined in membranes of microsomal and mitochondrial fractions.

To get more insight in the subunit composition of the dopamine receptor, a new approach using enzymatic treatment of striatal membranes was applied. In these experiments $^3$H-*N,n*-propylnorapomorphine (NPA) and $^3$H-haloperidol were used to label the stereospecific sites. NPA and apomorphine belong to the same group of catechol-like dopamine agonists, but NPA shows more potent agonistic activity (1) and proved to be a purer and more stable $^3$H-ligand. Haloperidol and spiperone are both butyrophenone-like dopamine antagonists, but haloperidol shows a greater selectivity for dopamine receptors than spiperone, which also interacts with serotonin receptors.

## MATERIALS AND METHODS

### Neuronal Lesions

Female Wistar rats (150 g) were anaesthetized with 2.5 mg/kg (i.p.) alfentanil, a short acting narcotic analgesic, kainic acid (2 µg/0.5 µl solution in saline buffered at pH 5–6) was injected over a 5-min period into the right striatum (coordinates A = 8.0, V = +1.4, L = 3.0 according to König and Klippel (6) using a microsyringe mounted on a David Kopf stereotaxic apparatus. Three groups of 40 rats were treated on different days. The animals were housed in groups of 10. Up to 4 days after the operation, the animals received Bactocilline (27 mg/kg i.m./day), and 7 ml Ringer solution was administered subcutaneously twice daily. At day 21 after the operation the animals were sacrificed by decapitation, brains removed from the skull and striata were rapidly dissected.

For cortical ablation the right front side of the skull was removed and the right cortex was sucked off from the prefrontal cortex to the bregma. Bleeding was controlled by gently pressing oxidized cellulose on the wound. After the operation animals were kept in individual cages for 5 days [a sufficiently long period to cause reduction of striatal $^3$H-haloperidol binding (12)] and were then sacrificed.

The controlateral side was used as control in both experiments.

Earlier studies on total membrane fractions had shown no difference in $^3$H-ligand binding between controlateral sides of lesioned rats, of sham-operated rats and of naive rats (8).

### Tissue Preparation

For lesioned animals, striata were rapidly dissected after decapitation; striata from the control or lesioned side were respectively pooled to form six groups of 11 to 13 kainic acid lesioned rats and three groups of 5 cortical ablated rats. Striata of naive female Wistar rats (150 g) were also freshly used. Preparations of the washed total particulate membrane fractions and washed membranes of various subcellular fractions were essentially as described in Leysen (8) and Leysen and Gommeren (10).

### Trypsin Pretreatment of Membranes

Unless otherwise indicated, membranes were suspended in Tris-EDTA buffer (see below) (12.5 mg tissue/ml). Trypsin was added to the ice-cold suspension followed either by immediate centrifugation at 0°C or by incubation at 37°C and then centrifugation. Thereafter, membranes were routinely washed once by resuspension in Tris buffer and centrifugation. Other membrane washings are indicated in the text. Controls were systematically run through a similar pretreatment procedure without trypsin.

The proteolytic degradation of $N^\alpha$-benzoyl-*L*-arginin-ethylester hydrochloride by trypsin in the Tris-EDTA buffer amounted to 0.066 µmoles·min$^{-1}$·U$^{-1}$ at 25°C; 1 U trypsin represented 4.1 µg protein.

## Binding Assay

Final membrane pellets were suspended in Tris buffers of varying composition as indicated. Composition of incubation mixtures is described in legends to tables and figures. Stereospecific binding is uniformly taken as the difference between total binding and nonspecific binding at 1000-fold excess (+)-butaclamol over the $^3$H-ligand. Incubations were run for 30 min at 25°C or 37°C, stopped by rapid filtration through glass fiber filters and completed as previously described (10).

## $^3$H-Ligands (Usual Concentration in Binding Assay)

$^3$H-Apomorphine (APO) (4 nM); (30 Ci/mmole, New England Nuclear); $^3$H-N-prophylnorapomorphine (NPAh) (0.5 nM); (58.5 Ci/mmole, New England Nuclear); $^3$H-haloperidol (2 nM); (12 Ci/mmole, IRE, Belgium); $^3$H-spiperone (25.5 Ci/mmole, New England Nuclear).

## Buffers

Tris-EDTA: Tris-HC1, 15 mM, pH 7.5, 1 mM EDTA, 0.01% ascorbic acid; Tris: Tris-HC1, 50 mM, pH 7.6; Tris-SALT: Tris-HC1, 50 mM, pH 7.6, 120 mM NaC1, 5 mM KC1, 2 mM CaCl$_2$, 1 mM MgCl$_2$, 0.1% ascorbic acid, 1 µM pargyline.

## RESULTS

### Lesion Studies

Twenty-one days after unilateral intrastriatal injection of kainic acid in rats, $^3$H-spiperone and $^3$H-apomorphine binding were investigated in membranes from the microsomal and the mitochondrial fraction of striata at the lesioned and the control site. The microsomal and the mitochondrial fractions were obtained each time from the same pool of striata. Scatchard plots of stereospecific binding to the microsomal membranes are shown in Fig. 1 and those of stereospecific binding to membranes from the mitochondrial fraction are presented in Fig. 2 (page 152). $^3$H-Spiperone binding, measured in its optimal assay conditions using Tris-SALT buffer, reveals linear Scatchard plots in all conditions; calculated $K_D$ and $B_{max}$ values, averaged for six independent experiments, are presented in the legends to Figs. 1 and 2. The binding affinity of $^3$H-spiperone is not affected by the lesion. The $B_{max}$ values in membranes at the lesioned side are reduced by 62% in membranes from the microsomal fraction and only by 30% in membranes from the mitochondrial fraction. It was noted that the reduction in binding measured at all $^3$H-spiperone concentrations separately, was over the entire concentration similar to the reduction in $B_{max}$.

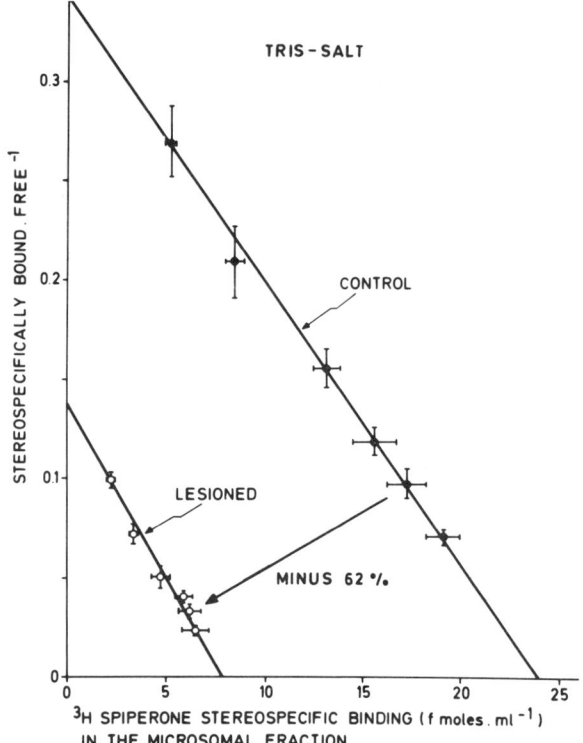
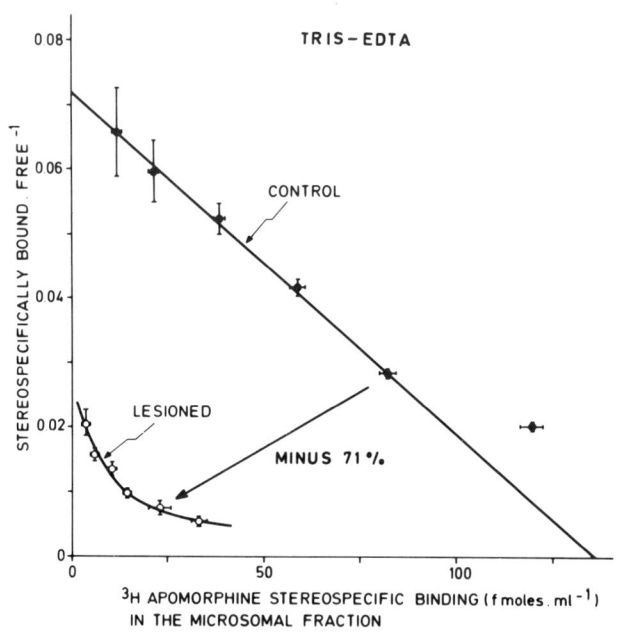

$^3$H-Apomorphine binding, assayed in its optimal conditions in Tris-EDTA buffer, revealed less linear Scatchard plots (Figs. 1 and 2). Some linearity was only obtained in microsomal membranes from striata at the control side, which is the tissue with the highest density in stereospecific binding sites. In the other membrane preparations (microsomal membranes at the lesioned side and membranes from the mitochondrial fraction) the amount of stereospecific binding is low compared with the high nonspecific binding. In these situations, systemic experimental errors or variations in total and nonspecific binding can have considerable effects on the appearance of Scatchard plots, therefore we think it is inappropriate to speculate on the nonlinearity of the plots. For evaluation of the effect of the lesion the reduction in stereospecific binding at all the $^3$H-apomorphine concentrations was checked. The reduction in binding at the lesioned side was similar over the entire concentration range and amounted to an average of 71% in the microsomal membranes and to an average of 40% in membranes from the mitochondrial fraction.

Biochemical measurements in the striata at the lesioned and the control side revealed in striata at the lesioned side a significant reduction by 43% of choline acetyl transferase (CAT) activity and by 38% of glutamic acid decarboxylase (GAD) activity. The protein content was reduced by 40% in the microsomal fraction and only by 10% in the mitochondrial fraction. No significant change in dopamine content was seen.

Similar investigations were done in striata of rats 5 days after unilateral cortical ablations, but $^3$H-ligands were used at a fixed concentration (0.25 nM for $^3$H-spiperone, 3 nM for $^3$H-apomorphine). In membranes from the striatal microsomal fraction, a significant reduction by 22% ($p < 0.05$) in stereospecific binding at the lesioned side, as compared with the control side, was found with both $^3$H-spiperone and $^3$H-apomorphine. With none of both ligands, a significant alteration in binding was observed in membranes from the mitochondrial fraction. Dopamine content,

---

FIG. 1. Scatchard plots of stereospecific $^3$H-spiperone binding (**above**) and stereospecific $^3$H-apomorphine binding (**below**) in microsomal membranes of rat striata at the control and lesioned side, 21 days after unilateral antrastriatal injection of kainic acid. $^3$H-Spiperone binding (0.025–0.3 nM) was assayed at 37°C in an incubation volume of 5.5 ml of Tris-SALT buffer containing 1.14 mg wet weight tissue/ml. $^3$H-Apomorphine binding (0.2–6 nM) was assayed at 25°C in an incubation volume of 1.1 ml in Tris-EDTA buffer containing 9.09 mg wet weight tissue/ml. Stereospecific binding (BOUND) was taken as the difference between total $^3$H-ligand binding and nonspecific binding in the presence of 1000-fold excess (+)-butaclamol. The free ligand concentration (FREE) was taken as the difference between the initial $^3$H-ligand concentration and the concentration totally bound. Points ± SEM represent mean values of six independent experiments. For linear Scatchard plots, binding parameters were calculated by linear regression analysis (methods of least squares) for separate experiments. Meaned values of six independent experiments are: $^3$H-spiperone, control: $K_D = 0.074 ± 0.005$ nM, $B_{max} = 21.5 ± 0.9$ fmoles/mg tissue, lesioned: $K_D = 0.063 ± 0.005$ nM, $B_{max} = 7.2 ± 0.8$ fmoles/mg tissue; $^3$H-apomorphine: control: $K_D = 2.3 ± 0.5$ nM, $B_{max} = 16.7 ± 1.8$ fmoles/mg tissue. The reduction in stereospecific binding in microsomal membranes at the lesioned side was similar at all ligand concentrations and amounted to 62 ± 1% for $^3$H-spiperone binding and to 71 ± 1% for $^3$H-apomorphine binding.

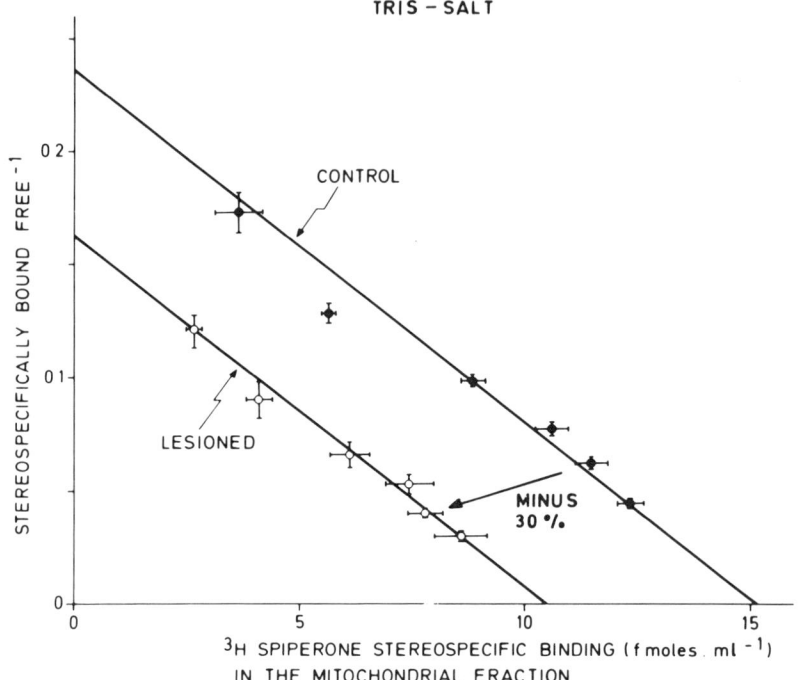

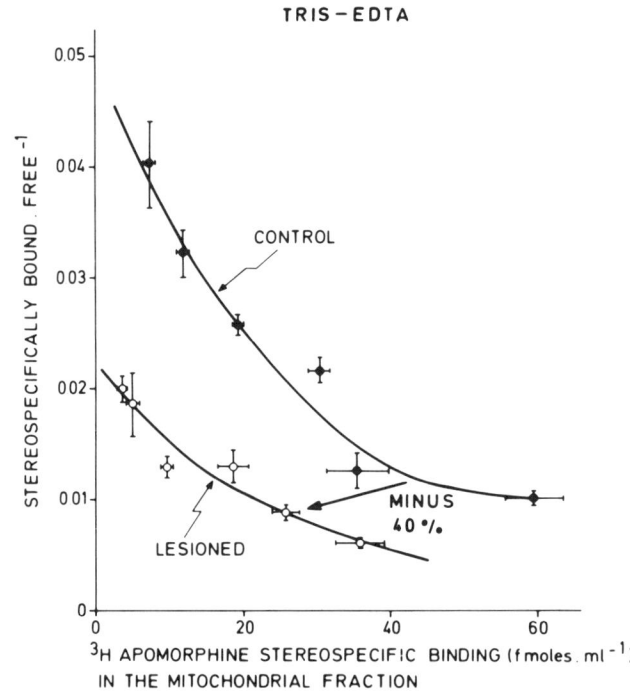

CAT activity and GAD activity in the striata were not affected by the lesion, demonstrating that the striata were apparently not injured by the ablation.

## Investigation of Enzyme Treatment

Microsomal membranes of rat striata were briefly pretreated with trypsin at 0°C (i.e., addition of the enzyme to the membrane suspension at 0°C followed by immediate centrifugation and washing) and thereafter stereospecific binding of $^3$H-NPA and $^3$H-haloperidol was measured. Table 1 shows results on binding assayed in various buffers after membrane pretreatment with trypsin in Tris-EDTA buffer in the absence and the presence of 120 mM NaCl. A marked reduction of stereospecific binding of both $^3$H-NPA and $^3$H-haloperidol was observed when binding assays were carried out in Tris-EDTA buffer. No effect of the trypsin pretreatment was apparent when the binding assays were carried out afterwards in the presence of 120 mM NaCl or SALT. Nevertheless, the reduction in binding in the Tris-EDTA buffer was seen after pretreatment with trypsin in the absence and the presence of 120 mM NaCl; in the latter case, the effect of the enzyme was only somewhat less pronounced.

Prolonged preincubation of the microsomal membranes with trypsin up to 1 hr at 37°C did not cause a marked further decrease in binding, as can be inferred from the data shown in Table 2. A small time-dependent effect was found following pretreatment in the absence of NaCl and was similarly observed in binding assays in Tris-EDTA and in Tris-SALT.

The pronounced reduction in stereospecific binding observed in binding assays in monovalent-ion-poor buffers, after brief trypsin pretreatment, was not reversed by extensive washing of the membranes with buffers containing 120 mM NaCl or KCl.

Since the most prominent effect of trypsin occurred very rapidly and additional time-dependent effects were very low, the trypsin effect was further explored by direct addition of the trypsin in the incubation medium during the binding assay.

Figure 3 shows inhibition curves of trypsin for $^3$H-NPA binding measured in Tris-EDTA and Tris buffer without additives and in the presence of NaCl or KCl or SALT. It is obvious that inhibition of binding occurs only in binding assays in Tris or Tris-EDTA buffer without additives. In the presence of 120 mM NaCl or KCl or SALT, no inhibition of binding by trypsin was seen.

Figures 4 and 5 show Scatchard plots of stereospecific $^3$H-NPA and $^3$H-haloperidol binding, respectively, to striatal microsomal membranes measured in the presence

---

**FIG. 2.** Similar experiments as described in Fig. 1, but using membranes of the mitochondrial fraction obtained from the same striata as used for experiments in Fig. 1. Calculated binding parameters are for $^3$H-spiperone: control: $K_D$ = 0.076 ± 0.005 nM, $B_{max}$ = 14.2 ± 0.4 fmoles/mg tissue, lesioned: $K_D$ = 0.070 ± 0.005 nM, $B_{max}$ = 9.5 ± 0.9 fmoles/mg tissue (mean values of six independent experiments). The reduction in stereospecific binding in membranes from the mitochondrial fraction at the lesioned side was similar at all ligand concentrations and amounted to 30 ± 1% for $^3$H-spiperone binding and to 40 ± 5% for $^3$H-apomorphine binding.

TABLE 1. *Effects of brief pretreatment with trypsin at 0°C of striatal microsomal membranes in the absence (A) and in the presence (B) of 120 mM NaCl on stereospecific binding of $^3$H-NPA (0.5 nM) and $^3$H-haloperidol (2 nM) assayed in various buffers*

| | Binding: fmoles/mg tiss. for controls, % of controls for trypsin-treated | | | | | |
|---|---|---|---|---|---|---|
| | $^3$H-NPA | | | $^3$H-Haloperidol | | |
| | Tris-EDTA | Tris-EDTA 120 mM NaCl | Tris-SALT | Tris-EDTA | Tris-EDTA 120 mM NaCl | Tris-SALT |
| A. Pretreatment in Tris-EDTA | | | | | | |
| Trypsin | | | | | | |
| 0 (control) | 6.6 ± 0.9 | 4.1 ± 0.7 | 3.9 ± 0.2 | 21.1 ± 0.8 | 10.8 ± 1.2 | 9.5 ± 1.4 |
| 0.01 U/ml | 41% | 105% | 103% | 64% | 111% | 104% |
| 0.1 U/ml | 18% | 85% | 92% | 37% | 103% | 105% |
| B. Pretreatment in Tris-EDTA + 120 mM NaCl | | | | | | |
| Trypsin | | | | | | |
| 0 (control) | 6.0 ± 1.0 | | 6.3 ± 0.5 | 17.9 ± 0.2 | | 9.5 ± 1.4 |
| 0.01 U/ml | 83% | | 99% | 87% | | 106% |
| 0.1 U/ml | 33% | | 94% | 50% | | 113% |

TABLE 2. *Effects of time of pretreatment with trypsin at 37°C of striatal microsomal membranes in the absence (A) and in the presence (B) of NaCl on stereospecific binding of $^3$H-NPA (0.5 nM) and $^3$H-haloperidol (2 nM) assayed in Tris-EDTA and Tris-SALT buffer*

| | | Percentage of binding in trypsin pretreated versus similarly pretreated membranes in the absence of trypsin | | | |
|---|---|---|---|---|---|
| | | $^3$H-NPA | | $^3$H-Haloperidol | |
| | Time (min) | Tris-EDTA (%) | Tris-SALT (%) | Tris-EDTA (%) | Tris-SALT (%) |
| A. Pretreatment in Tris-EDTA | | | | | |
| Trypsin | | | | | |
| 0.01 U/ml | 0 | 41 | 103 | 64 | 104 |
| | 30 | 31 | 77 | 37 | 94 |
| | 60 | 22 | 62 | 38 | 67 |
| 0.1 U/ml | 0 | 18 | 92 | 37 | 105 |
| | 30 | 14 | 62 | 25 | 80 |
| | 60 | 12 | 44 | 16 | 54 |
| B. Pretreatment in Tris-EDTA + 120 mM NaCl | | | | | |
| Trypsin | | | | | |
| 0.01 U/ml | 0 | 83 | 99 | 87 | 106 |
| | 30 | 65 | 110 | 72 | 104 |
| | 60 | 78 | 100 | 72 | 105 |
| 0.1 U/ml | 0 | 33 | 94 | 50 | 113 |
| | 30 | 40 | 102 | 43 | 99 |
| | 60 | 44 | 79 | 48 | 106 |

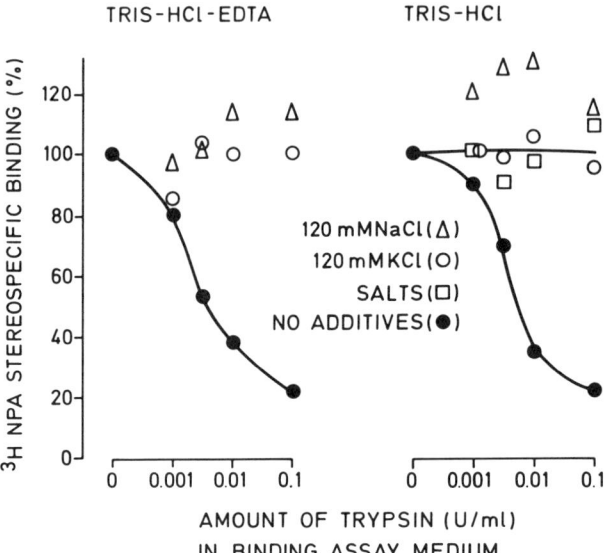

**FIG. 3.** Inhibition by trypsin directly added into the incubation medium of ³H-NPA binding to striatal microsomal membranes assayed in Tris-EDTA (a) and Tris-buffer (b) containing various additives as indicated. The incubation volume was 2.2 ml and contained 10.33 mg wet weight tissue/ml.

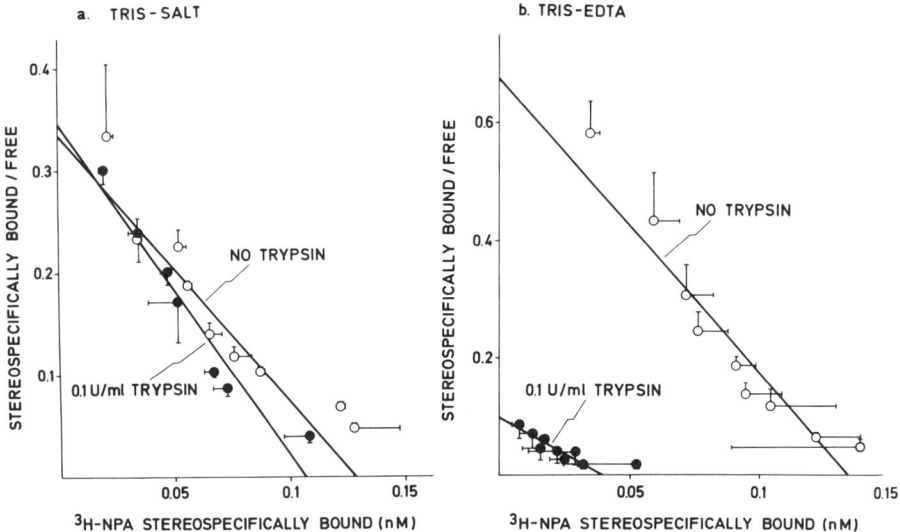

**FIG. 4.** Scatchard plots of stereospecific ³H-NPA binding (0.1–3.2 nM) to striatal microsomal membranes in Tris-SALT and Tris-EDTA buffer in the absence and the presence of trypsin. The incubation volume was 2.2 ml and contained 10.33 mg wet weight tissue/ml. Points are mean values of two independent experiments in duplicate. Binding parameters are presented in Table 3.

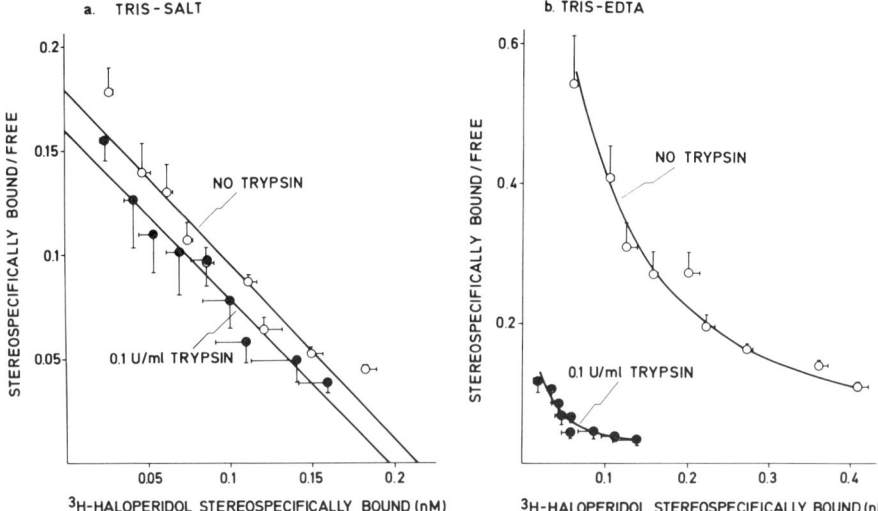

**FIG. 5.** Scatchard plots of stereospecific $^3$H-haloperidol binding (0.2–4.4 nM) to striatal microsomal membranes in Tris-SALT and Tris-EDTA buffer in the absence and the presence of trypsin. The incubation volume was 2.2 ml and contained 10.33 mg wet weight tissue/ml. Points are mean values of two independent experiments in duplicate. Binding parameters are presented in Table 3.

TABLE 3. *Binding parameters of $^3$H-NPA and $^3$H-haloperidol binding to membranes from microsomal (P) and mitochondrial (M + L) fractions of rat striatum measured in different buffers in the absence and the presence of 0.1 U/ml trypsin[a]*

| | | Tris-SALT | | Tris-EDTA | |
|---|---|---|---|---|---|
| | | $K_D$ (nM) | $B_{max}$ (fmoles/mg tiss.) | $K_D$ (nM) | $B_{max}$ (fmoles/mg tiss.) |
| NPA | | | | | |
| P | No trypsin | 0.37 ± 0.15 | 10.2 ± 0.6 | 0.14 ± 0.01 | 11.7 ± 0.4 |
| | Trypsin | 0.66 ± 0.47 | 11.0 ± 1.5 | 0.25 ± 0.04 | 3.1 ± 0.3 |
| M + L | No trypsin | 0.46 ± 0.16 | 14 ± 3 | 0.20 ± 0.07 | 13 ± 5 |
| | Trypsin | 0.29 ± 0.02 | 10 ± 1 | 0.33 ± 0.01 | 3.5 ± 1.5 |
| Haloperidol | | | | | |
| P | No trypsin | 1.25 ± 0.16 | 21 ± 1 | curved plot mean reduction | |
| | Trypsin | 1.30 ± 0.05 | 20 ± 3 | in binding: 69 ± 1% | |
| M + L | No trypsin | 1.23 ± 0.03 | 14 ± 4 | curved plot mean reduction | |
| | Trypsin | 1.95 ± 0.06 | 18 ± 3 | in binding: 64 ± 2% | |

[a] Scatchard plots for experiments with microsomal membranes are presented in Figs. 4 and 5. Experiments with membranes of the mitochondrial fractions were performed in exactly the same manner.

and the absence of trypsin in Tris-SALT and Tris-EDTA buffer. The derived binding parameters are presented in Table 3. Scatchard plots of $^3$H-NPA binding are linear in all conditions. Trypsin caused no effect on the binding measured in Tris-SALT buffer, but it reduced the $B_{max}$ value by 75% in Tris-EDTA buffer, the $K_D$ value was not significantly altered. The control experiments (no trypsin) revealed an apparently two times higher binding affinity of NPA for experiments in Tris-EDTA compared with Tris-SALT. The $B_{max}$ values in control assays were equal in both buffers. For $^3$H-haloperidol, Scatchard plots of stereospecific binding were linear in Tris-SALT buffer and no effect of trypsin was apparent. In Tris-EDTA buffer, Scatchard plots of stereospecific $^3$H-haloperidol binding were markedly curved in the absence and the presence of trypsin. In this buffer, trypsin produced an equal reduction in binding by 69% over the entire $^3$H-haloperidol concentration range. Completely similar findings were made in experiments using membranes from the mitochondrial fraction ($K_D$ and $B_{max}$ values are presented in Table 3, Scatchard plots are not shown).

Besides trypsin, other proteolytic and nonproteolytic enzymes were tested for their ability to inhibit $^3$H-NPA and $^3$H-haloperidol binding, assayed in Tris-EDTA and Tris-SALT buffer. Molar $IC_{50}$ values were derived from inhibition curves over enzyme concentrations between 1 and 1000 nM, and are shown in Table 4. None of the enzymes, except for the very basic lactoperoxidase, affected the binding assayed in Tris-SALT buffer. The serine-proteases, trypsin, and α-chymotrypsin, and the sulfhydryl-proteases, ficin and papain, revealed nanomolar $IC_{50}$ values for inhibition of $^3$H-NPA and $^3$H-haloperidol binding in Tris-EDTA buffer.

No inhibition of binding was caused by the proprotease, α-chymotrypsinogen, or proteases such as pepsin, carboxypeptidase, or collagenase. Also various non-proteolytic enzymes were ineffective.

## DISCUSSION

### Lesion Studies

Our investigations have shown that in rat striatum $^3$H-spiperone binding, measured in Tris-SALT buffer, and $^3$H-apomorphine binding, measured in Tris-EDTA buffer,

TABLE 4. *Inhibitory potency of enzymes ($IC_{50}$, nM) for stereospecific $^3$H-ligand binding to the rat striatal microsomal membranes*

| Enzymes | $^3$H-NPA (0.5 nM) binding in: | | $^3$H-Haloperidol (2 nM) binding in: | |
|---|---|---|---|---|
| | Tris-EDTA | Tris-SALT | Tris-EDTA | Tris-SALT |
| Trypsin | 1.3 | > 1,000 | 3.0 | > 1,000 |
| Ficin | 3.0 | > 1,000 | 2.8 | > 1,000 |
| Papain | 16 | 600 | 20 | > 1,000 |
| α-Chymotrypsin | 20 | > 1,000 | 32 | > 1,000 |
| Chymotrypsinogen-A | 2,000 | > 10,000 | 3,000 | > 10,000 |
| Pepsin | > 1,000 | > 10,000 | > 1,000 | > 1,000 |
| Collagenase | > 1,000 | > 1,000 | > 1,000 | > 1,000 |
| Carboxypeptidase-A | > 1,000 | > 1,000 | > 1,000 | > 1,000 |
| Lactoperoxidase | 200 | 140 | > 500 | > 500 |
| Catalase | > 1,000 | > 1,000 | > 1,000 | > 1,000 |
| Aldolase | > 500 | > 500 | > 500 | > 500 |
| Hyaluronidase | 6,000 | 17,000 | 17,000 | > 10,000 |

are similarly affected by striatal kainic acid lesions. It is, however, remarkable that the reduction in stereospecific binding of both ligands in membranes from the microsomal fraction is much more pronounced than the reduction in binding in membranes from the mitochondrial fraction. The parallelism in occurrence and reduction of the $^3$H-apomorphine and $^3$H-spiperone binding provides further evidence that agonist and antagonist binding sites occur concomitantly on different membranes. The findings described demonstrate that at least 60 to 70% of the receptors on membranes recovered in the microsomal fraction originate from intrastriatal neurons, which are destroyed by kainic acid. On the contrary, the major part of the receptors on membranes recovered in the mitochondrial fraction appear to originate from cellular structures, which are not affected by kainic acid. This suggests a different cellular origin for receptors in the microsomal and the mitochondrial fraction. It was a temptation to speculate that the receptors recovered in the mitochondrial fraction, which also contains synaptosomes, would represent dopamine receptors on corticostriatal afferents (12). However, this hypothesis is refuted by the lack of effect of cortical ablation on the stereospecific binding of $^3$H-apomorphine and $^3$H-spiperone to membranes of the mitochondrial fraction. It appears that dopamine receptors on corticostriatal afferents are also recovered in the microsomal fraction. These receptors represent approximately 22% of the total amount of dopamine receptors in this fraction, as shown by the reduction in binding after cortical ablation. The reduction in binding was again similar for $^3$H-apomorphine and $^3$H-spiperone, which further demonstrates the concomitant occurrence of the agonist and the antagonist binding sites; the cellular origin of the receptors in the mitochondrial fraction is still unknown. The above discussion is based on the parallelism in $^3$H-spiperone and $^3$H-apomorphine binding as regards detection in the different membrane preparations and degree of affection by the different lesions. We do not wish to speculate on the nonlinearity of Scatchard plots occasionally seen for $^3$H-apomorphine binding. Partly because of the reasons explained under Results and also because of the possible influence of surface phenomena, such as discussed previously (9,10).

## Investigation of Enzyme Treatment

An important observation in the investigations with enzymes is the marked and rapidly occurring inhibition by certain proteolytic enzymes, of stereospecific binding of $^3$H-NPA and $^3$H-haloperidol assayed in a monovalent-ion-poor buffer in contrast to a complete lack of effect of the enzymes in binding assays in the presence of monovalent ions. Inhibition of binding in a monovalent-ion-poor buffer is observed for the closely related serine proteases, trypsin and α-chymotrypsin (4,5) and of the sulfhydryl proteases, ficin and papain (3). The inhibition is enzyme-concentration dependent, it occurs readily at 0°C and is apparently not much further progressed by incubation at 37°C. The inhibition is irreversible by extensive membrane washing. An important observation is that when monovalent ions were present during the pretreatment of membranes with trypsin, the inhibition of binding measured afterwards in a monovalent-ion-poor buffer was still observed. This proves that the monovalent ions do not prevent the interaction between trypsin and the binding sites. The combination of the differentially observed effects of proteolytic enzymes in certain assay media and the influence of the monovalent ions suggest that two different types of stereospecific binding sites related to the dopamine receptor exist. One type of site is inhibited by the above-mentioned proteolytic enzymes; these sites are exposed for binding in the absence of monovalent ions, and they bind dopamine agonists and antagonists as well. These sites are denoted as protease-sensitive sites. The effect of the enzymes on binding to these sites is a reduction in the number of sites, which is equally observed in $^3$H-NPA and $^3$H-haloperidol binding. The mechanism of the major effect is apparently not by proteolytic breakdown of the receptor sites. It is supposed that it is due to the formation of a strong complex between the enzymes and probably a peptide chain of the protease-sensitive receptor sites. Such a complexation is to be compared to the well-known complexation between the proteolytic enzymes and the ubiquitous peptide-like protease inhibitions (7). The mechanism of the enzyme effect is discussed extensively elsewhere (11).

The second type of binding site is not affected by the proteolytic enzymes and becomes exposed for binding of dopamine agonists and antagonists in the presence of high concentrations of monovalent ions (120 mM NaCl or KCl or SALT). These sites are further called the protease-insensitive sites.

Protease-sensitive and protease-insensitive sites occur on membranes recovered in both microsomal and mitochondrial fractions and they show prominent common binding characteristics. They are both stereospecific and show high binding affinity for haloperidol and NPA. Preliminary observations revealed that $^3$H-apomorphine and $^3$H-spiperone binding are affected in the same way by the enzymes as $^3$H-NPA and $^3$H-haloperidol binding. Despite the major common features of the protease-sensitive and the protease-insensitive sites, the analysis in Scatchard plots of $^3$H-NPA and $^3$H-haloperidol binding in the buffers, which expose the sites respectively, revealed certain apparent differences in binding properties. From the linear Scatchard plots of $^3$H-NPA binding it appeared that the maximal number of protease-sensitive and protease-insensitive sites are approximately equal in both the microsomal and the mitochondrial fraction. NPA shows a somewhat higher binding affinity for the protease-sensitive than for the protease-insensitive sites. More marked differences in binding properties of haloperidol in the two buffers were noted. Scatchard plots of haloperidol binding are linear in the Tris-SALT buffer, but markedly curved in the Tris-EDTA buffer. This change in appearance of the Scatchard plots in different assay buffers is in agreement with previous observations in binding studies with $^3$H-spiperone in rat striatum. On that occasion, the contribution of surface phenomena on the binding equilibrium between ligands in solution and membrane micelles was discussed (9,10). It was argued that surface phenomena can considerably influence the appearance of Scatchard plots, especially for lipophilic and strongly surface active compounds such as haloperidol. Alterations in ionic strength of the medium, such as between the Tris-EDTA and the Tris-SALT buffer, will influence the surface activity of haloperidol and hence also the binding equilibrium. Thus, it is not yet possible to evaluate precisely the detailed differences in binding characteristics between the protease-sensitive and the protease-insensitive sites. More extensive research using a greater variety in buffers and investigation of binding affinities of several dopamine agonists and antagonists is required.

A pertinent question following the demonstration of protease-sensitive and protease-insensitive sites is whether they form part of the same dopamine receptor-macromolecular-complex or whether they represent distinct dopamine receptors. Indications about the localization of the binding sites can be derived from combining the results from the lesion studies and the investigations of binding and enzyme effects in different subcellular particles. In the above-described lesion studies, $^3$H-apomorphine binding was measured in Tris-EDTA buffer, which implies that it represented binding to the protease-sensitive sites. Otherwise, $^3$H-spiperone binding was assayed in Tris-SALT buffer, which means that in these assays the protease-insensitive sites were regarded. It can be inferred that the protease-sensitive and protease-insensitive sites are in the same way affected by the kainic acid lesions and cortical ablations. This indicates that they occur concomitantly on different types of membranes and neurons. Therefore it is reasonable to hypothesize that the protease-sensitive and protease-insensitive sites form part of the same unitary dopamine receptor complex. The role of monovalent ions lies apparently in the differential exposure of the sites.

By putting together findings from lesion studies and enzymatic treatment and by investigating the binding of several labeled ligands in different subcellular fractions and in several assay media, some insight could be achieved into the complex subunit composition of the dopamine receptor. It has appeared that simple analysis of binding isotherms or inhibition curves according to laws of mass action are inadequate to provide reliable information on the receptor properties and composition.

## ACKNOWLEDGMENT

This work was supported in part by a grant from I.W.O.N.L.

## REFERENCES

1. Canon, J. G., Costall, B., Laduron, P. M., Leysen, J. E., and Naylor, R. J. (1978): Effects of some derivatives of 2-aminotetralin on dopamine-sensitive adenylate cyclase and on the binding of [$^3$H]-haloperidol to neuroleptic receptors in the rat striatum. *Biochem. Pharmacol.*, 27:1417–1420.
2. Creese, I., and Sibley, D. R. (1979): Radioligand binding studies: evidence for multiple dopamine receptors. *Commun. Psychopharmacol.*, 3:385–395.
3. Glazer, A. N., and Smith, E. L. (1971): Papain and other plant sulfhydryl proteolytic enzymes. In: *The Enzymes, Hydrolysis Peptide Bounds, Vol. III*, edited by P. D. Boyer, pp. 502–505. Academic Press, New York, London.
4. Hess, G. P. (1971): Chymotrypsin—Chemical properties and catalysis. In: *The Enzymes, Hydrolysis Peptide Bounds, Vol. III*, edited by P. D. Boyer, pp. 213–222. Academic Press, New York, London.
5. Keil, B. (1971): Trypsin. In: *The Enzymes, Hydrolysis Peptide Bounds, Vol. III*, edited by P. D. Boyer, pp. 250–252. Academic Press, New York, London.
6. König, G. F. R., and Klippel, R. A. (1963): The rat brain. A stereotaxic atlas of the forebrain and lower parts of the brain stem. Williams and Wilkins, Baltimore.

7. Laskowski, M., Jr., and Sealock, R. W. (1971): Protein proteinase inhibitors—Molecular aspects. In: *The Enzymes, Hydrolysis Peptide Bounds, Vol. III*, edited by P. D. Boyer, pp. 376–383. Academic Press, New York, London.
8. Leysen, J. E. (1979): Unitary dopaminergic receptors composed of cooperatively linked agonist and antagonist sub-unit binding sites. *Commun. Psychopharmacol.*, 3:397–410.
9. Leysen, J. E. (1980): Localization and identification of multiple dopamine receptors: surface phenomena and anomalous kinetics of $^3$H-spiperone and $^3$H-apomorphine binding in rat striatum. In: *Psychopharmacology and Biochemistry of Neurotransmitter Receptors*, edited by Yamamura, Olsen, and Usdin, pp. 435–454. Elsevier/North-Holland, New York.
10. Leysen, J. E., and Gommeren, W. (1981): Optimal conditions for $^3$H-apomorphine binding and anomalous equilibrium binding of $^3$H-apomorphine and $^3$H-spiperone to rat striatal membranes: involvement of surface phenomena versus multiple binding sites. *J. Neurochem.*, 36:201–219.
11. Leysen, J. E., and Van Gompel, P. (1981): Effects of proteolytic enzymes and monovalent ions demonstrate protease-sensitive and protease-insensitive stereospecific binding sites on dopaminergic receptors in rat striatum. *Biochem. Pharmacol. (submitted)*.
12. Schwarcz, R., Creese, I., Coyle, G. T., and Snyder, S. H. (1978): Dopamine receptors localized on cerebral cortical afferents to rat corpus striatum. *Nature*, 271:766–768.
13. Seeman, P. (1980): Brain dopamine receptors. *Pharmacol. Rev.*, 32(3):229–313.

*Molecular Pharmacology of Neurotransmitter Receptors*, edited by T. Segawa et al.
Raven Press, New York © 1983.

# Two Distinct Classes of Dopamine Receptor Mediating Actions of Antipsychotics: Binding and Behavioral Studies

P. Sokoloff, M. P. Martres, *P. Protais, *J. Costentin, and J. C. Schwartz

*Unité 109 de Neurobiologie, Centre Paul Broca, rue d'Alésia 75014 Paris, France; *UER de Médecine et de Pharmacie, 76800 St. Etienne du Rouvray, France*

Neuroleptics are agents that antagonize the behavioral actions of dopamine (DA) mimetics, such as apomorphine (10,29,32), and increase DA turnover (7) in response to DA receptor blockade. These agents are currently used to alleviate schizophrenic symptoms but produce, to a variable degree, extrapyramidal motor side effects. Hence, there is considerable interest in isolating the DA receptors that are responsible for the various effects of neuroleptics—in behavioral and biochemical events in animals, for understanding mechanisms of DA neurotransmission, as well as in clinics for devising more selective therapeutical agents.

A large body of evidence now supports the existence of multiple DA receptors as possible sites of action for DA agonists and antagonists. Four classes of putative DA receptors displaying distinct pharmacological specificities have been identified recently in brain tissues either by measuring the stimulation of a specific adenylyl cyclase (D-1) or by studies with radioligands (D-2, D-3, and D-4) (20,37,38,40).

The criteria for identifying specific sites of neuroleptic actions include sensitivity to nanomolar concentrations, since therapeutic concentrations of the neuroleptics in plasma water are between 0.1 and 50 nM (36). The D-1 receptor is not likely to represent the common site of action for neuroleptics. Its pharmacological specificity does not correlate with biological actions of neuroleptics since agents like the butyrophenones, which are among the most potent in clinics, are active on the cyclase activity at concentrations in the micromolar range *in vitro* (9,19) and only at very high doses *in vivo* (28).

Furthermore, sulpiride, an antipsychotic drug, seems inactive as antagonist of the DA-stimulated cyclase activity (41). Also D-3 binding sites, which are likely to represent autoreceptors, are poorly recognized by all tested neuroleptics (micromolar affinities) (36–38,40) and therefore appear not to represent a site of action for these compounds.

In contrast, D-2 and D-4 binding sites, although pharmacologically distinct, are both recognized with high affinity (nanomolar range) by neuroleptics (38), and are therefore likely to represent the major sites of action. However, their identity as receptors remains putative as long as it cannot be demonstrated that they mediate biological responses. Because responses to dopamine in the central nervous system cannot yet be easily quantified in *in vitro* models (except those mediated by D-1 receptors), our approach has been to compare the pharmacology of D-2 and D-4 binding sites with that of carefully selected behavioral responses to apomorphine in rats, which are easily quantifiable.

## DEFINITION AND COMPARISON OF D-2 AND D-4 BINDING SITES

$^3$H-Butyrophenones such as $^3$H-haloperidol or $^3$H-spiperone have been used in most laboratories to study DA binding sites. However, they seem to present drawbacks such as relatively high nonspecific binding for the former and significant binding to non-DA receptors for the latter (12,14,18,23). We have recently developed the use of $^3$H-domperidone as a ligand with selectivity for DA receptors and low nonspecific binding (5). These properties are obviously critical in a study aimed at the distinction of subclasses of binding sites. The observation that prompted the distinction of two neuroleptic binding sites is that apomorphine and dopamine inhibited $^3$H-domperidone binding in a clearly biphasic manner (Fig. 1).

The Scatchard representations of these curves (38) showed that the high-affinity and low-affinity components for apomorphine and DA have similar capacities.

The plateau observed in these inhibition curves (Fig. 1) is not consistent with the idea that occupation of $^3$H-domperidone binding sites by agonists might progressively shift these sites into a state of low affinity for the agonists: this could have only resulted in a stretched out but monophasic inhibition curve (1). It is, on the contrary, consistent with the interpretation already suggested (4,6) that two classes of binding sites can be distinguished. The first one, which we call D-2, is characterized by a high affinity for apomorphine and DA ($IC_{50}$ = 5 and 35 nM, respectively). The second one, which we call D-4, is less readily recognized by apomorphine and DA ($IC_{50}$ = 790 nM and 14 µM, respectively).

The high discriminating property of apomorphine allowed us to use it for measuring separately the binding to D-2 sites and to D-4 sites by determining the fraction of $^3$H-domperidone binding inhibited either by 20 nM apomorphine (binding to D-2 sites) or by 50 µM apomorphine (binding to D-2 + D-4 sites).

In addition, the high affinity of apomorphine for D-2 sites suggested that these sites might also be labeled with $^3$H-apomorphine. We actually demonstrated that D-2 binding sites, evidenced as a fraction of $^3$H-domperidone binding, were identical to a fraction of $^3$H-apomorphine binding as indicated by their identical capacities, localizations or pharmacological specificities, as well as by the similar effects of both guanylnucleotides and heat exposure (38). Therefore, D-2 sites can be studied using either $^3$H-apomorphine (Table 1) or $^3$H-domperidone (Fig. 2) as ligand and their properties compared to those of D-4 sites labeled with $^3$H-domperidone (Table 1).

D-2 and D-4 binding sites are present in similar proportion only in brain regions where the density of DA innervation is high, as in the case of striatum, nucleus

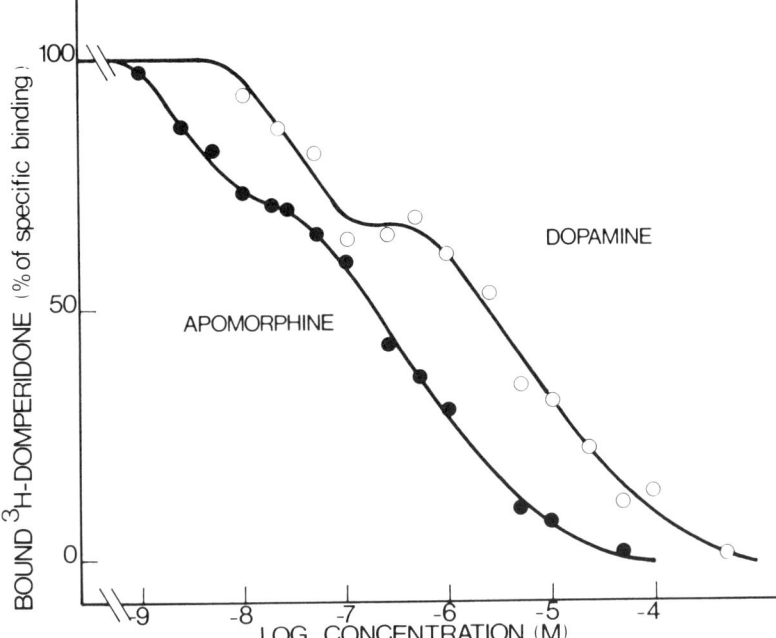

**FIG. 1.** Inhibition of ³H-domperidone binding to a particulate fraction of rat striatum. Striata were homogenized in 50 mM Tris-HCl buffer, pH 7.4. The pellet obtained after two successive centrifugations (5.10³ $g$ × min and 2.10⁵ $g$ × min, respectively) was incubated 12 min at 37°C. After centrifugation, membranes were resuspended in 50 mM Tris-HCl buffer containing 120 mM NaCl, 5 mM KCl, 1 mM CaCl₂, 1 mM MgCl₂, 0.1% ascorbic acid, and 10 μM pargyline. Following a 20-min preincubation, membranes were incubated for 30 min at 30°C with 4.5 nM ³H-domperidone (24.6 Ci.mmole⁻¹, IRE Belgium) and apomorphine and dopamine in increasing concentrations. Values are expressed as percentage of specific binding (100% corresponds to 343 ± 24 fmol.mg protein⁻¹) and are the mean of six to nine determinations.

accumbens, and olfactory tubercules (38). D-2 sites are mostly present on intrinsic neurons within the striatum, as indicated by their 57% decrease following intrastriatal injection of kainate and by their 39% increase after 6-OHDA-induced degeneration of DA neurons. These findings suggest that D-2 binding sites represent postsynaptic DA receptors exhibiting denervation hypersensitivity (4,13,27,34). The number of D-4 sites is modified in the same direction, but to a lesser extent by these lesions: 17% after kainate and 17% after 6-OHDA. This indicates that D-4 binding sites are mostly present on extrinsic neurons, probably on corticostriatal terminals where ³H-haloperidol binding sites were identified (35).

Addition of GTP in the incubation medium dramatically reduces the binding to D-2 sites whereas binding to D-4 sites is apparently increased. In fact, when measured solely with ³H-domperidone as ligand, the total specific binding (D-2 + D-4) is unchanged: the decrease in number of D-2 binding sites is exactly compensated (in fmol.mg protein⁻¹) by an increase in the apparent number of D-4 sites (38). The effect of an exposure to a moderate heat (45°C) is very similar:

TABLE 1. *Comparison of properties of D-2 and D-4 binding sites*

|  | D-2 binding sites[a] | D-4 binding sites[b] |
|---|---|---|
| Capacity in the striatum (fmol.mg prot.$^{-1}$) | 126 ± 11 | 203 ± 11 |
| Effects of lesions[c] |  |  |
| kainate into the striatum | − 57 ± 9% | − 17 ± 3% |
| 6-OHDA into the MFB | + 39 ± 10% | + 17 ± 5% |
| Effect of GTP (25 μM)[d] | − 77 ± 8% | + 21 ± 3% |
| Half-time at 45°C (min)[e] | 10.1 | > 30 |

[a] Binding to D-2 sites was measured using 6 nM $^3$H-apomorphine and defined as the difference between binding occurring in the absence and in the presence of 200 nM domperidone.

[b] Binding to D-4 sites was measured using 4.5 nM $^3$H-domperidone in the presence of 20 nM apomorphine to protect D-2 sites from labeling and defined as the excess over blank values obtained in the presence of 50 μM apomorphine.

[c] In kainate-lesioned animals, striatal glutamic acid decarboxylase activity decreased by 57%. In 6-OHDA-lesioned animals, striatal tryosine hydroxylase activity decreased by 95%.

[d] GTP (25 μM) was added at the start of incubations.

[e] Membranes were preincubated at 45°C during various periods and then incubated with $^3$H-ligands. Half-times were calculated assuming a monoexponential decrease.

binding to D-2 sites rapidly disappears (half-life about 10 min) whereas binding to D-4 sites is apparently increased and these two events follow the same kinetics (38). This might indicate that guanosine triphosphate (GTP) and a mild thermal exposure elicit a conformational change of D-2 sites by which they lose their high affinity for apomorphine but not for $^3$H-domperidone and are labeled and measured concurrently with D-4 sites. This accounts for the fact that the total specific binding of $^3$H-antagonists is not modified by either GTP or thermal exposure (15,22,42). It should be noted that the effect of GTP on D-2 binding sites is likely to reflect a physiological process (8) by which the number of receptors is regulated.

## PHARMACOLOGY OF D-2 AND D-4 BINDING SITES

D-2 and D-4 binding sites have a clearly distinct pharmacology regarding affinity for DA and agonists. Bromocriptine and *N*-propylnorapomorphine are less discriminating (Table 2).

In order to identify antagonists discriminating D-2 and D-4 binding sites, we have evaluated the inhibitory potencies of a number of neuroleptics belonging to various chemical classes (Fig. 2 and Table 2).

As shown in the case of haloperidol (Fig. 2), the affinities of most neuroleptics for D-2 and D-4 binding sites, respectively, did not greatly differ one from the other, the ratios of $K_I$ values being comprised between 0.6 (pimozide) and 1.9 (metoclopramide) (Table 2). One exception was sulpiride, which displayed approximately four times more affinity for D-4 than for D-2 sites, using either $^3$H-domperidone (Fig. 2) or $^3$H-apomorphine (Table 2) to label D-2 sites. The second exception was another substituted benzamide, LUR 2366, for which the selectivity

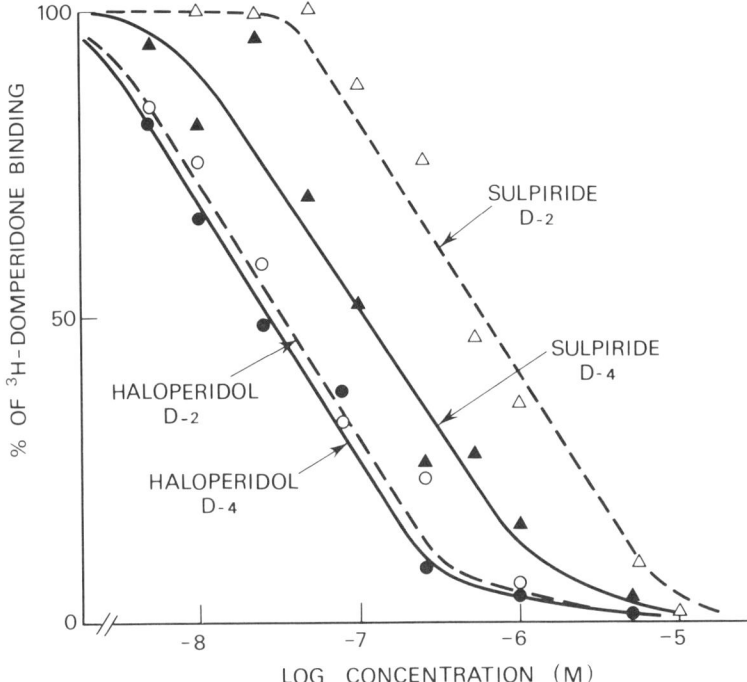

**FIG. 2.** Inhibition by haloperidol and sulpiride of ³H-domperidone binding to D-2 and D-4 sites from rat striatum. Total specific ³H-domperidone binding was measured in the presence of 4 nM ³H-ligand and defined as the excess over blank values obtained in the presence of 50 μM apomorphine. Binding to D-4 sites *(closed symbols)* was measured in the presence of 4 nM ³H-domperidone and 20 nM apomorphine to prevent labeling of D-2 sites. Binding to D-2 sites *(open symbols)* was evaluated as the difference between the binding occurring in the absence and in the presence of 20 nM apomorphine for each concentration of competing inhibitor. Values obtained in a typical experiment (means of triplicate determinations) are expressed in percentage of specific binding to each class of site. Uninhibited binding (100%) represented 94 ± 23 fmol.mg protein⁻¹ and 195 ± 15 fmol.mg protein⁻¹ to D-2 and D-4 sites, respectively.

for D-4 sites relative to D-2 sites was somewhat greater than that of sulpiride (Table 2). Although limited, these differences were statistically confirmed in independent experiments ($p < 0.005, N = 8$ and $p < 0.05, N = 3$ for sulpiride and LUR 2366, respectively). The $K_I$ value of sulpiride obtained for D-4 binding sites is in good agreement with the $K_D$ value of ³H-sulpiride for striatal binding sites (17,25,39). In addition, the effects of selective lesions on ³H-sulpiride binding are very similar to those on D-4 sites (25). This suggests that ³H-sulpiride mostly labels D-4 sites under the experimental conditions selected.

## COMPARISON OF NEUROLEPTICS IN ANTAGONISM OF APOMORPHINE-INDUCED BEHAVIORS

It had already been noticed that sulpiride differentially antagonizes various apomorphine-induced behaviors: for instance, while it clearly blocks the stereotyped

TABLE 2. *Inhibition constants of DA agonists and antagonists regarding binding to D-2 and D-4 sites*

| Agent | $K_i$ values (nM) | |
|---|---|---|
| | D-2 sites | D-4 sites |
| DA agonists | | |
| N-propylnorapomorphine | 0.40 ± 0.13 | 3.5 ± 0.8 |
| apomorphine | 0.58 ± 0.15 | 106 ± 8 |
| ADTN | 1.0 ± 0.3 | 80 ± 5 |
| bromocryptine | 7.2 ± 2.3 | 19 ± 2 |
| dopamine | 9.9 ± 2.8 | 1,830 ± 690 |
| DA antagonists | | |
| pimozide | 2.0 ± 0.5 | 3.2 ± 0.4 |
| haloperidol | 3.8 ± 1.4 | 3.2 ± 0.7 |
| thioproperazine | 2.2 ± 1.3 | 1.4 ± 0.2 |
| prochlorperazine | 10 ± 3 | 15 ± 2 |
| chlorpromazine | 19 ± 6 | 13 ± 1 |
| thioridazine | 32 ± 9 | 29 ± 1 |
| LUR 2366 | 4.6 ± 1.7 | 1.0 ± 0.4 |
| DAN 2163 | 5.7 ± 1.1 | 2.6 ± 0.5 |
| sultopride | 17 ± 5 | 20 ± 4 |
| sulpiride | 112 ± 20 | 29 ± 11 |
| metoclopramide | 158 ± 81 | 83 ± 16 |
| tiapride | 546 ± 113 | 377 ± 52 |
| mezilamine | 7.6 ± 3.1 | 9.2 ± 1.4 |
| clozapine | 154 ± 20 | 225 ± 25 |

Binding to D-2 sites was measured using 0.8 nM $^3$H-apomorphine and defined as the excess over blank values obtained in the presence of 200 nM domperidone. Binding to D-4 sites was measured using 2.5 nM $^3$H-domperidone in the presence of 20 nM apomorphine and defined as the excess over blank values obtained in the presence of 50 μM apomorphine.

Drugs were tested at 4 to 6 concentrations. $K_i$ values were derived from $IC_{50}$ values assuming a competitive inhibition and taking into account the $K_D$ values for each $^3$H-ligand: 0.92 nM and 0.70 nM for D-2 and D-4 sites, respectively. LUR 2366: N-{(1-cyclopropylmethyl-2-pyrolidinyl)methyl}2-methoxy-4-amino-5-ethylsulfonyl benzamide. DAN 2163: N-{(1-ethyl 2-pyrolidinyl)methyl}2-methoxy-4-amino-5-ethylsulfonyl benzamide.

climbing in mice (31,32), it has a low potency against head stereotypies in rats (10,24,32). Because the climbing behavior can also be elicited in selected rats of the Wistar strain (Protais et al., *in preparation*) by apomorphine at dosages for which head stereotypies like sniffing or licking (16) are simultaneously produced, it has been possible to compare in the same animals and, under strictly identical experimental conditions, the antagonist potencies of various neuroleptics towards different behaviors. Most neuroleptics like haloperidol (Fig. 3) antagonized the climbing and sniffing behaviors at similar dosages: thus the ratios of $ID_{50}$ ranged between 0.8 (pimozide) and 1.7 (sultopride) (Fig. 4). Again the exceptions were sulpiride and LUR 2366 which antagonized the two apomorphine-induced behaviors at clearly different dosages ($p < 0.001$). As shown in Fig. 3, the climbing behavior was almost suppressed in rats receiving 50 mg.Kg$^{-1}$ sulpiride, whereas sniffing

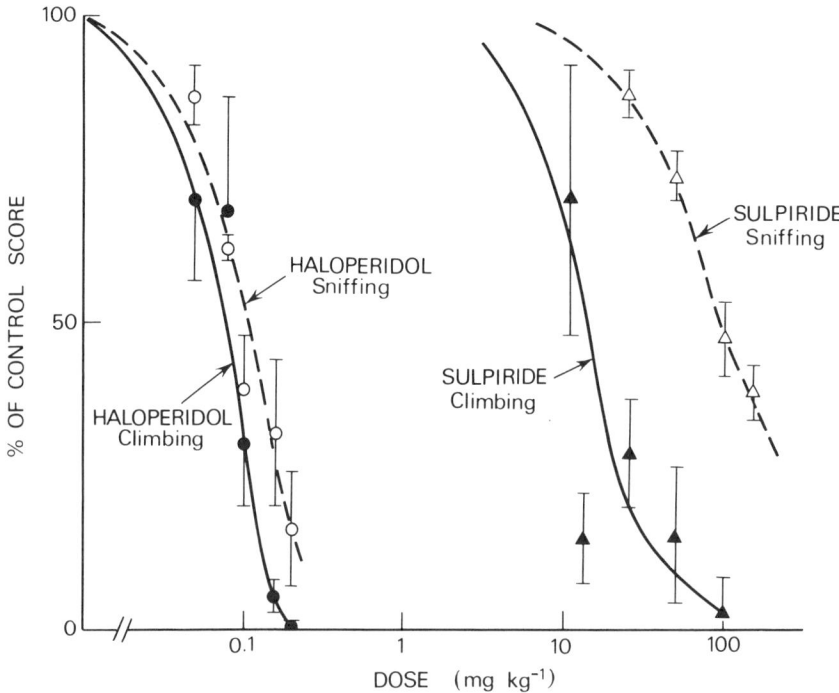

**FIG. 3.** Inhibition by haloperidol and sulpiride of two apomorphine-induced stereotyped behaviors in the rat. Male Wistar rats (200–250 g) responding to apomorphine administration (0.45 mg.kg$^{-1}$, s.c.) by a stereotyped climbing behavior analogous to that described in mice (31) were selected in a preliminary experiment. On the day of the test, they received haloperidol or sulpiride at the indicated dosages (i.p.) 30 and 90 min, respectively, before the administration of apomorphine (0.6 mg.kg$^{-1}$, s.c.) and were immediately introduced into individual wire mesh cages (L = 25 cm, W = 18 cm, H = 30 cm). Starting from 5 min after their introduction into the cages 6 animals were simultaneously scored for sniffing and climbing behaviors during 1 hr, by which time both stereotyped behaviors had vanished in controls. Sniffing was evaluated by measuring the time during which animals displayed this behavior (52 ± 2 min in rats non-pretreated with neuroleptics). Climbing was scored every 2 min as follows: 0 (the four paws on the floor), 1 (the forepaws on the wall), or 2 (the four paws on the wall); the final score of each animal represented the sum of the scores attributed during the 1-hr observation (20 ± 4 in rats non-pretreated with neuroleptics). Each value represents the mean (± SEM) of results obtained in experiments with 6–13 animals and is expressed as percentage of the control scores (saline-pretreated rats).

remained almost unaffected in these animals and could not even be totally antagonized at nontoxic dosages (below 150 mg.Kg$^{-1}$). It is important to stress that comparison is made by taking into account the ratios of ID$_{50}$ values of the drugs in the two behavioral tests and not their absolute *in vivo* potencies because this ensures that pharmacokinetic parameters, such as metabolism or access into brain, do not interfere. Under such conditions, the ratios of ID$_{50}$ values are likely to reflect selectivity of neuroleptics regarding two classes of central dopamine receptors with pharmacological specifities paralleling those of D-2 and D-4 binding sites. Thus, the ratios of ID$_{50}$ regarding sniffing and climbing for sulpiride and LUR 2366 were closely similar to the ratios of dissociation constants of these drugs for D-2 and D-4 binding sites, and the same parallelism can be drawn for the other neuroleptics

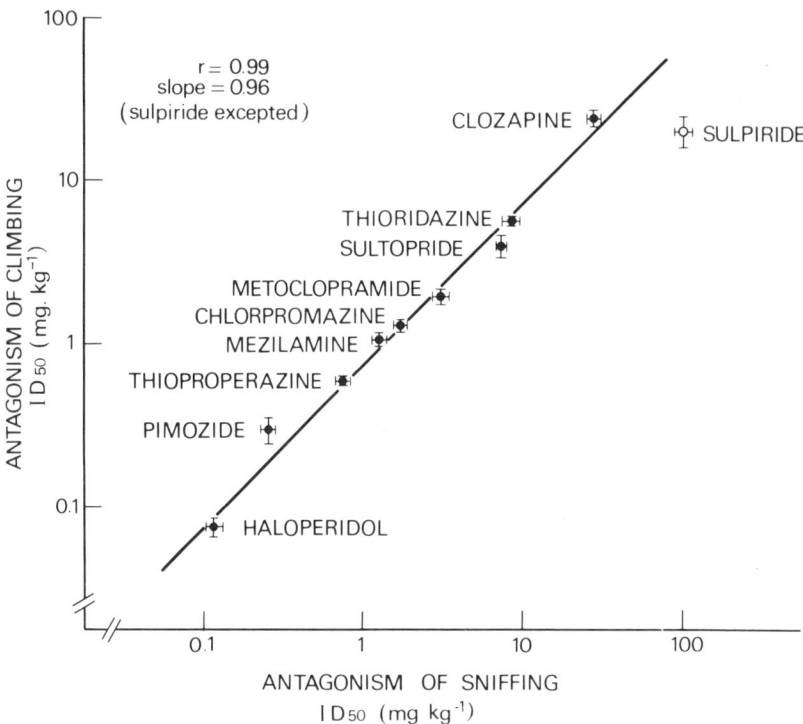

**FIG. 4.** Comparison of neuroleptic potencies towards sniffing and climbing behaviors. The sniffing and climbing behaviors elicited by apomorphine (0.6 mg. kg$^{-1}$,s.c.) were evaluated as described in the legend of Fig. 3. In each experiment, a group of 6 rats received saline or the neuroleptic in increasing dosage (30 min before apomorphine except for pimozide, sultopride, and sulpiride which were injected 90 min before). The ID$_{50}$ of the neuroleptics was calculated by log-probit analysis of data obtained in each experiment and the final ID$_{50}$ value represents the mean of values obtained in 6–13 experiments.

in spite of ratios closer to unity ($r = 0.92, N = 12, p < 0.001$; see Table 3). This strongly supports the view that these binding sites represent true receptors and indicates that stereotyped sniffing is triggered by stimulation of D-2 receptors, whereas stereotyped climbing results from D-4 receptor stimulation.

This pharmacological distinction does not imply any restrictive localization of the two classes of receptor to a brain area: although the present study was performed on striatal membranes, D-2 and D-4 binding sites are present in other dopaminergic regions of rat brain (38).

## CONCLUSIONS

We have identified two classes of DA binding sites—D-2 and D-4—which display clearly distinct properties regarding capacity, localization, effects of guanylnucleotides, and heat denaturation. These two classes of site show also different pharmacological specificities and the selectivity of neuroleptics regarding these

TABLE 3. Comparison between discriminating potencies of antagonists in binding and behavioral studies

| Neuroleptic | $K_i$ for D-2 binding sites / $K_i$ for D-4 binding sites | $ID_{50}$ for sniffing / $ID_{50}$ for climbing |
|---|---|---|
| Pimozide | 0.6 | 0.8 |
| Clozapine | 0.7 | 1.0 |
| Mezilamine | 0.8 | 1.1 |
| Sultopride | 0.9 | 1.7 |
| Thioridazine | 1.1 | 1.4 |
| Haloperidol | 1.2 | 1.4 |
| Chlorpromazine | 1.4 | 1.2 |
| DAN 2163 | 1.5 | 2.6[a] |
| Thioproperazine | 1.6 | 1.1 |
| Metoclopramide | 1.9 | 1.5 |
| Sulpiride | 3.7[b] | 4.7[c] |
| LUR 2366 | 4.7[a] | 10.2[c] |

Significantly different from unity at [a]$p < 0.05$, [b]$p < 0.005$, and [c]$p < 0.001$ by the one-tailed Student's $t$-test.

binding sites was correlated with their selectivity towards two apomorphine-induced behaviors.

The discriminating properties of sulpiride towards D-2 and D-4 receptors allow this agent to be used in identifying which of the two classes of receptor is involved in the various dopaminergic actions of neuroleptics. Thus, an effect can be ascribed to D-2 receptor blockade when produced by most neuroleptics in low dosage except sulpiride, for which doses above 100 mg.kg$^{-1}$ are required (blockade might not even occur when sulpiride is opposed to DA agonists in relatively high dosage). This seems to be the case of blockade of apomorphine-induced rotations (11,32) or head stereotypies (24) and production of catalepsy (10).

In contrast, D-4 receptors are likely to be involved when the effect is observed with all neuroleptics including sulpiride, the latter at dosages in the range of 20 mg.kg$^{-1}$. Apomorphine-induced climbing (31,32, *this chapter*) and hyperkinesia (21,24) seem to fulfill these criteria.

One difficulty in interpreting behavioral effects of neuroleptics is that most agents of this class have the ability to block non-DA receptors (26,30), properties which may modify one of the multiple events between DA receptor stimulation and behavioral response. For example, since there is a cholinergic link in extrapyramidal motor effects (2,3,10,33), the low potency of thioridazine and clozapine in producing catalepsy is likely to be related to the antimuscarinic properties of these drugs, and not to discrimination between D-2 and D-4 receptors. Nevertheless, sniffing and climbing behaviors appear, from the present study, to selectively reflect the stimulation of D-2 and D-4 receptors. Therefore, close comparison of some behavioral tests and binding assays may prove to be useful for devising antipsychotic agents with higher discriminating property than sulpiride and LUR 2366, the use of which may confirm the physiological role of D-2 and D-4 receptors.

## ACKNOWLEDGMENTS

This work is supported by Grants from Centre National de la Recherche Scientifique (Pharmacologie des récepteurs des neuromédiateurs). We thank Dr. A. Debay from Lab. Delagrange for the generous gifts of substituted benzamides LUR 2366 and DAN 2163.

## REFERENCES

1. Ariëns, E. J., Beld, A. J., Rodrigues de Miranda, J. F., and Simonis, A. M. (1978): The pharmacon-receptor-effector concept: a basis for understanding the transmission of information in biological systems. In: *The Receptors—A Comprehensive Treatise, Vol. 1: General Principles and Procedures*, edited by R. D. O'Brien, pp. 33–91. Plenum Press, New York, London.
2. Barbeau, A. (1973): Biochemistry of Huntington's chorea. In: *Advances in Neurology, Vol. 1*, edited by A. Barbeau et al., pp. 473–516. Raven Press, New York.
3. Bartholini, G., Lloyd K. G., and Stadler, H. (1974): Dopaminergic regulation of cholinergic neurons in the striatum: Relation to Parkinsonism. In: *Advances in Neurology, Vol. 5*, edited by F. H. McDowell and A. Barbeau, pp. 11–17. Raven Press, New York.
4. Baudry, M., Martres, M. P., and Schwartz, J. C. (1978): $^3$H-domperidone and $^3$H-pimozide: more specific ligands for dopamine receptors studied in vitro and in vivo. In: *Catecholamines: Basic and Clinical Frontiers, Vol. 1*, edited by E. Usdin, I. J. Kopin, and J. Barchas, pp. 565–567. Pergamon Press, New York.
5. Baudry, M., Martres, M. P., and Schwartz, J. C. (1979): $^3$H-domperidone: A selective ligand for dopamine receptors. *Naunyn Schmiedebers Arch. Pharmacol.*, 308:231–237.
6. Beld, A. J., Kuijer, B., Rodrigues de Miranda, J. F., and Wouterse, A. C. (1978): Ligand binding to dopamine receptors: analysis and interpretation. *Life Sci.*, 23:489–494.
7. Carlsson, A., and Lindqvist (1963): Effect of chlorpromazine or haloperidol on formation of 3-methoxytyramine and normetanephrine in mouse brain. *Acta Pharmacol. Toxicol.*, 20:140–144.
8. Chen, T. C., Cote, T. E., and Kebabian, J. W. (1980): Endogenous components of the striatum confer dopamine-sensitivity upon adenylate cyclase activity: the role of endogenous guanyl nucleotides. *Brain Res.*, 181:139–149.
9. Clement-Cormier, Y. C., Kebabian, J. W., Petzold, G. L., and Greengard, P. (1974): Dopamine-sensitive adenylate cyclase in mammalian brain: possible site of action of antipsychotic drugs. *Proc. Natl. Acad. Sci. USA*, 71 (4):1113–1117.
10. Costall, B., and Naylor, R. J. (1975): Detection of the neuroleptic properties of clozapine, sulpiride and thioridazine. *Psychopharmacologia (Berl.)*, 43:69–74.
11. Costall, B., Naylor, R. J., and Nohria, V. (1978): Differential actions of typical and atypical neuroleptic agents on two behavioral effects of apomorphine in the mouse. *Br. J. Pharmacol.*, 63:381–382.
12. Creese, I., Burt, D. R., and Snyder, S. H. (1975): Dopamine receptor binding: Differentiation of agonist and antagonist states with $^3$H-dopamine and $^3$H-haloperidol. *Life Sci.*, 17:993–1002.
13. Creese, I., Burt, D. R., and Snyder, S. H. (1977): Dopamine receptor binding enhancement accompanies lesion-induced behavioral supersensitivity. *Science*, 197:596–598.
14. Creese, I., and Snyder, S. H. (1978): $^3$H-spiroperidol labels serotonin receptors in rat cerebral cortex and hippocampus. *Eur. J. Pharmacol.*, 49:201–202.
15. Creese, I., Usdin, T. B., and Snyder, S. H. (1979): Dopamine receptor binding regulated by guanine nucleotides. *Mol. Pharmacol.*, 16:69–76.
16. Ernst, A. (1967): Mode of action of apomorphine and dexamphetamine on gnawing compulsion in rats. *Psychopharmacologia*, 10:316–323.
17. Freedman, S. B., and Woodruff, G. N. (1981): Effect of drugs on [$^3$H]-sulpiride binding in rat striatal synaptic membranes. *Br. J. Pharmacol.*, 72:129.
18. Howlett, D. R., and Nahorski, S. R. (1980): Quantitative assessment of heterogeneous $^3$H-spiperone binding to rat neostriatum and frontal cortex. *Life Sci.*, 26:511–517.
19. Iversen, L. L., Rogawski, M. A., and Miller, R. J. (1976): Comparison of the effects of neuroleptic drugs on pre- and postsynaptic dopaminergic mechanisms in the rat striatum. *Mol. Pharmacol.*, 12:251–262.
20. Kebabian, J. W., and Calne, D. B. (1979): Multiple receptors for dopamine. *Nature*, 277:93–96.

21. Kölher, C., Ögren, S. O., Haglund, L., and Ängeby, T. (1979): Regional displacement by sulpiride of $^3$H-spiperone binding in vivo. Biochemical and behavioral evidence for a preferential action on limbic and nigral dopamine receptors. *Neurosci. Lett.*, 13:51–56.
22. Lew, J. Y., and Goldstein, M. (1979): Dopamine receptor binding for agonists and antagonists in thermal exposed membranes. *Eur. J. Pharmacol.*, 55:429–430.
23. Leysen, J. E., Niemegeers, C. J. E., Tollenaere, J. P., and Laduron, P. M. (1978): Serotonergic component of neuroleptic receptors. *Nature*, 272:168–171.
24. Ljungberg, T., and Ungerstedt, U. (1978): Classification of neuroleptic drugs according to their ability to inhibit apomorphine-induced locomotion and gnawing: evidence for two different mechanisms of action. *Psychopharmacology*, 56:239–247.
25. Memo, M., Spano, P. F., and Trabucchi, M. (1981): Characterization and localization of dopamine-D-2 central receptors. *Br. J. Pharmacol.*, 72:124p.
26. Miller, R. J., and Hiley, C. R. (1974): Anti-muscarinic properties of neuroleptics and drug-induced Parkinsonism. *Nature*, 248:596–597.
27. Nagy, J. I., Lee T., Seeman, P., and Fibiger, H. C. (1978): Direct evidence for presynaptic and postsynaptic dopamine receptors in brain. *Nature*, 274:278–281.
28. Nakahara, T., Uchimara, H., Saito, M., Hirano, M., Kim, J. S., and Ito, M. (1978): Inhibition of dopamine-sensitive adenylate cyclase in rat striatum by neuroleptic drugs administered in vivo. *J. Neurochem.*, 31:1335–1337.
29. Niemegeers, C. J. E., and Janssen, P. A. J. (1979): A systematic study of the pharmacological activities of dopamine antagonists. *Life Sci.*, 24:2201–2216.
30. Peroutka, S. J., U'Prichard, D. C., Greenberg, D. A., and Snyder, S. H. (1977): Neuroleptic drug interactions with norepinephrine alpha receptor binding sites in rat brain. *Neuropharmacology*, 16:549–556.
31. Protais, P., Costentin, J., and Schwartz, J. C. (1976): Climbing behavior induced by apomorphine in mice: a simple test for the study of dopamine receptors in striatum. *Psychopharmacology*, 50:1–6.
32. Puech, A. J., Simon, P., and Boissier, J. R. (1978): Benzamides and classical neuroleptics: Comparison of their actions using 6 apomorphine-induced effects. *Eur. J. Pharmacol.*, 50:291–300.
33. Sayers, A. C., Bürki, H. R., Ruch, W., and Asper, H. (1976): Anticholinergic properties of antipsychotic drugs and their relation to extrapyramidal side-effects. *Psychopharmacology*, 51:15–22.
34. Schwartz, J. C., Costentin, J., Martres, M. P., Protais, P., and Baudry, M. (1978): Modulation of receptor mechanisms in the CNS: hyper-and hyposensitivity to catecholamines. *Neuropharmacology*, 17:665–685.
35. Schwarcz, R., Creese, I., Coyle, J. T., and Snyder, S. H. (1978): Dopamine receptors localised on cerebral cortical afferents to rat corpus striatum. *Nature*, 271:766–768.
36. Seeman, P. (1980): Brain dopamine receptors. *Pharmacol. Rev.*, 32:229–313.
37. Sokoloff, P., Martres, M. P., and Schwartz, J. C. (1980): $^3$H-Apomorphine labels both dopamine post-synaptic receptors and autoreceptors. *Nature*, 288:283–286.
38. Sokoloff, P., Martres, M. P., and Schwartz, J. C. (1980): Three classes of dopamine receptors (D-2, D-3, D-4) identified by binding studies with $^3$H-apomorphine and $^3$H-domperidone. *Naunyn Schmiedebergs Arch. Pharmacol.*, 315:89–102.
39. Theodorou, A., Crockett, M., Jenner, P., and Marsden, C. D. (1979): Specific binding of $^3$H-sulpiride to rat striatal preparations. *J. Pharm. Pharmacol.*, 31:424–426.
40. Titeler, M., List, S., and Seeman, P. (1979): High affinity dopamine receptors (D3) in rat brain. *Comm. Psychopharmacol.*, 3:411–420.
41. Trabucchi, M., Longoni, R., Fresia, P., and Spano, P. F. (1975): Sulpiride: A study of the effects on dopamine receptors in rat neostriatum and limbic forebrain. *Life Sci.*, 17:1551–1556.
42. Zahniser, N. R., and Molinoff, P. B. (1978): Effect of guanine nucleotides on striatal dopamine receptors. *Nature*, 275:453–454.

Molecular Pharmacology of Neurotransmitter
Receptors, edited by T. Segawa et al.
Raven Press, New York © 1983.

# Dopamine Receptor System Involving Adenylate Cyclase in Canine Caudate Nucleus

Hiroo Maeno, Kenji Sano, Koji Nishikori, Osamu Noshiro, Akiko Sato, Takashi Yoneda, Shinji Usuda, and Sumio Iwanami

*Department of Pharmacology and Biochemistry, Central Research Laboratories, Yamanouchi Pharmaceutical Co. Ltd., Tokyo 174, Japan*

The presence of multiple dopamine receptors in the central nervous system has been demonstrated by electrophysiological, pharmacological, and biochemical studies (1,6,14). We have recently characterized two distinct dopamine binding sites with low and high affinity in the synaptic membrane fractions of canine caudate nucleus by means of [³H]dopamine binding (9,12). The low and high affinity sites are referred to as $D_1$ and $D_2$, respectively. Their equilibrium dissociation constant is 3.6 μM for $D_1$ and 0.012 μM for $D_2$. Of catecholamines dopamine can displace more specifically [³H]dopamine at either site. Classical neuroleptics such as haloperidol and chlorpromazine inhibit [³H]dopamine binding to $D_1$ and $D_2$ to an approximately equal extent. Furthermore, we have provided evidence demonstrating that $D_1$ is associated with adenylate cyclase (11).

In this chapter, the following results are shown: (a) inhibitory effects of 28 2-methoxy-benzamide derivatives on [³H]dopamine binding to $D_1$ and $D_2$ in the canine caudate nucleus as well as on apomorphine-induced stereotypy in rats; (b) separation of [³H]dopamine-labeled $D_1$ from $D_2$ after solubilization; (c) dissociation and reconstitution of guanine nucleotide-sensitive adenylate cyclase; and (d) cyclic adenosine monophosphate- (cAMP)-dependent endogenous protein phosphorylation.

## INHIBITORY EFFECTS OF 2-METHOXY-BENZAMIDE DERIVATIVES ON [³H]DOPAMINE BINDING TO $D_1$ AND $D_2$

It has been reported that YM-09151-2 is a very potent $D_1$-selective dopamine antagonist, whereas sulpiride is a $D_2$-selective antagonist (11,15). Since both compounds are 2-methoxy-benzamide derivatives, it is of interest to view the structure-inhibition relationship of the benzamide derivatives. For this purpose, twenty-eight 2-methoxy benzamide derivatives with the basic structure as illustrated in Table 1 have been synthesized in our laboratories.

TABLE 1. *Structure-selectivity relationship of benzamide derivatives*

R1, OCH3, CONH-R3, R2 (benzamide structure)

| | | | | Selectivity [-log Kd($D_1$)/Kd($D_2$)] | | | | |
|---|---|---|---|---|---|---|---|---|
| | $R_1$ | NHCH$_3$ | NHCH$_3$ | NH$_2$ | NH$_2$ | N(CH$_3$)$_2$ | H | H |
| $R_3$ | $R_2$ | SO$_2$CH$_3$ | Cl | SO$_2$CH$_3$ | Cl | Cl | SO$_2$C$_2$H$_5$ | SO$_2$NH$_2$ |
| CH$_3$-N-pyrrolidine-CH$_2$-phenyl | | 2.75 (5) | 2.30 (2) | 2.12 (4) | 2.26 (1) | 0.97 (3) | | 1.51 (6) |
| -CH$_2$-N-pyrrolidine-CH$_2$-phenyl | | 2.50 (14) | 2.32 (12) | > 2.20 (13) | 1.34 (11) | | | 0.16 (15) |
| N-pyrrolidine-CH$_2$-phenyl | | | 2.04 (8) | | 0.94 (7) | 1.44 (9) | 0.09 (10) | |
| -CH$_2$CH$_2$N(CH$_3$)(CH$_2$-phenyl) | | | 1.35 (17) | | -0.24 (16) | | | 0.08 (18) |
| -CH$_2$CH$_2$H(C$_2$H$_5$)$_2$ | | | -0.05 (28) | | -0.11 (27) | | | |
| N-pyrrolidine-C$_2$H$_5$ | | 0.23 (21) | -2.0 (20) | | -0.23 (19) | | | |
| -CH$_2$-N-pyrrolidine-C$_2$H$_5$ | | -0.67 (24) | -0.73 (22) | -0.67 (23) | | | -1.11 > (25) | -1.92 > (26) |

[$^3$H]Dopamine binding was determined using the synaptic membrane fraction of canine caudate nucleus as described previously (9). The compound numbers 2, 8, 25, 26, and 27 are YM-09151-2, YM-08050, sultopride, sulpiride, and metoclopramide, respectively.

Substitution at benzene ring ($R_1$ and $R_2$) and amino moiety ($R_3$) of the benzamide compounds results in marked effects on both potency and selectivity in the inhibition of [$^3$H]dopamine binding to $D_1$ and $D_2$. Of particular importance in the selective binding to $D_1$ are the methylamino group at $R_1$ and the $N$-benzyl group in $R_3$, as examplified by YM-09151-2. To the contrary, $N$-ethyl group in $R_3$ and sulfamoyl moiety at $R_2$ seem to be more influential on the increase in the inhibition of $D_2$ binding as represented by sulpiride.

## INHIBITORY EFFECTS OF 2-METHOXY-BENZAMIDE DERIVATIVES ON APOMORPHINE-INDUCED STEREOTYPY IN RATS

Since YM-09151-2, which is so far the most potent and highly $D_1$-selective dopamine antagonist, still blocks $D_2$ site with the affinity of one-hundredth as much as that for $D_1$, it is desirable to obtain a more $D_1$-selective antagonist than YM-09151-2, particularly from the aspect of determining biological activities relevant to $D_1$. At present, when no such strictly $D_1$-selective antagonist is found, we have attempted to see which type of dopamine sites are more closely correlated with the occurrence of stereotypy in animals: to this end we have compared a number of dopamine antagonists, with different relative affinities for $D_1$ and $D_2$, for their ability to inhibit [$^3$H]dopamine binding and to reduce the apomorphine-induced stereotypy in rats. As shown in Fig. 1, the antagonistic effect on stereotypy is apparently more closely correlated with the inhibitory effect on [$^3$H]dopamine binding to $D_1$ ($\gamma = 0.69$, $p < 0.003$) than to $D_2$ ($\gamma = 0.41$, $p < 0.05$). However, when the compounds under investigation exhibit little effect on the behaviors, one has to be cautious in the interpretation of the results, because of the possiblity of their poor passage through the blood-brain barrier. In fact, sulpiride, which lacks cataleptogenicity and inhibition of the stereotypy by systemic administration, has recently been demonstrated to induce the catalepsy and to inhibit the stereotypy when administered intraventricularily (5). Our preliminary experiments have indicated that $D_1$-selective YM-09151-2 inhibits the apomorphine-induced stereotypy at noncataleptogenic doses by intraventricular administration, whereas $D_2$-selective sulpiride is cataleptogenic rather than inhibitory on the stereotypy. These data also support the view that $D_1$ is more closely associated with apomorphine-induced stereotypy than $D_2$. Other dopamine-related responses such as emesis, locomotor activity, and prolactin level may occur primarily through stimulation of $D_2$, since sulpiride and some ergot alkaloids, which are virtually ineffective on dopamine-sensitive adenylate cyclase, considerably alter these responses (2,3,7,8,13).

## SEPARATION OF [$^3$H]DOPAMINE-LABELED $D_1$ AND $D_2$

In order to show that $D_1$ and $D_2$ are distinct entities, photoaffinity labeling with [$^3$H]dopamine has been utilized (9,16). When the synaptic membranes are incubated with [$^3$H]dopamine under ultraviolet light, [$^3$H]dopamine, free or bound, is converted to a free radical. The bound radical reacts spontaneously with a certain amino acid in the binding site with subsequent formation of a covalent bond. Thus, it

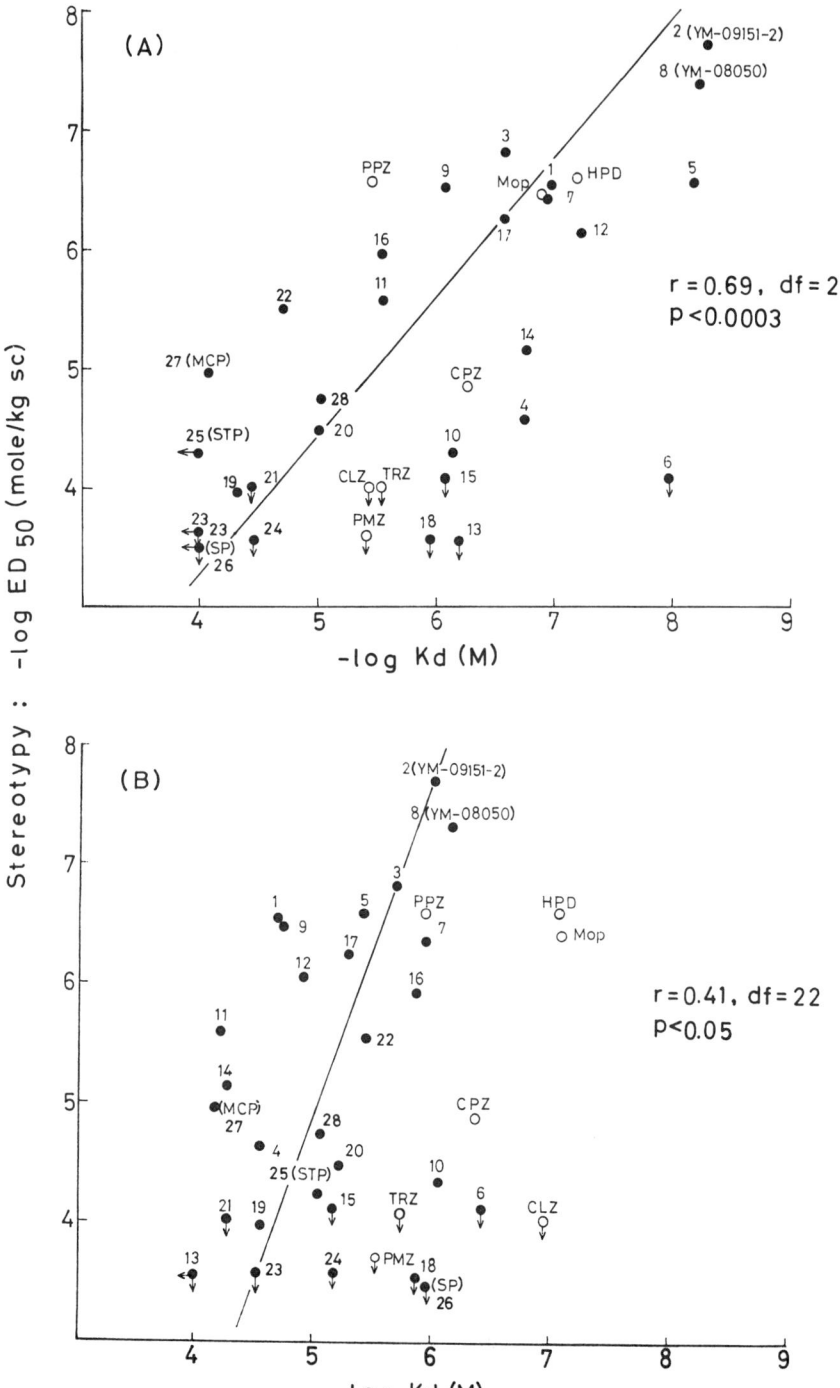

would be possible to separate [$^3$H]dopmaine-labeled $D_1$ and $D_2$ from one another after solubilization with detergents.

Under the $D_1$ binding conditions, the synaptic membrane fraction of canine caudate nucleus is incubated with [$^3$H]dopamine under ultraviolet lamp, washed thoroughly to remove free radioactivities, and then solubilized with 2% Lubrol PX. The extract is then subjected to gel filtration through a Sephadex G-200 column. Figure 2 shows elution patterns of protein, Lubrol PX micelle, and radioactivity. Most of the radioactivity is found in the same fraction as Lubrol PX, and its Stokes radius is computed to be 4.5 nm by comparing with the elution volume of several marker proteins. This incorporation of [$^3$H]dopamine into the membranes can be completely abolished by the addition of a $D_1$-selective antagonist, YM-09151-2, at 0.1 μM which is a noneffective concentration for $D_2$ binding, while a $D_2$-selective α-ergocryptine at 10 μM shows no effect. When the membranes are photochemically labeled under the $D_2$ binding conditions, the Stokes radius of the labeled proteins is 6.5 nm. The incorporation of [$^3$H]dopamine is not affected by 0.1 μM YM-09151-2, but almost entirely inhibited by 10 μM α-ergocryptine. These data indicate that $D_1$ and $D_2$ are obviously distinct entities.

## BIOCHEMICAL EVENTS SUBSEQUENT TO DOPAMINE BINDING TO $D_1$

It has been reported from this laboratory that $D_1$ is associated with adenylate cyclase in the synaptic membrane fraction of canine caudate nucleus and that dopamine sensitivity of the adenylate cyclase requires GTP strictly (11). In analogy to other hormone-sensitive adenylate cyclase (10), the solubilized and partially purified adenylate cyclase of the caudate nucleus which is unresponsive to dopamine but stimulatable by guanylyl imidodiphosphate [Gpp(NH)p] is dissociable into a nucleotide binding unit (N) and a catalytic unit (C) by the treatment with GTP-Sepharose affinity resin. The catalytic unit with no affinity for the GTP-Sepharose shows no responsiveness to Gpp(NH)p. The nucleotide binding unit which is adsorbed by the resin and elutable with 1 mM GTP exhibits no adenylate cyclase activity even in the presence of $Mn^{2+}$. When incubated for 60 min at 27°C with the nucleotide binding unit from which GTP has been removed by ultrafiltration, the catalytic unit can restore the sensitivity to Gpp(NH)p. The nucleotide binding unit which confers Gpp(NH)p-sensitivity is heat-labile and inactivated by trypsin (Table 2). These results indicate that Gpp(NH)p-sensitive adenylate cyclase of

---

**FIG. 1.** Relationship between the inhibitory activities of the benzamide derivatives *(solid circles)* and other structurally different neuroleptics *(open circles)* in apomorphine-induced stereotypy and [$^3$H]dopamine binding to $D_1$ **(A)** and $D_2$ **(B)**. The compounds with *horizontal* and *vertical arrows* do not inhibit the stereotypy and [$^3$H]dopamine-binding, respectively, at the illustrated doses. The regression line does not include the compound with the *arrow*. The number indicates the compound number that is identical to that in Table 1. HPD, haloperidol; Mop, moperone; CPZ, chlorpromazine; PPZ, perphenazine; TRZ, thioridazine; CLZ, clozapine; SP, sulpiride; STP, sultopride; MCP, metoclopramide.

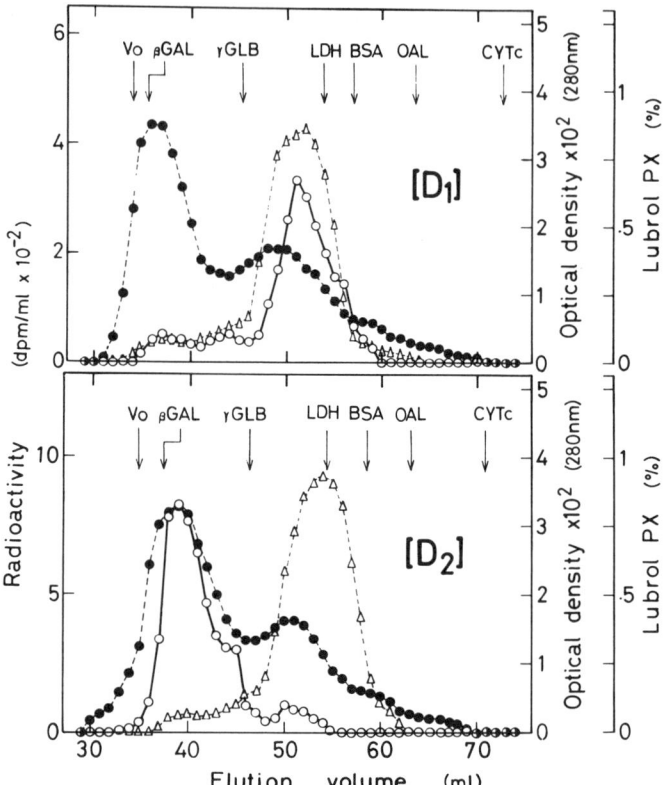

**FIG. 2. Top:** Sephadex G-200 column chromatography of solubilized $D_1$ labeled with [$^3$H]dopamine by the photoaffinity method. Following a photochemical incubation under the $D_1$ binding conditions, the synaptic membrane fraction was solubilized with 2% Lubrol PX and chromatographed on a Sephadex G-200 column. Specifically incorporated radioactivity *(open circles)* Lubrol PX *(open triangles)* and optical density at 280 nm (solid circles) are shown for each eluate. Specifically incorporated radioactivity is expressed as the difference between total and nonspecific incorporation. The *arrows* locate the elution peak of marker proteins. βGAL, β-galactosidase; γGLB, γ-globulin; LDH, lactic dehydrogenase; BSA. bovine serum albumin; OAL, ovalbumin; CYTc cytochrtome C. **Bottom:** Sephadex G-200 column chromatography of solubilized $D_2$ labeled with [$^3$H]dopamine. Following photochemical incubation under the $D_2$ binding conditions, the synaptic membranes were processed as described for $D_2$.

canine caudate nucleus is composed of the catalytic unit and the guanine nucleotide binding protein. Thus, a signal of the first messenger, dopamine, is transmitted from $D_1$ to the catalytic unit via an intermediary action of the nucleotide binding unit and generates the second messenger, cAMP.

The role of cAMP in the nervous system has been studied in depth by Greengard (4). The primary action of cAMP which is generated by certain neurotransmitters is to stimulate cAMP-dependent protein kinase which then elevates phosphorylation of membrane protein Ia (MW 86,000) and Ib (MW 80,000). The protein Ia and Ib

TABLE 2. Reconstitution of Gpp(NH)p-sensitive adenylate cyclase from C and N

| Experiment | Preincubation | | Adenylate cyclase activity | | |
| --- | --- | --- | --- | --- | --- |
| | Amounts of N (μg) | Temp. (°C) | None | Gpp(NH)p (pmol cAMP/min) | $Mn^{2+}$ |
| 1. | 0 | 0 | 2.74 | 2.86 | 5.98 |
| | 18.7 | 0 | 2.80 | 2.85 | 8.19 |
| | 9.13 (GTP removed) | 0 | 1.47 | 2.11 | 3.76 |
| | 9.13 (GTP removed) | 27 | 1.02 | 1.91 | 3.71 |
| 2. | 7.23 | 27 | 0.846 | 2.24 | 2.20 |
| | 7.23 (heated) | 27 | 0.675 | 0.850 | 1.53 |
| | 7.23 (trypsin-treated) | 27 | 0.654 | 0.833 | 1.64 |

In experiment 1, 60 μg protein of C was preincubated with indicated amounts of N at 0°C for 20 min or at 27°C for 60 min in a total volume of 1.5 ml of 0.1 M glycylglycine buffer (pH 7.4) containing 0.1 M NaCl, 1 mM EDTA, 3 mM dithiothreitol, 5 mM $MgSO_4$, and 0.67 mM GTP. When N was used, from which GTP was removed by ultrafiltration (Amicon PM-10), GTP was not added to the preincubation mixture. Following preincubation, 240 μl of the preincubated mixture was used to determine the activity under the standard assay conditions (12) except for the incubation time of 12 min instead of 4 min at 30°C in the absence and presence of 50 μM Gpp(NH)p. $Mn^{2+}$-sensitive activity was determined in the presence of 16 mM $MnSO_4$ and 2.4 mM $MgSO_4$. In the experiment 2, 70 μg protein of C was preincubated with indicated amounts of GTP-free N at 27°C for 30 min. Other experimental conditions were the same as in the experiment 1. Heated N was prepared by placing in boiling water bath for 10 min. Proteolysis of N with trypsin (1 μg/500 μl) was carried out for 35 min at 27°C and terminated by incubation with soybean trypsin inhibitor (3 μg/500 μl) for another 20 min. Heated or trypsin-treated N was preincubated as in the experiment 1.

are mostly found in the postsynaptic membranes as well as in the synaptic vesicles by an immunohistochemical technique. Phosphorylation of these two proteins is presumed to be responsible for the diverse effects of neurotransmitters. In the synaptic membrane fractions from canine caudate nucleus, protein Ia and Ib can be endogenously phosphorylated by [γ-$^{32}$P]ATP in the presence of cAMP as shown by the autoradiography in Fig. 3. The low level of this phosphorylation may be at least partly responsible for a neuroleptic-induced increase in dopamine turnover (data not shown) and the inhibition of stereotypy.

## BIOCHEMICAL EVENTS SUBSEQUENT TO DOPAMINE BINDING TO $D_2$

Biochemical changes subsequent to $D_2$ stimulation by dopamine are totally unknown. Metabolism of certain phospholipids and movement of $Ca^{2+}$ may be the target for such studies. What we certainly know is that hypolocomotion, hyperlocomotion, catalepsy, emesis, and prolactin release are apparently correlated with $D_2$ and it is very unlikely that these behavioral changes are associated to $D_1$.

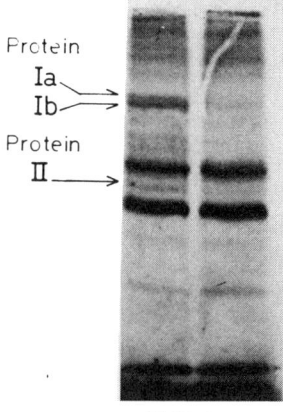

**FIG. 3.** Effect of cAMP on endogenous phosphorylation of the synaptic membranes from canine caudate nucleus. After an incubation of the membranes with [γ-$^{32}$P]ATP for 10 sec at 30°C in the presence and in the absence of 5 μM cAMP, the reaction was terminated by the addition of sodium dodecyl sulfate. The mixture is then subjected to slab acrylamide gel electrophoresis and then to autoradiography.

## SUMMARY

Two distinct dopamine binding sites, referred to as $D_1$ and $D_2$, exist in canine caudate nucleus, as characterized by [$^3$H]dopamine binding to the synaptic membrane fraction. $D_1$ has the low affinity for dopamine with the dissociation constant of a few micromolar, whereas the affinity for $D_2$ is about two orders of magnitude greater. Classical neuroleptics such as haloperidol and chlorpromazine have no selectivity in the inhibition of $D_1$ and $D_2$ binding, whereas a number of 2-methoxy benzamide derivatives which have been synthesized in our laboratories exhibit rather different selectivity. Correlation between the selectivity of those benzamide derivatives for the two sites and the inhibition of apomorphine-induced stereotypy in rats suggests that $D_1$ is more responsible for the stereotypy. Photoaffinity labeling of $D_1$ and $D_2$ with [$^3$H]dopamine demonstrates that the two sites are distinct entities.

In the $D_1$ system, the adenylate cyclase which is responsive to Gpp(NH)p can be dissociable by the treatment with GTP-Sepharose into a guanine nucleotide binding unit and a catalytic unit which is insensitive to Gpp(NH)p. The catalytic unit restores the responsiveness to Gpp(NH)p after preincubation with the nucleotide binding unit. Furthermore, endogenous cAMP-dependent phosphorylation of two particular proteins (protein Ia and Ib) is shown, which may be at least partly responsible for stereotypy and dopamine turnover in the caudate nucleus.

## REFERENCES

1. Cools, A. R., and Van Rossum, J. M. (1980): Multiple receptors for brain dopamine in behaviour regulation; concept of dopamine E and dopamine I receptors. *Life Sci.*, 27:1237–1253.
2. Costall, B., Funderburk, W. H., Leonard, C. A., and Naylor, R. J. (1978): Assessment of the neuroleptics potential of some novel benzamide, butyrophenone, phenothiazine and indole derivatives. *J. Pharm. Pharmacol.*, 30:771–778.
3. Fuxe, K., Feldholm, B. B., Agnati, L. F., Ogren, S.-O., Everitt, B. J., Jonsson, G., and Gustafsson, J.-Å. (1978): Interaction of ergot drugs with central monoamine systems. *Pharmacology (Suppl. 1)*, 16:99–134.

4. Greengard, P. (1978): *Cyclic Nucleotides, Phosphorylated Proteins, and Neuronal Function.* Raven Press, New York.
5. Honda, F., Satoh, Y., and Simomura, K. (1977): Dopamine receptor blocking; Activity of sulpiride in the central nervous system. *Jpn. J. Pharmacol.*, 27:397–411.
6. Kebabian, J. W., and Calne, D. B. (1979): Multiple receptors for dopamine. *Nature*, 277:93–96.
7. Lee, H. K., Chung, P. M., and Wang, S. C. (1978): Mechanisms of antiemetic action of penfluridol in the dog. *Eur. J. Pharmacol.*, 53:29–38.
8. Meltzer, H. Y., So, R., Miller, R. J., and Fang, V. S. (1979): Comparison of the effects of substituted benzamides and standard neuroleptics on the binding of $^3$H-spiroperidol in the rat pituitary and striatum with in vivo effects on rat prolactin secretion. *Life Sci.*, 25:573–584.
9. Nishikori, K., Noshiro, O., Sano, K., and Maeno, H. (1980): Characterization, solubilization, and separation of two distinct dopamine receptors in canine caudate nucleus. *J. Biol. Chem.*, 255:10909–10915.
10. Rodbell, M. (1980): The role of hormone receptors and GTP-regulatory proteins in membrane transduction. *Nature*, 284:17–22.
11. Sano, K., Nishikori, K., Noshiro, O., and Maeno, H. (1979): Reconstitution of dopamine-sensitive adenylate cyclase from dissociated components in canine caudate nucleus. *Arch. Biochem. Biophys.*, 197:285–293.
12. Sano, K., Noshiro, O., Katsuda, K., Nishikori, K., and Maeno, H. (1979): Dopamine receptors and dopamine-sensitive adenylate cyclase in canine caudate nucleus: characterization and solubilization. *Biochem. Pharmacol.*, 28:3617–3627.
13. Schachter, M., Bédard, P., Debono, A. G., Jenner, P., Marsden, C. D., Price, P., Parkes, J. D., Keenan, J., Smith, B., Rosenthaler, J., Horowski, R., and Dorow, R. (1980): The role of D-1 and D-2 receptors. *Nature*, 286:157–159.
14. Seeman, P., Titeler, M., Tedesco, J., Weinreich, P., and Sinclain, D. (1978): Brain receptors for dopamine and neuroleptics. *Advances in Biochemical Pharmacology, Vol. 19*, edited by P. J. Roberts, G. N. Woodruff, and L. L. Iversen, pp. 167–176. Raven Press, New York.
15. Usuda, S., Nishikori, K., Noshiro, O., and Maeno, H. (1981): Neuroleptic properties of cis-N-(1-benzyl-2-methylpyrrolidin-3-yl)-5-chloro-2-methoxy-4-methylaminobenzenamide (YM-09151-2) with selective antidopaminergic activity. *Psychopharmacology*, 73:103–109.
16. Yoshioka, M., Kirino, Y., Tamura, Z., and Kwan, T. (1977): Semiquinone radicals generated from catecholamines by ultraviolet irradiation. *Chem. Pharm. Bull.*, 25:75–78.

# Modification of Dopaminergic Transmission by Thyrotropin-Releasing Hormone

Shigehiko Narumi and Yuji Nagawa

*Central Research Division, Takeda Chemical Industries, Ltd., Osaka 532, Japan*

Thyrotropin-releasing hormone (TRH) is present in the hypothalamus and elicits the release of thyroid stimulating hormone (TSH) (5,7) and prolactin (2) from the anterior pituitary. In the mammalian brain this hormone is widely distributed outside the hypothalamus (3,6,9,17). Plotnikoff et al. (15) reported that TRH potentiated the excitatory action of L-DOPA in the presence of pargyline (a monoamine oxidase inhibitor) in hypophysectomized and in normal mice. Inoue et al. (8) and Miyamoto and Nagawa (14) suggested the important role of the mesolimibic dopamine (DA) system in mediating the TRH-stimulated spontaneous motor activity (SMA) in mice and rats. These findings led to the idea that TRH may have some neuroregulatory effect on the catecholaminergic system in SMA or emotional activity, in addition to its well-established endocrine function.

DA is localized in the nigrostriatal and the mesolimbic pathways. There are reports (1,11) suggesting that stereotypy and locomotor stimulation induced by certain drugs are mediated via the nigrostriatal and mesolimbic DA system, respectively. In the present study, we found that TRH enhanced the SMA in rats by systemic or direct injection of TRH into the nucleus accumbens, one of the nerve terminal sites of the mesolimbic DA system, and also enhanced the effect of TRH on circling behavior by DA agonist in mice with unilateral striatal lesion induced by 6-hydroxydopamine (6-OHDA). We now report the apparent participation of the DA and $3',5'$-adenosine monophosphate (cyclic AMP) systems in these effects of TRH.

## MATERIALS AND METHODS

### Unilateral Striatal Lesioning and Intracerebral Administration of Drugs

Jcl:ICR mice (28–35 g, 5–6 weeks old) anesthetized with chloral hydrate were fixed on a stereotaxic apparatus, and a needle with 0.4 mm outer and 0.2 mm inner diameters was inserted unilaterally into the caudate nucleus. 6-OHDA (4 $\mu g/\mu l$) was injected into the unilateral caudate nucleus using a microsyringe connected with the injection needle.

## Unilateral Lesioning of the Nigrostriatal DA System by Injection of 6-OHDA and Intracerebral Injection of Drugs

Jcl:SD rats (200–300 g, 7–8 weeks old) were anesthetized with chloral hydrate, and an injection needle with 0.4 mm outer and 0.2 mm inner diameters was stereotaxically inserted unilaterally into the nigrostriatal DA pathway (16) at coordinates of A:4.6, L:1.8, and H:2.2, according to the atlas of König and Klippel (12) for the injection of 8 µg/µl of 6-OHDA. The animals that responded to an intraperitoneal dose of 0.25 mg/kg of apomorphine with contralateral circlings 5 days after the lesioning were used for further experiments at weekly intervals for 8 weeks at the longest.

Some of these lesioned or normal rats were anesthetized with pentobarbital Na, and stainless steel guide cannulae with 0.5 mm inner and 0.8 mm outer diameters were implanted bilaterally into the caudate nucleus at the coordinates of A:8.2, L:2.8, and H:2.5, or into the nucleus accumbens (ACB) at the coordinates of A:9.4, L:1.6, and H:1.0, according to the atlas of De Groot (4). The cannulae were fixed on the skull with dental cement, and stainless steel stylets, 0.4 mm in diameter and extending 1 mm below the tips of the guide cannulae, were retained to prevent occlusion of the lumen by blood and tissue. These animals were used for experiments 1–6 weeks later. The test drug in a volume of 2 µl was injected over 1 min, into the caudate nucleus or ACB by means of a microsyringe which extended into the brain tissue 1.5 mm below the tip of the guide cannula.

## Measurement of SMA

Each rat was placed in a perspex cage (26 × 42 × 15 cm) mounted on the top of a Varimex meter, which was tuned to a sensitivity 20 µA in order to count mainly large vertical and horizontal movements consisting of locomotion, rearing, head-movement, etc. The SMA counts were automatically recorded on a printer at 10-min intervals. After the rat was well acclimated to the activity cage, until the counts were less than 50 during a 10-min period, SMA was measured for 60 or 90 min following the drug injection. All experiments were performed between 8:00 a.m. and 6:00 p.m. in a sound-proof, uniformly illuminated room maintained at 22 ± 2°C.

## Measurement of Circling

The mice with the striatal lesion were placed individually in 1-liter glass beakers. Thirty minutes later, they were given an i.p. injection of the test drug, or saline. Circling in both directions as counted for 1 min every 10 min after the drug administration. The circling counts in the above three-to-nine determinations were totaled in each animal and the average group value was expressed as total circling count. Similarly, circling in the rats with unilateral nigrostriatal DA pathway lesion induced by 6-OHDA was counted after placing the rats in a transparent plastic cage, at 5- or 10-min intervals from 5 to 60 min after the drug administration. The number of circlings was expressed as an average per time unit or the total circling count for a total period of 55 min. The direction of circling was expressed as ipsilateral (toward the lesioned side) or contralateral (toward the intact side) in reference to the lesioned side, regardless of the side of the drug injection.

## Measurement of Cyclic AMP Levels in Slices of Mouse Striatum

Cyclic AMP was determined according to the method of Krueger et al (16). Left and right striata of mice were pooled and suspended in Krebs-Ringer phosphate buffer (KRPB) containing 10 mM theophylline. The 2.5-mm thick slices, prepared by chopping using a McIlwain tissue chopper, were suspended in KRPB, centrifuged at 1,000 × $g$ for 10 min and then rinsed with KRPB. The wet slices were weighed and resuspended in fresh KRPB to a final volume of 15 ml. The 0.2-ml aliquots of these suspensions were added to tubes containing 0.1 ml KRPB with various concentrations of DA and the preparations incubated for 15 min at 37°C. After the reaction was terminated by placing the tube in boiling water for 3 min, the supernatant obtained by centrifugation (1,000 × $g$ for 10 min) and assayed for cyclic AMP by the radioimmunoassay method using a Yamasa cyclic AMP assay kit.

## Measurement of DA Release from Rat ACB and Striatal Slices

Jcl:SD rats (300–450 g, 8–10 weeks old) were decapitated, and ACB and striata were excised. The ACB and striatal tissues were sliced in 0.5-mm thick sections with a McIlwain tissue chopper and were dispersed in 95% $O_2$-5% $CO_2$ saturated KRPB containing 0.1 mM pargyline, 1 mM ascorbic acid, and 10 mM glucose, and were centrifuged at 2,000 × $g$ for 5 min at 4°C. The slices of 40 mg wet weight were put into each test tube containing 2 ml KRPB, incubated with 1 μCi/3.7 × $10^{-8}$M of 3,4-[7-$^3$H$(N)$]-DA([$^3$H]-DA) for 60 min at 37°C, then repeatedly rinsed with fresh KRPB and centrifuged three times. The slices thus preloaded with [$^3$H]DA were superfused with KRPB at a constant rate of 0.2–0.3 ml/min in the superfusion apparatus. The radioactivities of $^3$H in the superfusate effluents collected every 10 min for 30 min and every 5 min from 30 to 100 min, and in supernatant (3,000 × $g$ for 10 min at 4°C) of 5% trichloroacetic acid homogenized slices were counted using a liquid scintillation spectrometer with ACS® II scintillation.

## RESULTS

### Effect of TRH on the Mesolimbic DA Nerve Terminals

#### Effects on SMA

As shown in Fig. 1, TRH (20 mg/kg, i.p.) produced no significant increase in SMA in cage-nonadapted rats, but the cage-well-adapted rats given the same dose of TRH did show a mild acceleration of motor activity during the initial 30-min periods. On the other hand, methamphetamine (MAP, 1 mg/kg, i.p.) produced

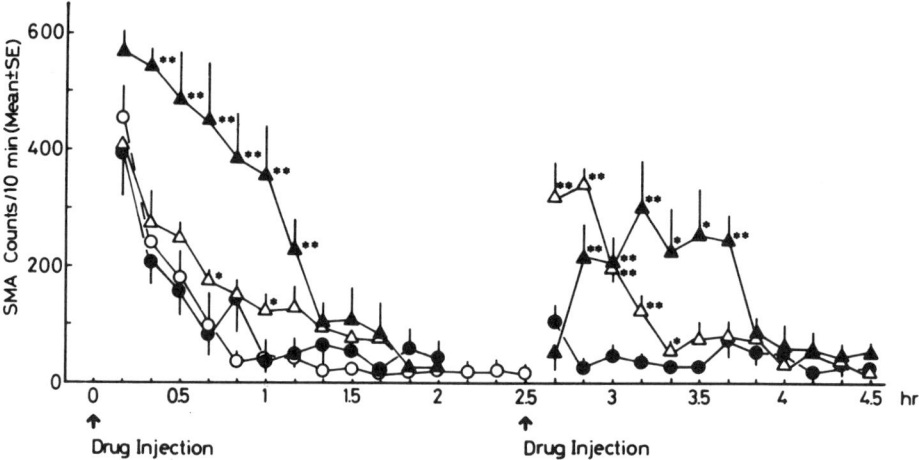

FIG. 1. Effects of TRH and MAP on SMA in cage-nonadapted and -adapted rats. SMA was measured by a Varimex meter. TRH or MAP was given i.p. immediately before rats were placed in an activity cage (nonadapted) or after being placed in an activity cage for a long period (adapted). *Vertical rules* represent SEM. *Open circles*, normal; *open triangles*, TRH 20 mg/kg, i.p.; *closed circles*, saline; *closed triangles*, MAP 1 mg/kg, i.p. *$p < 0.05$, **$p < 0.01$ vs saline control.

significant motor hyperactivity, regardless of cage-adaptation. These observations would suggest that TRH and MAP have different effects on the motor activity. The cage-well-adapted rats were used in the following experiments. TRH given i.p. 10 to 20 mg/kg or 5 to 10 µg bilaterally into the ACB or tuberculum olfactorium (TUO) showed a similar dose-dependent motor hyperactivity, whereas TRH (50 µg) given into the caudate-putamen (CPU) had little effect on SMA (Fig. 2).

## Effects of Various Inhibitors on TRH-Induced SMA Stimulation

The effects of DA receptor antagonists, pimozide (PMZ) and haloperidol (HPD), a tyrosine hydroxylase inhibitor, α-methyl-*p*-tyrosine (α-MT), anticholinergic drugs, atropine (AT) and atropine methylbromide (ATMB), and a monoamine oxidase inhibitor, pargyline (Parg), on the spontaneous motor stimulatory action of TRH were studied (Fig. 3). Pretreatment with PMZ (0.5–2 mg/kg, i.p., 4 hr before), α-MT (250 mg/kg, i.p., 4 hr before) or bilateral intra-ACB injection of HPD (5 µg, 15 min before) significantly reduced the effect of TRH given i.p. or into ACB. On the contrary, pretreatment with Parg (100 mg/kg, 16–20 hr before) produced no significant SMA stimulation, yet significantly enhanced the spontaneous motor stimulatory action of TRH (10 mg/kg, i.p.). Lesioning of the mesolimbic DA pathway by local injection of 6-OHDA (8 µg, 14 days before) did not modify the SMA stimulatory action of TRH injected into the ACB. In contrast, the SMA stimulatory action of DA injected into similar brain site was markedly enhanced. This result suggests that TRH had no direct stimulatory action on the DA receptor. The intracerebroventricular (i.c.v.) injection of AT or ATMB did not modify the TRH effect (Fig. 3).

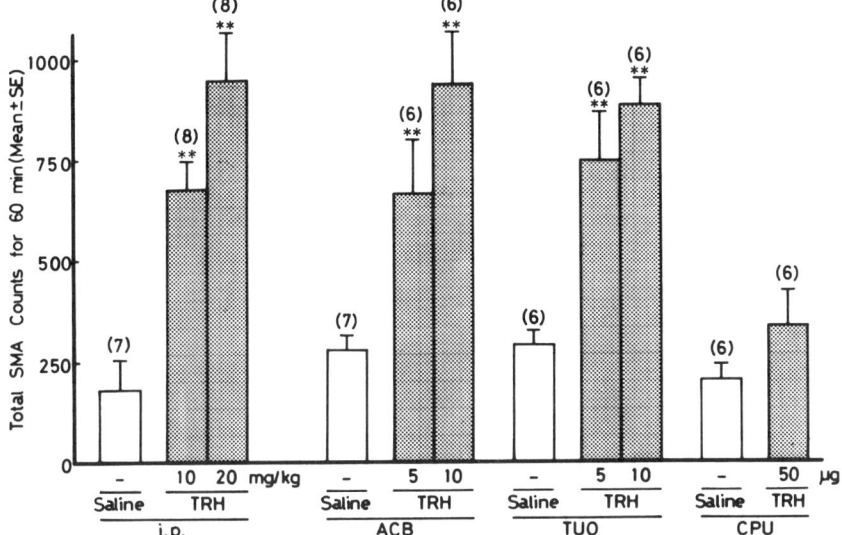

**FIG. 2.** Effects of TRH administered i.p. or i.c. on SMA in rats. SMA was measured by a Varimax meter. TRH was injected i.p. or bilaterally into ACB (n. accumbens), TUO (tuberculum olfactorium), or CPU (n. caudate-putamen). *Vertical rules* represent SEM. *Parentheses* indicate number of rats. ** $p < 0.01$ vs saline control.

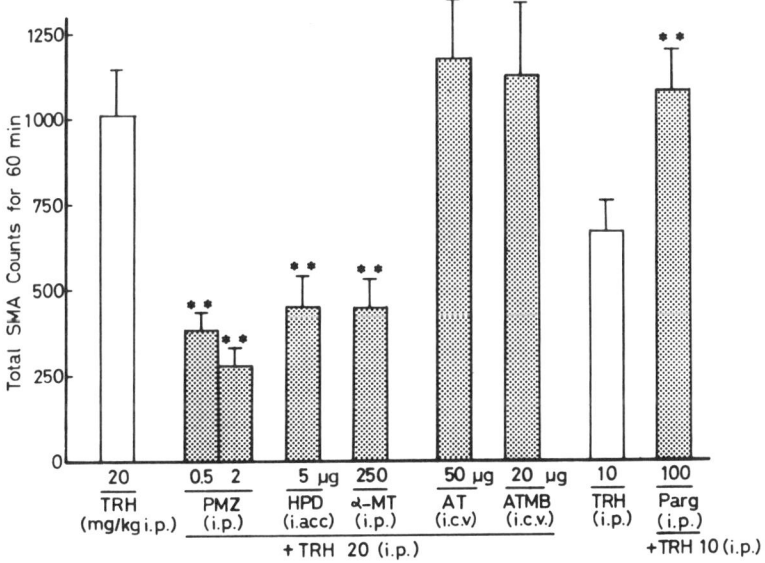

**FIG. 3.** Influence of DA receptor antagonists, catecholamine synthesis inhibitor, monoamine oxidase inhibitor, and anticholinergic drugs on TRH-induced hyperactivity in rats. SMA was measured by a Varimex meter. TRH was given i.p., and inhibitors were pretreated i.p. or by injection into n. accumbens (i.acc) or into a cerebroventricle (i.c.v.). PMZ, pimozide; HPD, haloperidol; α-MT, α-methyl-*p*-tyrosine; AT, atropine; ATMB, atropine methylbromide. **$p < 0.01$ vs TRH control.

These results suggest that TRH may activate presynaptically neurons in the ACB to release DA from the nerve terminals. This is supported by the *in vitro* result that TRH enhances the release of [³H]DA from the superfused ACB slices after a stable spontaneous DA release was established, as shown in Fig. 4a.

## Effect of TRH on Nigrostriatal DA Nerve Terminals

### Effects on Presynaptic Sites

TRH in dose of 20 or 50 mg/kg (i.p.) did not induce circling in rats with 6-OHDA lesions in the unilateral nigrostriatal DA pathway. A higher dose of TRH (100 mg/kg, i.p.), however, resulted in ipsilateral circling behavior at a peak frequency of 12.5 min during the first 5 min. Thereafter, the frequency of the ipsilateral circlings gradually decreased and disappeared 50 min later (Fig. 5A). Apomorphine in a dose of 0.125 or 0.25 mg/kg i.p. induced contralateral circling behavior 5 min after administration to these lesioned rats. MAP in doses of 1 and 2 mg/kg i.p. induced ipsilateral circling behavior 5 min after administration.

Injection of 50 µg of TRH into the lesioned side of caudate nucleus did not elicit circling behavior, whereas a dose of 5 µg of MAP elicited contralateral circlings only during the first 10 min. On the other hand, the injection of 20 or 50 µg of TRH into the intact side of the caudate nucleus induced ipsilateral circlings that reached a peak in frequency during the early period and gradually decreased to a complete disappearance 40 min later. The ipsilateral circling induced by the unilateral injection of 5 µg of MAP into the intact side of the caudate nucleus was longer lasting than that caused by 50 µg of TRH (Fig. 5A and B). The ipsilateral circlings induced by systemic injection of 100 mg/kg i.p. of TRH or by injection

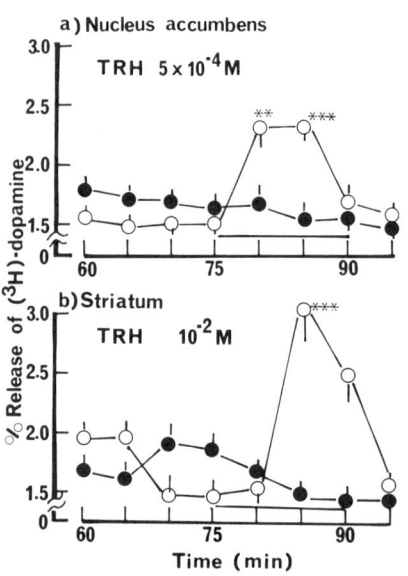

**FIG. 4.** Effects of TRH on the release of [³H]DA from nucleus accumbens **(a)** and striatal **(b)** slices of rats by superfusion. Nucleus accumbens and striatal slices were pre-labeled with $3.7 \times 10^{-8}$M [³H]DA at 37°C for 60 min. Drug was added from 75 to 90 min after the start of the superfusion, as indicated by the *bar*. Control *(closed circles)*, TRH *(open circles)*. Mean ± SE of five experiments. **$p < 0.01$, ***$p < 0.001$ vs control.

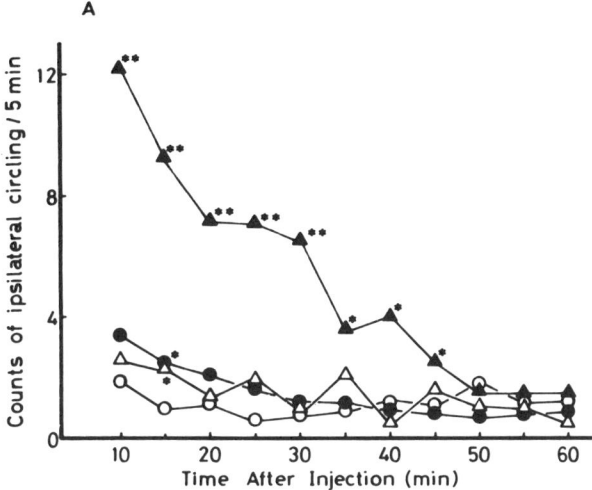

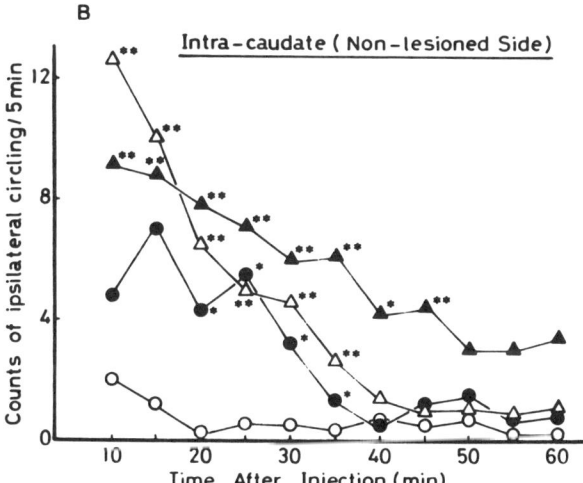

**FIG. 5.** Circling-inducing effect of TRH in the rats with unilateral striatal lesion produced by 6-OHDA. Circling induced by TRH or MAP was directed toward the lesioned side (ipsilateral). **A**: TRH was given i.p. *Open circles*, saline (9); *closed circles*, TRH 20 mg/kg, i.p. (6); *open triangles*, TRH 50 mg/kg, i.p. (6); *closed triangles*, TRH 100 mg/kg, i.p. (6). **B**: TRH or MAP was injected into the intact, nonlesioned side of the caudate nucleus (striatum). *Open circles*, saline; *closed circles*, TRH 20 μg (6); *open triangles*, TRH 50 μg (8); *closed triangles*, MAP 5 μg (5). *$p < 0.05$, **$p < 0.01$ vs saline control.

of 50 μg of TRH into the intact caudate nucleus were markedly attenuated or blocked either by 0.1 mg/kg of haloperidol or by 250 mg/kg of α-MT.

These results suggest that TRH may presynaptically activate neurons in the intact striatum to release DA from the nerve terminals and that the ipsilateral circling would then follow. The *in vitro* study demonstrated that higher concentration ($10^{-2}$M) of TRH enhanced the release of preloaded [$^3$H]DA from the striatal slices, as shown in Fig. 4b.

## Effects on Postsynaptic Sites

From the above findings, we postulate that TRH has no direct stimulating action on the DA receptor. However, Plotnikoff et al. (15) found the enhancing effect of TRH on the excitation induced by L-DOPA in mice pretreated with Parg. Thus, TRH may modify the action of DA in the process of postsynaptic transmission.

The effect of TRH itself was investigated in mice with unilateral striatal lesion induced by 6-OHDA. In the 6-OHDA lesioned mice, TRH in doses of 10–100 mg/kg i.p. given 2 weeks after the lesioning induced no predominant circling toward either side. However, the contralateral circling behavior induced by 1 mg/kg i.p. of apomorphine or by 400 mg/kg i.p. of L-DOPA in the 6-OHDA lesioned mice 2–3 weeks after the lesioning was significantly enhanced by 2.5–10 mg/kg i.p. of TRH injected 30 min before (Fig. 6, p.194).

The basal cyclic AMP levels in the caudate nucleus slices taken from the 6-OHDA lesioned side and intact side 3 weeks after 6-OHDA injection were 19.0 ± 4.3 and 41.0 ± 8.0 pmol/g wet weight, respectively. Further, the basal cyclic AMP levels in the caudate nucleus slices of mice treated with 10 mg/kg of TRH were 15.5 ± 3.9 and 33.5 ± 3.9 pmol/g in the lesioned and intact sides, respectively.

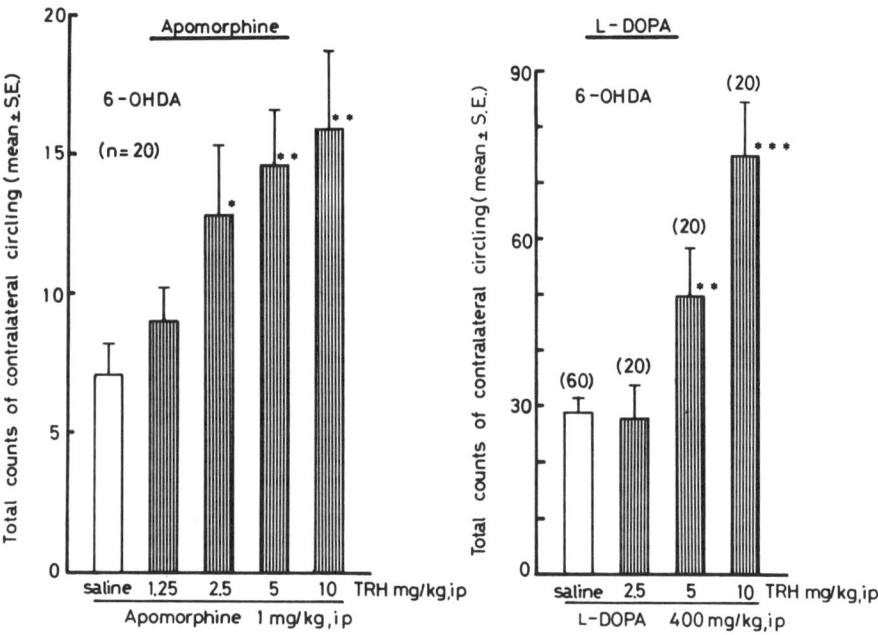

**FIG. 6.** Enhancement of circling response to apomorphine **(left)** and L-DOPA **(right)** by TRH in mice with unilateral striatal 6-OHDA lesion. *Parentheses* indicate number of mice. *$p < 0.05$, **$p < 0.01$, ***$p < 0.001$ vs saline control.

The values of lesioned side were about half those of the intact side in the mice given or not given TRH. Figure 7 (p. 194) shows the effects of TRH pretreatment or nontreatment on the action of DA on cyclic AMP contents of the caudate nucleus slices taken from the intact and lesioned sides of the mice with unilateral lesions. The patterns of DA-induced cyclic AMP formation in the caudate nucleus slices of the intact side were almost the same irrespective of pretreatment with TRH. In contrast, DA-stimulated cyclic AMP formation in the caudate nucleus slices taken from 6-OHDA lesioned side was mildly augmented in a concentration-dependent manner. Furthermore, pretreatment with TRH markedly enhanced the DA-stimulated cyclic AMP formation in the 6-OHDA lesioned caudate nucleus slices.

These results indicate that the enhancing effect of TRH on DA agonist-induced circling behavior in mice is probably closely associated with the enhancement of DA-stimulated cyclic AMP formation.

Figure 8 shows the proposed mode of action of TRH at presynaptic and postsynaptic sites in the striatum. TRH at higher doses facilitates the DA presynaptic transmission by increasing the DA release from the striatum and at low doses facilitates the DA postsynaptic transmission with an increase in DA-stimulated cyclic AMP formation in the striatum, under conditions of supersensitization of the DA receptor.

## DISCUSSION

TRH enhanced the SMA by systemic injection or direct microinjection of TRH into the nucleus accumbens in rats. Prevention of this TRH effect by pretreatment with haloperidol or pimozide, a DA receptor blocker, or $\alpha$-MT, an inhibitor of tyrosine hydroxylase, suggested that the SMA stimulant action of TRH is mediated by enhancing the release of DA from nerve terminals of the mesolimbic DA system. In fact, the *in vitro* study demonstrated that TRH ($5 \times 10^{-4}$M) enhanced the release of preloaded [$^3$H]DA from the slices of nucleus accumbens. In the nigrostriatal system, the DA content of caudate nucleus taken from the lesioned side decreased to about 30% of intact side from 1 to 3 weeks after the 6-OHDA injection. Cyclic AMP content in the 6-OHDA injected side was about half that of the nonlesioned side, 3 weeks later. Apomorphinc-induced contralateral circlings were observed from 1 to 3 weeks after the 6-OHDA injection, and were correlated with the degree of decrease in DA or cyclic AMP content. Thus, the receptor supersensitivity to DA agonists clearly occurred for some period after 6-OHDA injection, and the duration of supersensitivity depended on the degree of degeneration of the DA nerve terminals induced by 6-OHDA. The enhancing effect of TRH on apomorphine or L-DOPA-induced circling was marked from 1 to 3 weeks after 6-OHDA injection in which the supersensitivity to apomorphine or L-DOPA occurred, but the TRH effect disappeared 5 weeks later. These results suggest that the receptor supersensitivity to DA is important for the enhancing effect of TRH on DA agonist-induced circling behavior.

The striatal DA-sensitive adenylate cyclase may be closely related to the DA receptor (10), suggesting that cyclic AMP may be involved in the DA transmission

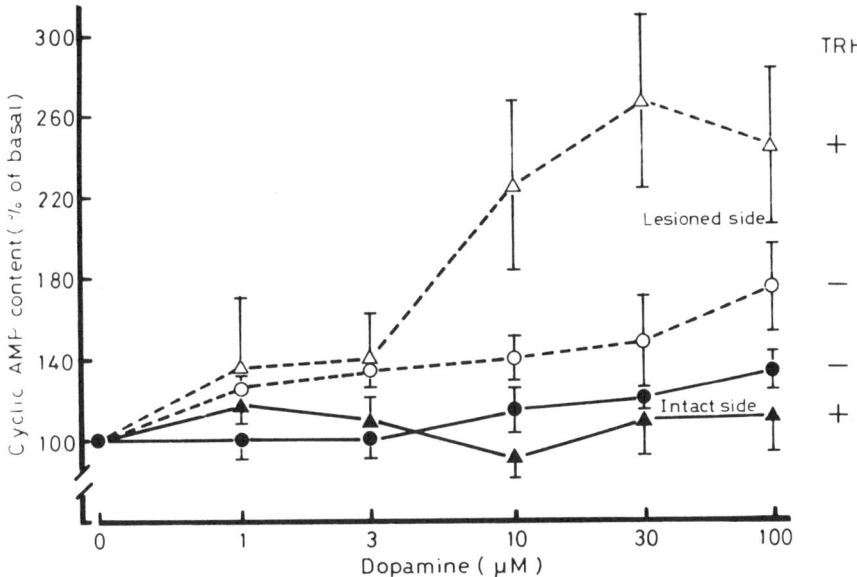

**FIG. 7.** Effects of various concentrations of DA on cyclic AMP content of the caudate nucleus slices taken from intact and lesioned sides of mice with unilateral striatal 6-OHDA lesion. TRH-nontreated (−): intact side *(closed circles)*, lesioned side *(open circles)*. TRH (10 mg/kg i.p.) pretreated (+): intact side *(closed triangles)*, lesioned side *(open triangles)*. Cyclic AMP levels were represented as percentage of the basal cyclic AMP levels obtained in the absence of added DA in terms of mean ± SE of 12 to 16 samples.

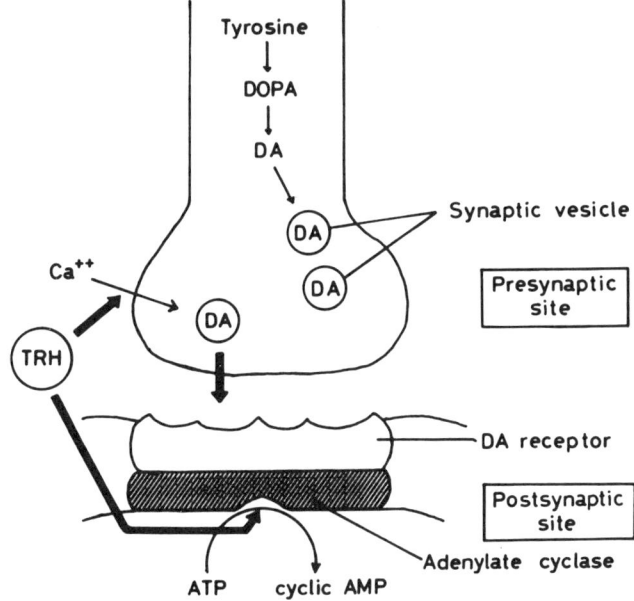

**FIG. 8.** Proposed mode of action of TRH at presynaptic and postsynaptic sites in the striatum.

in striatal system. The present experiment also demonstrated that the 6-OHDA injection not only sensitized the DA receptor but also enhanced adenylate cyclase activity: DA-induced cyclic AMP formation was significantly greater in the 6-OHDA injected side than in the intact side. Therefore, we thought that TRH raised the cyclic AMP formation due to DA in association with enhancement of the DA agonist-induced circling under supersensitization of the DA receptors caused by 6-OHDA injection. In fact, an increase in the ability of DA to stimulate cyclic AMP formation was markedly observed in the caudate nucleus slices taken from the 6-OHDA lesioned side of the mice pretreated with TRH, but not in the caudate nucleus slices from the intact side. An attempt to explain the probable mechanism of the enhancing effect of TRH on DA-stimulated cyclic AMP formation is made as follows: Supersensitization would render TRH more accessible to the site of action and (a) TRH further increases the binding affinity of DA to the receptor or adenylate cyclase, (b) TRH enhances the DA-induced cyclic AMP formation by acting on some process of cyclic AMP formation. In the present *in vitro* study, the enhancing effect of TRH on DA release from rat striatal slices was $Ca^{2+}$-dependent. Also, TRH might enhance the cyclic AMP formation by affecting the $Ca^{2+}$ movements. Thus it is supposed that the enhancing effect of TRH on DA agonist-induced circling behavior is closely related with the enhancement of DA-stimulated cyclic AMP formation.

The bilateral microinjection into the nucleus accumbens of small dose of TRH (10 or 20 μg) markedly enhanced the SMA of intact rats, whereas the unilateral intracaudate injection of TRH (50 μg) did not induce any circling behavior in intact rats. These observations suggest the differential affinity of TRH to the presynaptic neurons in the mesolimbic and nigrostriatal DA system. In the present investigation, however, an intraperitoneal administration of a large dose of TRH (100 mg/kg, i.p.) produced mild circling behavior ipsilateral to the lesioned side in rats with unilateral nigrostriatal DA pathway lesions induced by 6-OHDA injection. Furthermore, unilateral injection of 20 of 50 μg of TRH into the caudate nucleus on the lesioned side produced no circling, while a similar injection of the same dose of TRH into the intact side clearly caused the circling behavior directed to the lesioned side. Such circling was blocked by haloperidol or α-MT. Also a high concentration of TRH enhanced the [$^3$H]DA release from rat striatal slices *in vitro*. These observations strongly suggest that TRH produces the circling behavior by acting on the presnyaptic site of striatal neurons to stimulate the DA release from the nerve terminals, but that TRH does not act directly on the DA receptors.

## SUMMARY

TRH may act on the brain independently of its effects on the pituitary, and some of the CNS actions of TRH are probably closely related to brain catecholamines.

TRH enhanced SMA by systemic injection (20 mg/kg, i.p.) or direct microinjection (10 μg) of TRH into the nucleus accumbens (ACB), one of the nerve terminal sites of the mesolimbic dopaminergic system, in rats. Prevention of this TRH effect by pretreatment with haloperidol or pimozide, a DA receptor blocker, or α-MT, an inhibitor of tyrosine hydroxylase, indicated that the SMA stimulatory action of TRH was the result of an enhancement of the release of DA from the nerve terminals. In rats lesioned unilaterally in the nigrostriatal DA pathway by 6-OHDA, high doses of TRH given i.p. (100 mg/kg) or into the nonlesioned caudate nucleus (50 µg) produced a circling toward the lesioned side which was suppressed by haloperidol or α-MT. The *in vitro* study demonstrated that TRH ($5 \times 10^{-4}$M) enhanced the release of preloaded [$^3$H]DA from the slices of ACB after stable spontaneous DA release was established under superfusion, while a higher concentration ($10^{-2}$M) was required to enhance the DA release from striatal slices. These *in vitro* studies supported the findings in investigation *in vivo*. In addition, TRH (2.5–20 mg/kg) markedly enhanced the circling behavior induced by L-DOPA or apomorphine in mice with unilateral caudate nucleus lesions induced by injection of 6-OHDA. In the 6-OHDA lesioned mice treated with TRH, DA-induced cyclic AMP formation was clearly enhanced in the striatal slices taken from the lesioned side but not from the intact side.

In conclusion, TRH in low doses facilitates the DA presynaptic transmission by increasing the release of this amine from the ACB and also the DA postsynaptic transmission by increasing DA-stimulated cyclic AMP formation in striatum supersensitized with 6-OHDA. Endogenous TRH may play a physiological role as a modulator on DA transmission in CNS.

## ACKNOWLEDGMENTS

We are grateful to Dr. Y. Saji, Dr. N. Fukuda, M. Miyamoto, and Y. Nagai for invaluable technical assistance, and M. Ohara, Kyusu University, for advice on the manuscript.

## REFERENCES

1. Asher, I. M., and Aghajanian, G. K. (1974): 6-Hydroxydopamine lesions of olfactory tubercles and caudate nuclei: Effect on amphetamine-induced stereotyped behavior in rats. *Brain Res.*, 82: 1–12.
2. Bowers, C. Y., Freiesen, H. G., Hwang, P., Guyda, H. J., and Folkers, K. (1971): Prolactin and thyrotropin release in man by synthetic pyroglutamyl-histidyl-prolinamide. *Biochem. Biophys. Res. Commun.*, 45:1033–1041.
3. Brownstein, M. J., Palkovits, M., Saaverdra, J. M., Bassiri, R. M., and Utiger, R. D. (1974): Thyrotropin-releasing hormone in specific nuclei of rat brain. *Science*, 185:267–269.
4. De Groot, J. (1959): The forebrain in stereotaxic coordinates. *Verh. K. Acad. Wet.*, 52:1–40.
5. Fleischer, N., Burgus, R., Vale, W., Dunn, T., and Guillemin, R. (1970): Preliminary observation on the effect of synthetic thyrotropin releasing factor on plasma thyrotropin levels in man. *J. Clin. Endocrinol. Metab.*, 31:109–112.
6. Hökfelt, T., Fuxe, K., Johansson, O., Jeffcoate, S., and White, N. (1975): Distribution of thyrotropin-releasing hormone (TRH) in the central nervous system as revealed with immunohistochemistry. *Eur. J. Pharmacol.*, 34:389–392.
7. Hollander, C. S., Mitsuma, T., Shenkman, L., Woolf, P., and Gershengorn, M. C. (1972): Thyrotropin-releasing hormone: Evidence for thyroid response to intravenous injection in man. *Science*, 175:209–210.
8. Inoue, M., Miyamoto, M., Fujitani, H., Suhara, I., and Nagawa, Y. (1976): Relation of stimulant action of thyrotropin releasing hormone (TRH) on spontaneous motor activity to the central catecholaminergic system. *J. Takeda Res. Lab.*, 35:194–203.

9. Jackson, I. M. D., and Reichlin, S. (1974): Thyrotropin releasing hormone (TRH): Distribution in the brain, blood and urine of the rat. *Life Sci.*, 14:2259–2266.
10. Kebabian, J. W., Petzold, G. L., and Greengard, P. (1972): Dopamine-sensitive adenylate cyclase in caudate nucleus of rat brain, and its similarity to the dopamine receptor. *Proc. Nat. Acad. Sci. USA*, 69:2145–2149.
11. Kelly, P. H., Serviour, P. W., and Iversen, S. D. (1975): Amphetamine and apomorphine responses in the rat following 6-OHDA lesions of the nucleus accumbens septi and corpus striatum. *Brain Res.*, 94:507–522.
12. König, J. F., and Klippel, R. A. (1963): *The Rat Brain Stereotaxic Atlas*. Williams and Wilkins, Baltimore.
13. Krueger, B. K., Forn, J., Walters, J. R., Roth, R. H., and Greengard, P. (1976): Stimulation of dopamine of adenosine cyclic 3′,5′-monophosphate formation in rat caudate nucleus: Effect of lesions of the nigrostriatal pathway. *Mol. Pharmacol.*, 12:639–648.
14. Miyamoto, M., and Nagawa, Y. (1977): Mesolimbic involvement in the locomotor stimulant action of thyrotropin-releasing hormone (TRH) in rats. *Eur. J. Pharmacol.*, 44:143–152.
15. Plotnikoff, N. P., Prange, A. J., Jr., Breese, G. R., Anderson, M. S., and Wilson, I. C. (1972): Thyrotropin releasing hormone: Enhancement of Dopa activity by a hypothalamic hormone. *Science*, 178:417–418.
16. Ungerstedt, U. (1971): Stereotaxic mapping of the monoamine pathways in the rat brain. *Acta Physiol. Scand. (Suppl.)*, 367:1–48.
17. Winokur, A., and Utiger, R. D. (1974): Thyrotropin-releasing hormone: Regional distribution in rat brain. *Science*, 185:265–267.

# Inhibition of VIP-Sensitive Adenylate Cyclase by Dopamine in Rat Anterior Pituitary

Pierluigi Onali, Joan P. Schwartz, and E. Costa

*Laboratory of Preclinical Pharmacology, National Institute of Mental Health, Saint Elizabeths Hospital, Washington, D.C. 20032*

The coupling of dopamine (DA) receptors to adenylate cyclase has been used as a criterion to distinguish two classes of DA receptors: those linked to a stimulation of the enzyme (D-1) and those not coupled to adenylate cyclase (D-2) (14). The DA receptors present on mammotrophs of anterior pituitary have been considered as a representative example of D-2 DA receptors. These receptors mediate the inhibitory action of DA on prolactin release and synthesis (17,19). Whether or not the pituitary DA receptors are entirely dissociated from adenylate cyclase is controversial: reports vary from inhibition (9) to stimulation (1) to ineffectiveness (25,27,30). Since the heterogeneity of the cell population of anterior pituitary could have been a limiting factor in detecting consistent responses of basal adenylate cyclase activity to DA, we have investigated the effect of DA when the enzyme was activated by vasoactive intestinal peptide (VIP). Previous studies have shown that, *in vitro*, this peptide stimulates only the release of prolactin from anterior pituitary cells (22,24), antagonizes the inhibitory action of DA on prolactin release (13), and is a potent activator of adenylate cyclase of pituitary gland (4). These results indicate that VIP acts directly on the mammotrophs of anterior pituitary. Thus, the VIP-sensitive adenylate cyclase could be a useful model to ascertain whether the D-2 receptors of these cells are coupled to adenylate cyclase. In the present report we show that stimulation of pituitary DA receptors inhibits the VIP-sensitive adenylate cyclase, thus suggesting that D-2 receptors in anterior pituitary are linked in an inhibitory way to adenylate cyclase.

## CHARACTERISTICS OF DA INHIBITION OF VIP-SENSITIVE ADENYLATE CYCLASE

The adenylate cyclase activity of male rat anterior pituitary is stimulated by VIP in a dose-dependent manner (Fig. 1). The maximal activation was obtained with concentrations of VIP ranging from $5 \times 10^{-7}$ M to $10^{-6}$ M and corresponded to a threefold increase of the basal enzyme activity. Half-maximal activation was reached at a concentration of VIP of approximately $10^{-7}$ M. In the presence of DA, the

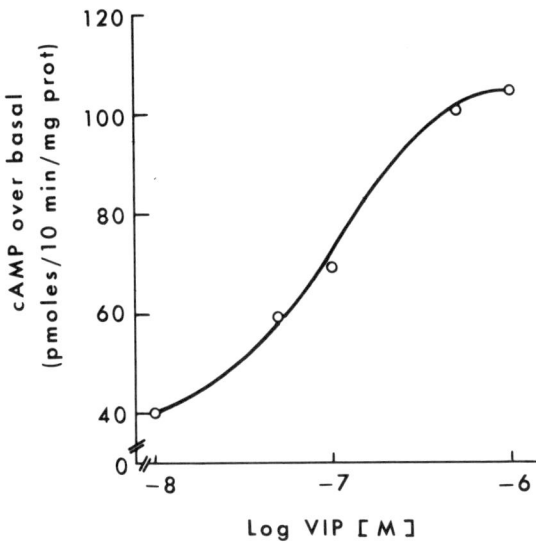

**FIG. 1.** Dose-response curve for VIP on male rat anterior pituitary adenylate cyclase. Basal enzyme activity (64 ± 1.3 pmoles of cAMP/10 min/mg prot. ± SEM) was subtracted from each point. The profile is representative of eight experiments. Anterior pituitaries from male rats (170–250 g) were homogenized manually in ice cold buffer (1:30 wt/vol) containing 10 mM HEPES (pH 7.4 at 4°C), 1 mM dithiothreitol (DTT), 1 mM EGTA, and 0.32 M sucrose. The homogenate was then centrifuged at 400 × $g$ for 5 min. Unless otherwise specified, adenylate cyclase activity was assayed at 30°C for 10 min in a reaction mixture (150 μl) containing 53 mM HEPES (pH 7.4 at 30°C), 0.3 mM EGTA, 1 mM DTT, 2 mM MgCl$_2$, 1 mM cyclic AMP, 0.5 mM l-methyl-3-isobutylxanthine, 10 μM bacitracin, 50 μg of bovine serum albumin, 10 μM GTP, 0.5 mM [α-$^{32}$P]ATP (25–50 cpm/pmol), 20 mM creatine phosphate, 100 U/ml creatine phosphokinase, and 50 μl of 400 × $g$ supernatant (150–200 μg of protein). [$^{32}$P]Cyclic AMP was isolated by sequential chromatography on Dowex 50W-X4 and alumina according to Salomon et al. (23). Protein was assayed according to the method of Bohlen et al. (3).

activation of the adenylate cyclase by VIP was markedly reduced (Fig. 2). A concentration of DA of $10^{-5}$ M inhibited the activation of the enzyme by approximately 50% at all the concentrations of VIP tested. At this concentration DA failed to affect either the basal enzyme activity or the activation of adenylate cyclase by prostaglandin E$_1$, a hormone which does not stimulate prolactin release (11,18) (results not shown). The inhibitory effect of DA occurred without an apparent lag phase, being already evident after 2 min of incubation, and remained constant up to 15 min (Fig. 3). This inhibition was dependent on the concentration of DA (Fig. 4). The maximal effect was observed with a concentration of $10^{-5}$ M and the apparent IC$_{50}$ value was approximately 4 × $10^{-7}$ M.

The kinetic nature of this inhibition was investigated by testing the effect of different concentrations of DA on the activation of the enzyme elicited by increasing concentrations of VIP. A double reciprocal plot of the data (Fig. 5) shows that DA decreased primarily the maximum velocity of the activated enzyme with only a slight effect on the apparent affinity constant of VIP, indicating that the inhibition was noncompetitive.

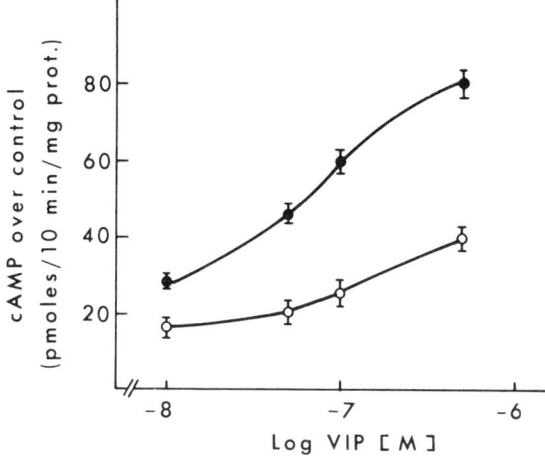

**FIG. 2.** DA inhibition of the adenylate cyclase activity stimulated by VIP. VIP was tested at the reported concentrations alone *(closed circles)* and in the presence of 10 μM DA *(open circles)*. Adenylate cyclase stimulation was calculated by subtracting the control values for each compound. Control values, expressed as pmoles of cAMP formed in 10 min/mg prot (mean ± SEM) were: basal activity, 70 ± 2.8; DA, 69 ± 5.2.

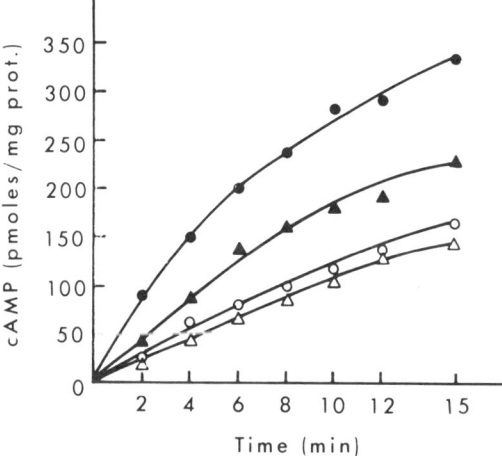

**FIG. 3.** Time course of DA inhibition of VIP sensitive adenylate cyclase. Aliquots of 400 × $g$ supernatant were incubated for the indicated times in the presence of vehicle *(open circles)*, VIP 0.1 μM *(closed circles)*, DA 10 μM *(open triangles)*, and DA + VIP *(closed triangles)*. Values were obtained from one experiment performed in duplicate and confirmed by an additional experiment.

## PHARMACOLOGICAL PROPERTIES OF THE DA RECEPTOR MEDIATING THE INHIBITION OF VIP-SENSITIVE ADENYLATE CYCLASE

The inhibitory effect of DA was mimicked by dopaminergic agonists. Figure 6 shows that apomorphine and A-6, 7-DTN inhibited the VIP-sensitive adenylate cyclase in a dose-dependent manner. These compounds were more potent than DA, in agreement with their rank order of potency in inhibiting prolactin release *in vivo*

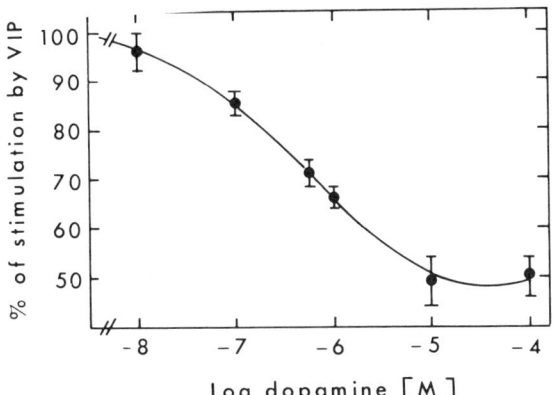

**FIG. 4.** Dose-dependent inhibition of VIP-sensitive adenylate cyclase by DA. DA was tested alone and in the presence of 0.1 μM VIP. The VIP stimulation of the enzyme was determined by subtracting the respective control value. Inhibition is expressed as a percentage of the enzyme stimulation produced by VIP. Control values as pmoles of cAMP/mg prot./10 min (means ± SEM) were: basal activity, 55 ± 1.2; 0.1 μM VIP, 118.0 ± 2.3. The enzyme activity assayed in the presence of DA alone was not significantly different from the basal activity. ($N = 6$).

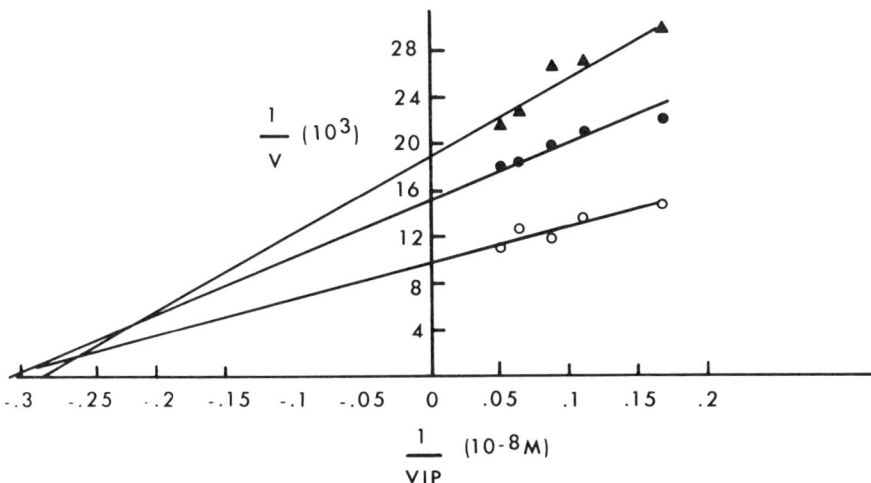

**FIG. 5.** Noncompetitive inhibition of VIP-sensitive adenylate cyclase by DA. Enzyme activity was assayed in the presence of VIP alone (from 3 to 20 × $10^{-8}$ M) *(open circles)* and VIP plus DA at 5 × $10^{-7}$ M *(closed circles)* and at $10^{-5}$ M *(triangles)*. Incubations were carried out at 30°C for 6 min. Enzyme velocities are expressed as total pmoles of cAMP/mg of protein formed during the incubation time and were corrected by subtracting the respective control values. These values were (mean ± SEM): basal, 77 ± 0.7; DA 5 × $10^{-7}$, 69 ± 0.4; DA $10^{-5}$, 65 ± 0.6. $V_{max}$ values of the stimulated enzyme were: VIP alone, 97.7; VIP + DA 5 × $10^{-7}$, 63.5; VIP + DA $10^{-5}$, 52.6.

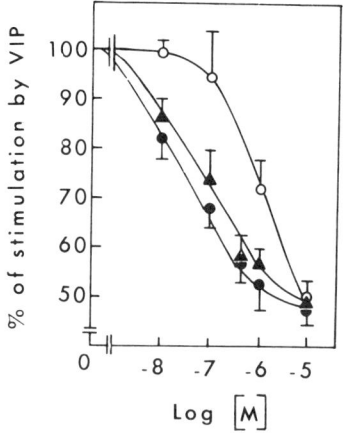

**FIG. 6.** Effect of different concentrations of A-6,7-DTN *(closed circles)*, apomorphine *(triangles)*, and noradrenaline *(open circles)* on VIP-sensitive adenylate cyclase. Each compound was tested alone and in the presence of 0.1 μM VIP. Enzyme activities were determined as described in the legend of Fig. 4. The observed $IC_{50}$ values were approx.: A-6,7-DTN $4 \times 10^{-8}$ M; apomorphine, $10^{-7}$ M; noradrenaline, $10^{-6}$ M. ($N = 4$).

and *in vitro* (7,20). We also tested the effect of three ergot alkaloids, 2-bromo-α-ergocriptine, lergotrile, and lisuride, which are potent inhibitors of prolactin release (2,7,12,15). These compounds were weaker than DA in inhibiting the VIP-sensitive adenylate cyclase. Moreover, lisuride behaved like a partial agonist *(results not shown)*. One possible explanation of the lower activity of the ergot alkaloids could be their poor solubility in aqueous solutions. However, two binding sites for DA with differing affinities have been described in bovine anterior pituitary (6) and in human pituitary adenomas (5); additionally, it has been shown that guanine nucleotides decrease the affinity of pituitary recognition sites for DA and dopaminergic agonists, but not that for 2-bromo-α-ergocriptine (26). It has also been reported that dihydroergocryptine, a potent inhibitor of prolactin release, did not displace the binding of a DA agonist, RU 24213, to rat anterior pituitary (10). Thus, it is possible that different subtypes of D-2 DA receptors are present on mammotrophs and that those which inhibit the adenylate cyclase activity lack the high affinity for DA agonists such as the ergot alkaloids.

Among α- and β-adrenergic agonists tested, only noradrenaline in micromolar concentrations significantly inhibited the VIP stimulation of adenylate cyclase activity (Fig. 6, Table 1), whereas *l*-phenylephrine and *l*-isoproterenol were ineffective *(results not shown)*. The inhibitory effect of noradrenaline was probably due to a stimulation of DA receptors rather than α-adrenergic receptors because, as shown in Table 1, it was antagonized by (−)sulpiride, a D-2 DA receptor blocker (14,28,29), but not by phentolamine; phentolamine failed to reverse the inhibitory effect of DA.

To further establish that the DA inhibition was mediated by stimulation of specific recognition sites for DA, we investigated the effect of different antagonists of DA receptors. As shown in Fig. 7, these compounds counteracted the inhibitory effect of DA on VIP-sensitive adenylate cyclase. At a concentration of $10^{-6}$ M the antipsychotic drugs failed to affect the activation of the enzyme by VIP, but completely

TABLE 1. *Effect of phentolamine and (−)sulpiride on the DA and noradrenaline inhibition of the VIP-sensitive adenylate cyclase activity of anterior pituitary*

| Experimental condition | cAMP (pmoles/10 min/mg prot.) over control |
|---|---|
| VIP[a] | 108.6 |
| VIP + NA | 59.3 |
| VIP + NA + (−)sulpiride, $10^{-6}$ M | 92.9 |
| VIP + NA + phentolamine $10^{-6}$ M | 65.7 |
| VIP[b] | 75.4 |
| VIP + DA | 43.7 |
| VIP + DA + phentolamine, $10^{-5}$ M | 45.5 |

*l*-Noradrenaline (NA) and DA were tested at a concentration of $10^{-5}$ M alone, in the presence of 0.1 μM VIP, and in the presence of VIP plus the receptor blocking agents. The stimulation produced by VIP was measured by subtracting the respective control value. These values (pmoles of cAMP/mg prot./10 min; mean ± SEM) were:
[a] basal, 47 ± 1.2; NA, 55 ± 0.8.
[b] basal, 52 ± 2.1; DA, 46 ± 0.6. (N = 4.)

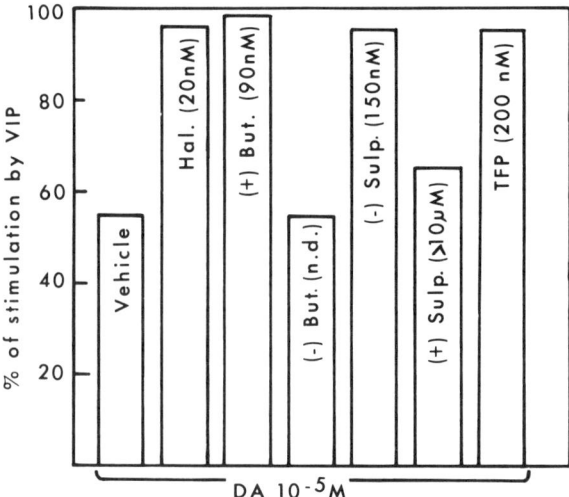

**FIG. 7.** Reversal of DA inhibition of VIP-sensitive adenylate cyclase by antipsychotic drugs. Each antagonist was tested at a concentration of 1 μM alone and in the presence of 0.1 μM VIP or VIP plus $10^{-5}$ M DA. The stimulation caused by VIP was measured by subtracting the respective control value; the effect of DA is reported as percentage of the stimulation obtained with VIP alone. Abbreviations: haloperidol, Hal.; (+)butaclamol, (+) But.; (−)butaclamol, (−)But.; (−)sulpiride, (−) Sulp.; (+)sulpiride, (+)Sulp.; trifluoperazine, TFP. Numbers in parentheses indicate the $IC_{50}$ value for each DA antagonist, the concentration required to half-maximally reverse the inhibitory effect of 10 μM DA. These values were obtained from experiments in which each antagonist was tested at concentrations ranging from 10 nM to 10 μM.

reversed the inhibitory effect of DA. This antagonism was stereospecific, as demonstrated by the weaker effect of the less active enantiomers, $l$-butaclamol and $d$-sulpiride, and was dose-dependent. The rank order of potency of these antipsychotic drugs in reversing the inhibitory effect of DA on VIP-sensitive adenylate cyclase agrees with their ability to displace dopaminergic agonist bound to pituitary DA recognition sites and to antagonize the inhibitory action of DA on prolactin release (6–8).

## EFFECT OF GUANINE NUCLEOTIDES ON DA INHIBITION OF VIP-SENSITIVE ADENYLATE CYCLASE

Guanine nucleotides play an important role in regulating the activity of the adenylate cyclase system (21). In rat anterior pituitary, the activation of adenylate cyclase by VIP was dependent on the concentration of guanosine triphosphate (GTP) (Table 2). The potentiating effect of GTP on the hormonal activation of the enzyme is mediated through the regulatory component of the adenylate cyclase (16). To investigate whether this regulatory component was also involved in the mechanism of action of DA, we tested the effect of GTP on the inhibition of the enzyme by DA. As shown in Table 2, in the absence of added GTP, VIP significantly stimulated the enzyme but DA was completely ineffective. At a concentration of GTP of $10^{-7}$ M, VIP increased the enzyme activity threefold whereas DA still had no effect on this activation. Only when the concentration of GTP was raised to $10^{-5}$ M could the DA inhibition be detected. These results indicate that the inhibitory effect of DA was dependent on the presence of GTP and that the concentration of the guanine nucleotide necessary for this inhibition was higher than that required for the activation of the enzyme by VIP.

We next investigated whether a less hydrolyzable analog of GTP, GMP imidodiphosphate [GMPP(NH)P] could substitute for GTP in supporting the inhibitory

TABLE 2. *GTP dependency of DA inhibition of VIP-sensitive adenylate cyclase in rat anterior pituitary*

| Experimental conditions | cAMP (pmoles/10 min/mg prot. ± SEM) formed in the presence of: | | |
|---|---|---|---|
| | −GTP | GTP $10^{-7}$ M | GTP $10^{-5}$ M |
| Basal | 23.8 ± 0.6 | 32.2 ± 0.4 | 80.1 ± 1.7 |
| VIP, $10^{-7}$ M | 43.6 ± 1.5 | 97.8 ± 1.8 | 289.7 ± 2.6 |
| DA, $10^{-5}$ M | 25.5 ± 0.4 | 34.3 ± 0.6 | 75.3 ± 4.7 |
| VIP ($10^{-7}$ M) + DA ($10^{-5}$ M) | 43.9 ± 1.0 | 106.61 ± 4.6 | 203.6 ± 4.3 |

Anterior pituitaries were homogenized in 30 vol (wt/vol) of homogenizing buffer. The homogenate was centrifuged at 400 × $g$ for 5 min. The supernatant was centrifuged at 30,000 × $g$ for 20 min. The pellet was washed once by resuspension and centrifugation at 30,000 × $g$ for 20 min. The final pellet was resuspended in homogenizing buffer and was used for enzyme assay. Reaction mixtures contained 0.1 mM ATP, 7mM creatine phosphate, 33 U/ml of creatine phosphokinase, and 0.33 mg of protein/ml. The values reported were obtained from one experiment carried out in triplicate and were confirmed by an additional experiment.

TABLE 3. *Different effects of GTP and GMPP(NH)P on DA inhibition of VIP-sensitive adenylate cyclase in rat anterior pituitary*

| Experimental conditions | cAMP (pmoles/10 min/mg prot. ± SEM) formed in the presence of: | |
|---|---|---|
| | GTP, $10^{-5}$ M | GMPP(NH)P, $10^{-5}$ M |
| Basal | 117.7 ± 3.1 | 205.3 ± 4.8 |
| DA, $10^{-5}$ M | 111.7 ± 2.2 | 225.5 ± 1.9 |
| VIP, $10^{-7}$ M | 427.4 ± 5.7 | 440.2 ± 8.0 |
| VIP ($10^{-7}$ M) + DA ($10^{-5}$ M) | 295.8 ± 1.25 | 444.5 ± 7.9 |

Anterior pituitaries were homogenized in 30 volumes (wt/vol) of homogenizing buffer. The homogenate was then centrifuged at 400 × $g$ for 5 min. The supernatant was centrifuged at 30,000 × $g$ for 20 min. The pellet was resuspended in homogenizing buffer and used for adenylate cyclase assay. Protein concentration in the reaction mixture was 0.8 mg/ml. The values reported were obtained from one experiment carried out in triplicate and were confirmed by an additional experiment.

effect of DA. As shown in Table 3, when GMPP(NH)P is substituted for GTP, DA failed to affect the stimulation of adenylate cyclase by VIP, suggesting that the hydrolysis of GTP to GDP was somehow required for the inhibition.

## CONCLUSIONS

The results of the study reported in this chapter show that DA and dopaminergic agonists inhibit the stimulation of pituitary adenylate cyclase by VIP. This inhibition is mediated by stimulation of specific dopamine receptors, is noncompetitive, and is specific for VIP-sensitive adenylate cyclase. The DA effect requires GTP, suggesting an interaction of the DA-receptor complex with the regulatory component of the adenylate cyclase system. On the basis of these results, we conclude that both classes of DA receptors (D-1 and D-2) are coupled to adenylate cyclase; however, they exert opposite effects on the activity of the enzyme. This difference may depend either on the molecular nature of the coupling device or on the different properties of the two classes of DA receptors or on both factors.

## REFERENCES

1. Ahn, H. S., Gardner, E., and Makman, M. (1979): *Eur. J. Pharmacol.*, 53:313–317.
2. Besser, G. M., Parke, L., Edwards, C. R. W., Forsyth, I. A., and McNeilly, A. S. (1972): *Br. Med. J.*, 3:669–672.
3. Bohlen, P., Stein, S., Dairman, W., and Udenfriend, S. (1973): *Arch. Biochem. Biophys.*, 155:213–220.
4. Borghi, C., Nicosia, S., Giachetti, A., and Said, S. I. (1979): *FEBS Lett.*, 108:403–406.
5. Bression, D., Brandi, A. M., Martes, M. P., Nousbaum, A., Cesselin, F., Racadot, J., and Peillon, F. (1980): *J. Clin. Endocrinol. Metab.*, 51:1037–1043.
6. Calabro, M. A., and MacLeod, R. M. (1978): *Neuroendocrinology*, 25:32–46.
7. Caron, M. G., Beaulieu, M., Raymond, V., Gagne, B., Drouin, J., Lefkowitz, R. J., and Labrie, F. (1978): *J. Biol. Chem.*, 253:2244–2253.
8. Cronin, M. J., Roberts, J. M., and Weiner, R. I. (1978): *Endocrinology*, 96:302–309.
9. De Camilli, P., Macconi, D., and Spada, A. (1979): *Nature*, 278:252–254.

10. Di Paolo, T., Calmichael, R., Labrie, F., and Raynaud, J.-P. (1979): *Mol. Cell. Endocrinol.*, 16:99–113.
11. Drouin, J., and Labrie, F. (1976): *Prostaglandins*, 11:355–364.
12. Graf, K.-J., Neumann, F., and Horowski, R. (1976): *Endocrinology*, 98:598–605.
13. Kato, Y., Iwasaki, Y., Iwasaki, J., Abe, H., Yanaihara, N., and Imura, H. (1978): *Endocrinology*, 103:554–558.
14. Kebabian, J. W., and Calne, D. B. (1979): *Nature*, 277:93–96.
15. Lemberg, L., Crabtree, R., Clemens, J., Dyke, R. W., and Woodburn, R. T. (1974): *J. Clin. Endocrinol. Metab.*, 39:579–584.
16. Limbird, L. E. (1981): *Biochem. J.*, 195:1–13.
17. MacLeod, R. M. (1976): In: *Frontiers in Neuroendocrinology*, edited by L. Martini, and G. Ganong, pp. 169–194. Raven Press, New York.
18. MacLeod, R. M., and Lehmeyer, J. E. (1970): *Proc. Natl. Acad. Sci. USA*, 67:1172–1179.
19. Maurer, R. A. (1980): *J. Biol. Chem.*, 255:8092–8097.
20. Rick, J. R., Szabo, M., Payne, P., Kovathana, N., Cannon, J. G., and Frohman, L. A. (1979): *Endocrinology*, 104:1234–1242.
21. Rodbell, M. (1980): *Nature*, 284:17–22.
22. Rotsztejn, W. H., Bernoist, L., Besson, J., Beraud, G., Bluet-Pajot, M. T., Kordon, C., Rosselin, G., and Duval, J. (1980): *Neuroendocrinology*, 31:282–286.
23. Salomon, Y., Londos, C., and Rodbell, M. (1974): *Anal. Biochem.*, 58:541–548.
24. Samson, W. K., Said, S. I., Snyder, G., and McCann, S. M. (1980): *Peptides*, 1:325–332.
25. Schmidt, M. J., and Hill, L. E. (1977): *Life Sci.*, 20:789–798.
26. Sibley, D. R., and Creese, I. (1979): *Eur. J. Pharmacol.*, 55:341–343.
27. Spano, P. F., Govoni, S., and Trabucchi, M. (1977): *Adv. Biochem. Pharmacol.*, 19:155–166.
28. Theodorou, A. E., Hall, M. D., Jenner, P., and Marsden, C. D. (1980): *J. Pharm. Pharmacol.*, 32:441–444.
29. Trabucchi, M., Longoni, R., Fresia, P., and Spano, P. F. (1975): *Life Sci.*, 17:1551–1556.
30. Zor, U., Kaneko, T., Schneider, H. P. G., McCann, S., Lowe, P. I., Bloom, G., Borland, B., and Field, J. B. (1969): *Proc. Natl. Acad. Sci. USA*, 63:918–925.

Molecular Pharmacology of Neurotransmitter
Receptors, edited by T. Segawa et al.
Raven Press, New York © 1983.

# The Benzodiazepine Receptor: Complex Binding Properties and the Influence of GABA

Frederick J. Ehlert, William R. Roeske, Susan H. Yamamura, and Henry I. Yamamura

*Departments of Pharmacology, Internal Medicine, Biochemistry, and Psychiatry, The University of Arizona Health Sciences Center, Tucson, Arizona 85724*

The concept of benzodiazepine receptors has gained acceptance during the past few years largely through advances made in ligand binding studies with benzodiazepines. Following the initial demonstration by Squires and Braestrup (30) of specific [$^3$H]diazepam binding sites in the brain, several investigators have provided additional evidence for the existence of neuronally localized benzodiazepine receptor-loci within the mammalian brain (2,6,19,20,29,32). As a result of these studies, a reasonably consistent picture of the nature of benzodiazepine-receptor interactions has emerged that satisfies several criteria thought to be important for defining receptor-specific binding. For example, the binding of benzodiazepines is stereospecific, saturable, and in most cases it is consistent with mass action behavior (6,19,20,30). Moreover, the binding is sensitive to inhibition by pharmacologically active benzodiazepines but not by drugs that are thought to interact with other neurotransmitter receptors (6,19,20,30). The regional distribution of the clonazepam-sensitive high-affinity component of [$^3$H]flunitrazepam ([$^3$H]FLU) or [$^3$H]diazepam binding is restricted to the central nervous system (6) and retina (26), and within the brain, it has a distribution that could account for the pharmacological effects of benzodiazepines (6). Perhaps the most convincing evidence demonstrating that [$^3$H]benzodiazepine binding represents a specific interaction with a pharmacologically relevant receptor is the good correlation between the behavioral doses of a series of benzodiazepines and their respective affinities for [$^3$H]benzodiazepine binding sites in the brain (19,30).

## HETEROGENEOUS BINDING PROPERTIES

Initially, it seemed as if benzodiazepine receptors were homogeneous, since the displacement of [$^3$H]FLU or [$^3$H]diazepam binding by several nonlabeled benzodiazepines always resembled simple competitive inhibition. However, evidence soon appeared which indicated that benzodiazepine receptors were not simply a homogeneous class of independent binding sites. In 1979, Squires et al. (29) found that a new class of compounds, the triazolopyridazines, inhibited [$^3$H]FLU binding in a manner that was characterized by shallow competition curves with Hill coefficients in the range of 0.5 to 0.7. One member of this class of compounds, CL 218,872 (3-methyl-6-[3-(trifluoromethyl)phenyl]-1,2,4-triazolo[(4,3-b]pyridazine), was reported to displace [$^3$H]FLU binding with a potency that was comparable to that of benzodiazepines (12,13). In addition to the novel binding properties of the triazolopyridazines, these compounds displayed a unique spectrum of pharmacological effects as well. CL 218,872 was found to be as potent as diazepam in preventing behavior reenforced by punishment (anticonflict test) and in preventing metrazol-induced convulsions in animals (12,13). In contrast to the benzodiazepines, however, CL 218,872 did not cause ataxia or sedation at doses 5 to 10 times greater than those which were effective in the conflict and convulsive tests (12,13). Thus, the triazolopyridazines may represent a class of selective anxiolytic drugs which lack the sedative properties of the benzodiazepines.

Complexities in the nature of ligand-interactions with the benzodiazepine receptor have also been observed in studies of the binding of alkyl derivatives of β-carboline-3-carboxylate (4,22). During an attempt to identify an endogenous ligand for the benzodiazepine receptor, Braestrup et al. (4) found that the ethyl ester of β-carboline-3-carboxylate was a potent inhibitor of [$^3$H]FLU binding ($IC_{50}$ = 4 nM) and that the nature of the displacement of binding was more complex than that of simple competitive inhibition (4,22). Subsequent studies have shown that the competition curves for the inhibition of [$^3$H]FLU binding by alkyl β-carboline-3-carboxylates are characterized by Hill coefficients that are less than one (22). However, unlike the triazolopyridazines, ethyl β-carboline-3-carboxylate (ECC) has been shown to be pharmacologically antagonistic to benzodiazepines, particulary with regard to its convulsive effects (15,24,34). In addition to the 3-carboxilic acid ester derivatives of β-carboline, harmane and similar β-carboline compounds have been shown to inhibit [$^3$H]FLU binding (27) in a manner that is sometimes described by low Hill coefficients (21). It has been known for quite some time that these compounds have pharmacological properties that are qualitatively antagonisitic to benzodiazepines. A cursory overview of the progress made toward an understanding of neurotransmitter-receptor interactions will reveal that the identification of differences between the binding properties of agonists and antagonists has played a central role in the formulation of elegant theories for receptor function and the significance of receptor heterogeneity (1,8). Therefore, it seems likely that studies of the interaction of β-carboline compounds with benzodiazepine receptors may provide insight into fundamental molecular mechanisms of benzodiazepine receptor heterogeneity and function.

In the foregoing studies concerning the inhibition of [$^3$H]benzodiazepine binding by β-carbolines and triazolopyridazines, the shallow competition curves with low Hill coefficients have been interpreted as evidence for multiple benzodiazepine receptors. In general, the data have been consistent with the presence of two major populations of receptors which have come to be known as type 1 and type 2 receptors (13,14,20). Moreover, studies of the competitive inhibition of [$^3$H]FLU binding by

ECC and CL 218,872 showed that their respective $IC_{50}$ values varied from low, 1 and 37 nM in the cerebellum, to high, 7 and 330 nM in the hippocampus, suggesting that the proportions of these receptor subtypes vary in different regions of the brain (5,12). Regression analysis of the ECC/[$^3$H]FLU competition data suggested that the cerebellum contains predominantly type 1 receptors (91%) whereas the cerebral cortex and hippocampus contain somewhat smaller proportions of 75% and 50 to 60%, respectively (3). The difference in the affinity of the type 1 and type 2 receptors is not particularly great; the potency ratio of ECC for these two sites is approximately 10 (3).

## THE BINDING OF [$^3$H]PROPYL β-CARBOLINE-3-CARBOXYLATE

The complex binding characteristics of β-carboline-3-carboxilic acid esters have also been detected by direct measurements of the binding of [$^3$H]propyl β-carboline-3-carboxylate ([$^3$H]PCC). The initial studies of Nielsen et al. (23) showed that [$^3$H]PCC binding exhibited characteristics of saturability and a pharmacological specificity and regional distribution remarkably similar to that of [$^3$H]FLU binding (23). Subsequently, we investigated the interaction of [$^3$H]PCC with benzodiazepine receptors in the cerebral cortex of the rat and identified additional complexities in the nature of benzodiazepine receptor binding that were not apparent in previous studies (10). Figure 1 shows the results of a study in which the binding of PCC to membrane preparations of the cerebral cortex was determined by direct measurements of [$^3$H]PCC binding and by competitive inhibition of [$^3$H]FLU binding. It can be seen that PCC receptor occupancy measured by competitive inhibition of [$^3$H]FLU binding (open symbols) is inconsistent with simple mass action behavior, as indicated by the large nonrandom deviations between the mean binding values, and the dotted line, which represents the best fit to the data assuming only one major binding site for PCC. Regression analysis revealed that the competition data were adequately described by the presence of high (H) and low (L) affinity binding sites having dissociation constants of 0.54 and 10 mM and relative densities of 55 and 45%, respectively. The good agreement between the mean binding values and the regression equation for two major binding sites is illustrated graphically in Fig. 1 by the solid line. The high- and low-affinity sites described above most likely correspond to the type 1 and 2 receptors identified by other investigators. When direct measurements of [$^3$H]PCC binding (solid symbols) are scaled to the capacity of the [$^3$H]FLU sites and compared with receptor occupancy determined by inhibition of [$^3$H]FLU binding, there is good agreement between the two independent sets of data up to about 60% receptor occupancy. Above this level, [$^3$H]PCC binding is greater, suggesting the existence of a population of receptors labeled by [$^3$H]PCC in the nanomolar range which have low affinity for [$^3$H]FLU.

Additional complexities in the nature of PCC binding are shown in Fig. 2, which illustrates direct measurements of [$^3$H]PCC binding in the cerebral cortex of the rat. Scatchard analysis of the data clearly shows deviations from simple mass action behavior and suggests the presence of a small component of binding having an

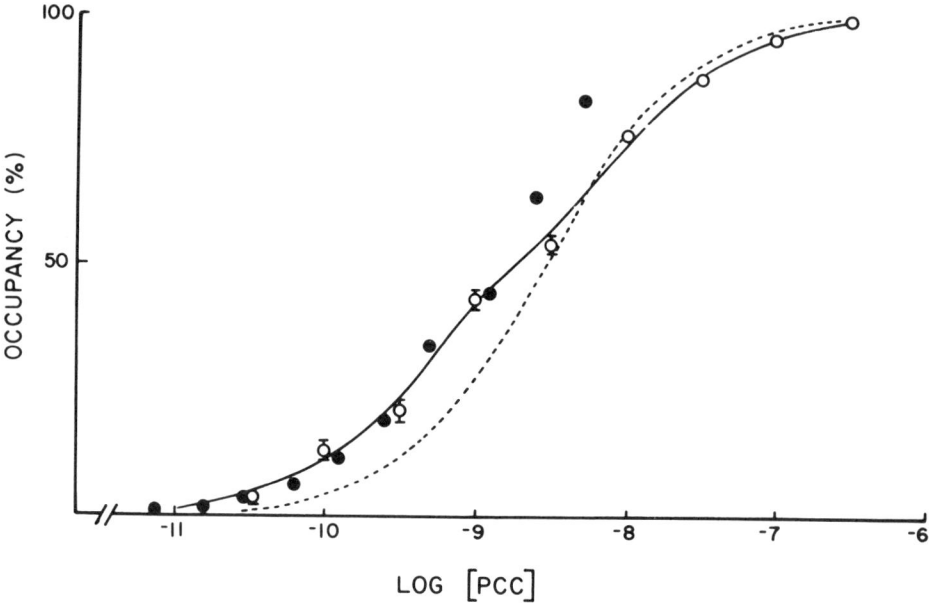

**FIG. 1.** Comparison of the binding of PCC measured directly *(closed circles)* or by inhibition of [$^3$H]FLU binding *(open circles)*. Mean specific [$^3$H]PCC binding values *(closed circles)* are plotted as a percentage of the total number of [$^3$H]FLU sites. Mean specific binding values ± SEM *(open circles)* from six PCC/[$^3$H]FLU competition experiments are plotted with percentage occupancy equaling the percentage of specifically bound [$^3$H]FLU displaced. The competition curve is corrected for occupancy of receptors by [$^3$H]FLU. Assays were carried out in 50 mM Na-K/phosphate buffer, pH 7.4, for 90 min at 0°C on three times washed homogenates of the rat cerebral cortex. Other experimental details are described by Ehlert et al. (10). The theoretical curves represent a mass action curve *(dotted line)* and a two site curve *(solid line)*. (From Ehlert et al., ref. 10, with permission.)

affinity much higher than that of the rest of the sites. Regression analysis of the data by a two site mass action equation yielded a dissociation constant of 100 pM and a relative abundance of 6% for these super high-affinity sites (SH). Very low [$^3$H]ligand concentrations as well as long equilibration times (60 min) are required to detect these SH affinity sites which makes them easy to overlook in cursory studies of [$^3$H]PCC binding.

In spite of our efforts to measure with care [$^3$H]PCC binding at low ligand concentrations, it seemed likely that the dissociation constant and receptor density of the SH site were overestimated when computed by regression analysis of the [$^3$H]PCC binding isotherm according to a site binding equation. This conclusion is based on the following information: (a) the relative density of the SH site is quite low; (b) collectively, the [$^3$H]PCC binding isotherm and PCC/[$^3$H]FLU competition curve suggest a total of three sites for PCC (SH, H, and L), making the use of a two site model inappropriate; and (c) it is well known that errors in parameter estimates are correlated. Thus, we attempted to measure the SH site more carefully by selectively labeling it with a very low concentration of [$^3$H]PCC (50 pM) and

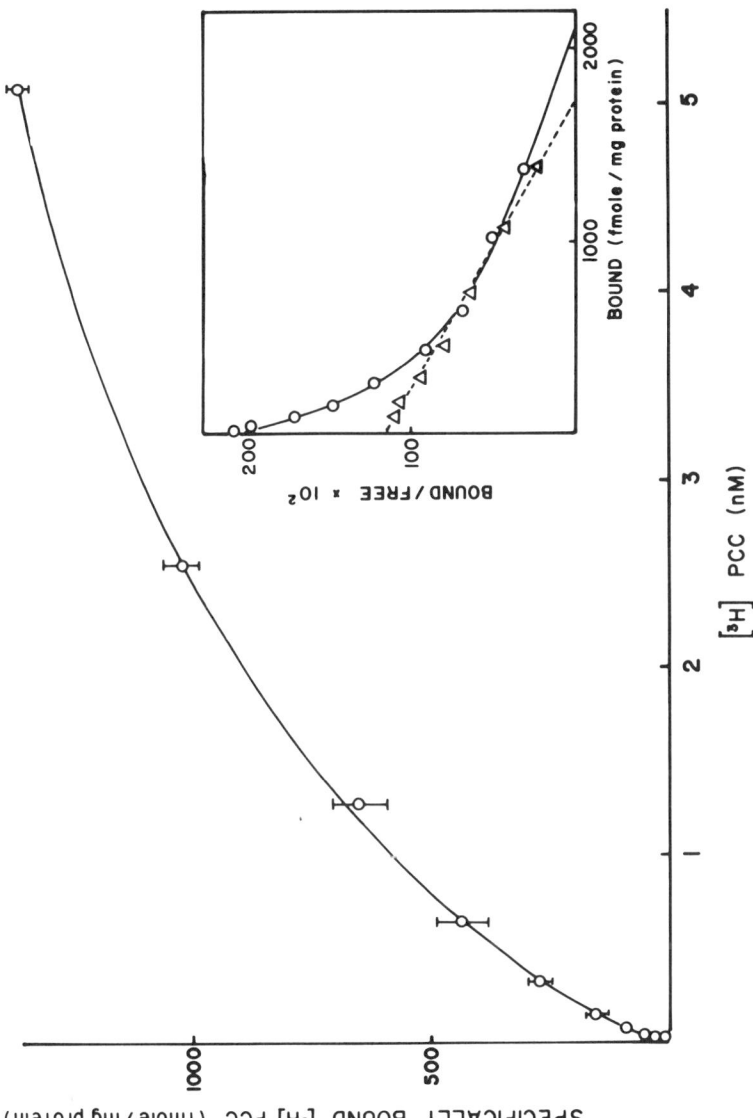

**FIG. 2.** Specific [³H]PCC binding to homogenates of the cerebral cortex of the rat. Mean specific binding values ± SEM (circles) were determined from three equilibrium binding experiments. The theoretical curve represents the weighted least squares fit to the data. Inset: Scatchard analysis of the mean specific binding values for [³H]PCC (circles) and [³H]FLU (triangles). Experimental conditions are the same as those described in the legend to Fig. 1. (The data are from Ehlert et al., ref. 10, with permission.)

competitively inhibiting the binding with nonlabeled PCC. The results of such an experiment are shown in Fig. 3. Scatchard analysis of the data shows that a large proportion (46%) of the sites labeled by [³H]PCC at a concentration of 50 pM have a very high affinity. When these data were analyzed by regression analysis, a value of 30 pM was calculated for the dissociation constant of the SH site which had a relative abundance of 3%. These latter estimates of the binding parameters of the SH site are probably more accurate than those measured by analysis of the [³H]PCC binding isotherm.

## MODULATION OF BENZODIAZEPINE RECEPTOR BINDING BY GABA

Although systemic administration of benzodiazepines has been shown to affect a variety of neurotransmitter systems, there is convincing evidence that the pharmacological effects of benzodiazepines are mediated, at least in part, by primary effects on the neurotransmission of GABA (33). Several electrophysiological studies, for example, have shown that benzodiazepines potentiate GABA-mediated

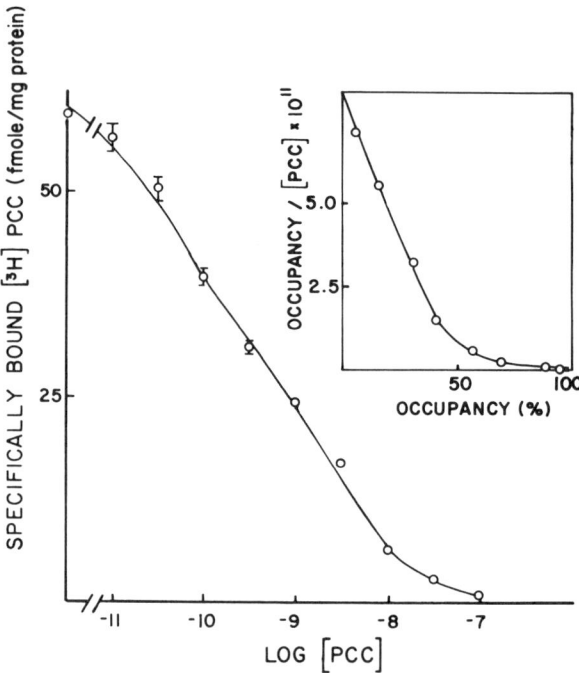

**FIG. 3.** Competitive inhibition of [³H]PCC binding by nonlabeled PCC. Mean specific binding values ± SEM *(circles)* of three experiments are shown. The concentration of [³H]PCC used in the competition experiments was 50 pM. The theoretical curve represents the weighted least squares fit to the data. *Inset:* Scatchard analysis of the mean binding values. The experimental conditions are the same as those described in the legend to Fig. 1. (The data are from Ehlert et al., ref. 10, with permission.)

transmission in a variety of neuronal systems, and binding studies have revealed that GABA enhances the binding of [$^3$H]FLU and [$^3$H]diazepam, suggesting that GABA receptors are coupled to benzodiazepine receptors [see review by Tallman et al. (32)]. The selective effects of chloride on [$^3$H]diazepam and [$^3$H]FLU binding (7,16,17,18,31) also implicate a close association of GABA receptors and benzodiazepine receptors since GABA receptors are thought to be coupled to chloride channels. Direct biochemical evidence for the close association of receptors for GABA and benzodiazepines comes from a study in which the co-purification of benzodiazepine and GABA binding was demonstrated in experiments on solubilized fractions from brain membranes (11).

Since pharmacological studies have indicated that β-carboline derivatives are antagonistic to benzodiazepines (15,24,34), it was of interest to compare the effects of GABA on the binding of PCC and FLU. During an initial study of the effects of GABA on the binding of [$^3$H]FLU and [$^3$H]PCC at [$^3$H]ligand concentrations of 0.5 nM we noted that GABA caused a maximal 180% increase in [$^3$H]FLU binding with the $ED_{50}$ for this effect being $10^{-6}$ M, whereas no significant effects of GABA ($10^{-7}$–$10^{-4}$ M) on PCC binding were detected (9,10). These experiments were carried out at 37°C in 50 mM Na-K/phosphate buffer plus 100 mM NaCl. When the experiments were carried out in the absence of 100 mM NaCl, similar results were obtained except that the maximal stimulation and $ED_{50}$ of GABA for enhancing [$^3$H]FLU binding were less (95% and $3 \times 10^{-7}$ M, respectively) (9,10).

The effects of GABA on the competitive inhibition of [$^3$H]FLU binding by PCC and FLU are shown in Fig. 4. An important feature of this type of experiment is that the binding of PCC to all the receptor subtypes is monitored, and not just the binding to the higher affinity sites which were selectively labeled, presumably, in the experiments described in the previous paragraph. As illustrated by the data in Fig. 4, GABA ($10^{-5}$ M) caused a modest threefold increase in the potency of FLU when assays were done at 37°C in the presence of 100 mM NaCl, whereas no significant effect of GABA ($10^{-5}$ M) on the binding of PCC was detected. It should be noted that the concentration of [$^3$H]FLU used in these experiments was low (0.5 nM) with respect to the $IC_{50}$ values of FLU; thus, correction from $IC_{50}$ to $K_I$ is unnecessary and the competition curves represent intrinsic binding isotherms for the ligands. A summary of the effects of GABA ($10^{-5}$ M) on the binding of FLU and PCC as measured by [$^3$H]ligand competition is given in Table 1. Inspection of the data indicates that at 37°C GABA enhances the potency of FLU in a manner that is potentiated by NaCl, whereas no significant effects on the binding of PCC were detected. It is interesting to note that the GABA-induced increase in the potency of FLU is also demonstrable by competitive inhibition of [$^3$H]PCC binding. This finding is consistent with the idea that PCC and FLU interact competitively at the same receptor locus.

## CONCLUSIONS

The PCC binding data described in the present report are consistent with previous notions of benzodiazepine receptor heterogeneity and illustrate additional com-

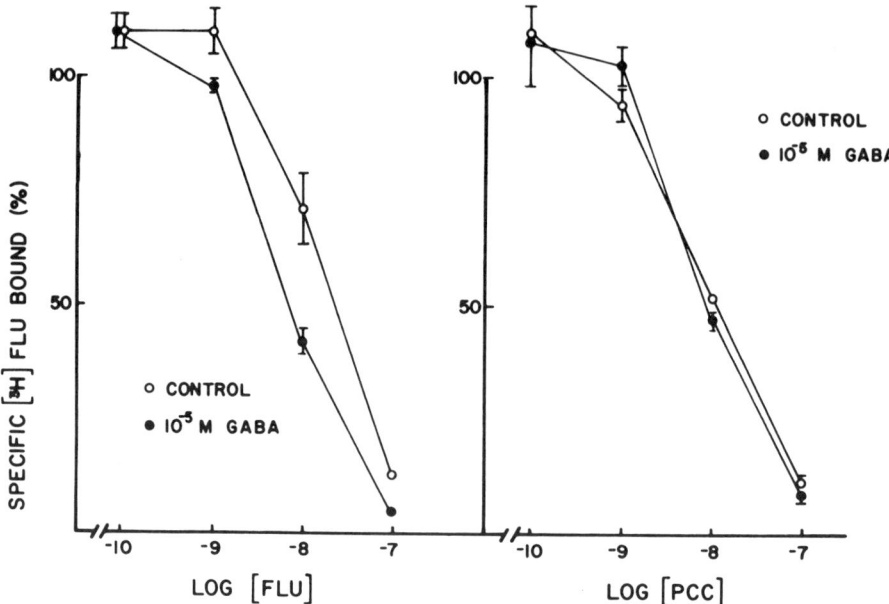

**FIG. 4.** Effect of GABA on the competitive inhibition of [³H]FLU binding by FLU and PCC. The competitive inhibition of [³H]FLU binding by FLU and PCC was determined in the presence *(closed circles)* and absence *(open circles)* of $10^{-5}$ M GABA. Assays were carried out at 37°C for 30 min in 50 mM Na-K/phosphate buffer, pH 7.4, containing 100 mM NaCl. Five times washed homogenates of the rat cerebral cortex were used.

plexities that were not apparent in previous studies—namely, the existence of a super high affinity site of low capacity. The implications of the various benzodiazepine binding sites are not readily apparent although it has been suggested that the type 1 and type 2 receptors selectively mediate different pharmacological effects (12,13). Direct evidence for molecular heterogeneity of the benzodiazepine receptor has been reported in a study of solubilized benzodiazepine receptors that were labeled irreversibly with [³H]FLU by uv irradiation. When the labeled receptors were examined by SDS polyacrylamide gel electrophoresis, two major molecular weight species of 51,000 and 55,000 daltons were apparent which had a regional distribution in the brain that correlated generally with the distribution of the type 1 and 2 receptors, respectively (28). Moreover, protection of the type 1 receptor from irreversible labeling by addition of CL 218,872 during uv irradiation resulted in a selective reduction in the labeling of the 51,000-dalton species (28). If the primary structure of the receptive loci of the two receptors are different, then selective type 1 and type 2 ligands should be possible. If future research fails to identify such ligands, then the difference in molecular weight probably corresponds to structural differences not associated with the binding region of the receptor.

The modulation of the benzodiazepine receptor by GABA may provide the basis for correlating binding measurements with pharmacological activity. We have proposed elsewhere (10) that the differential effects of GABA on the binding of FLU and PCC might be rationalized on the basis of a two state model for benzodiazepine

TABLE 1. *Effect of GABA on the competitive inhibition of [$^3$H]FLU and [$^3$H]PCC binding by FLU and PCC*

| Drugs | IC$_{50}$ | | K$_\mathrm{I}$ (control) |
| --- | --- | --- | --- |
| | Control (nM) | 10 μM GABA (nM) | K$_\mathrm{I}$ (GABA) |
| [$^3$H]FLU competition experiments | | | |
| FLU | 22.4 | 14.0$^a$ | 1.9 |
| FLU (100 mM NaCl) | 28.2 | 12.6$^a$ | 3.1 |
| PCC | 15.0 | 13.0 | 1.3 |
| PCC (100 mM NaCl) | 16.0 | 16.0 | 1.2 |
| [$^3$H]PCC competition experiments | | | |
| FLU | 17.9 | 18.0 | 1.0 |
| FLU (100 mM NaCl) | 35.0 | 7.9$^a$ | 4.4 |

$^a$Significantly different from control, $p < 0.05$.
Each IC$_{50}$ represents the geometric mean of values determined from four experiments. For an individual experiment, IC$_{50}$ values of a drug for inhibition of [$^3$H]FLU or [$^3$H]PCC binding were determined simultaneously in the same tissue in the presence and absence of GABA (10 μM). The IC$_{50}$ values of FLU and PCC for inhibition of [$^3$H]FLU binding were corrected to $K_\mathrm{I}$ values by the following relationship $K_\mathrm{I} = \mathrm{IC}_{50}/(1 + X/K)$ in which $X$ equals the concentration of [$^3$H]FLU and $K$ equals the dissociation constant of [$^3$H]FLU. The values in the third column represent the ratio of $K_\mathrm{I}$'s calculated from the IC$_{50}$ values shown in the first two columns. Since GABA had no effect on [$^3$H]PCC binding, the ratio of $K_\mathrm{I}$ values for FLU, determined by competitive inhibition of [$^3$H]PCC binding in the presence and absence of GABA were assumed to be equal to the corresponding ratio of IC$_{50}$ values. All competition experiments were carried out at 37°C for 30 min. As indicated in parentheses, some assays were done in the presence of 100 mM NaCl. The concentrations of [$^3$H]FLU and [$^3$H]PCC used in the competition experiments were 5.0 and 0.5 nM, respectively. The data are from Ehlert et al. (10).

receptor function. It is reasonable to assume that the benzodiazepine receptor is part of a macromolecular complex which includes the chloride ionophore and GABA receptor. It follows that, in the absence of ligands, the complex is in a ground state characterized by a nonconductive chloride channel. If the binding of GABA and benzodiazepines stabilizes an activated state of the complex in which the chloride channel is open, then these ligands must have higher affinity for their receptors when the complex is in the activated state, and GABA should potentiate the binding of benzodiazepines. If the nature of the interaction of PCC with the benzodiazepine receptor is different from that of FLU, such that it cannot distinguish between the ground and activated states, then the binding of PCC will be insensitive to GABA. Moreover, the lack of sensitivity of PCC for the activated state of the complex predicts that PCC would pharmacologically antagonize the effects of benzodiazepines. These two predictions have been fulfilled as described above. A representation of this model is shown in Fig. 5. The model also predicts a correlation between the GABA-modulation of binding and pharmacological activity of a series of drugs that interact with the benzodiazepine receptor.

Interestingly, we have found recently that the binding of CL 218,872 is enhanced by GABA (26), although the magnitude of this effect is not as great as that seen with FLU (Ehlert et al., *unpublished observations*). This smaller GABA effect may

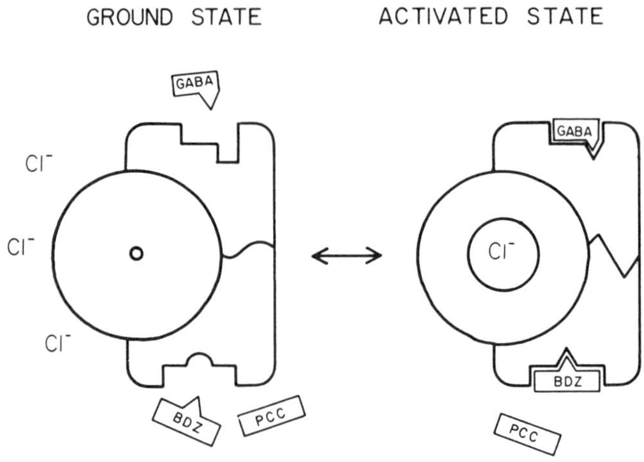

**FIG. 5.** Hypothetical model for the benzodiazepine receptor-GABA receptor-chloride ionophore complex. The macromolecular complex is in equilibrium between "ground" (G) and "activated" (A) states that correspond respectively to the closed and open states of the chloride channel. The equilibrium between the two states of the complex can be described by a constant ($K$ = [A]/[G]). It is plausible to assume that, in the absence of ligands, the ground state of the complex predominates ($K \ll 1$). GABA and benzodiazepines (BDZ's) bind preferentially to the activated state of the complex as indicated by the greater complementarity between the BDZ and GABA molecules and their respective receptors when the complex is in the activated state. The greater selectivity of these ligands for the activated state of the complex enables them to stablize the complex in the activated state. It also follows that GABA should act as a positive heterotropic allosteric effector of BDZ binding. It is proposed that PCC cannot discriminate between the G and A states of the complex; thus, the binding of PCC should be insensitive to GABA, and PCC should antagonize the pharmacological effects of BDZ's.

indicate that CL 218,872 doesn't potentiate GABA transmission to as great an extent as that observed with high doses of benzodiazepines. This interpretation may provide the basis for the lack of sedative properties of CL 218,872 as compared with benzodiazepines. Although the two-state model described above does not explain many of the complex interactions of the benzodiazepine receptor, it may provide the framework for an accurate model of benzodiazepine receptor function.

## ACKNOWLEDGMENTS

We thank Andy Chen for technical assistance. Portions of our work described in this chapter were supported by Public Health Service Grants MH-27257, MH-30626, HL-21486, and Program Project Grant HL-20984. Henry I. Yamamura is a recipient of USPHS Research Scientist Development Award, Type II (MH-00095) from the National Institute of Mental Health, and William R. Roeske is a recipient of a USPHS Research Scientist Development Award (HL-00776) from the National Heart Lung and Blood Institute.

## REFERENCES

1. Birdsall, N. J. M., Burgen, A. S. V., and Hulme, E. C. (1977): Correlation between the binding properties and pharmacological responses of muscarinic receptors. In: *Cholinergic Mechanisms and Psychopharmacology*, edtied by D. J. Jenden, pp. 25–33. Plenum Press, New York.

2. Braestrup, C., Albrechtsen, R., and Squires, R. F. (1977): High densities of benzodiazepine receptors in human cortical areas. *Nature*, 269:702–704.
3. Braestrup, C., and Nielsen, M. (1980): Multiple benzodiazepine receptors. *Trends Neurosci.*, 3:301–303.
4. Braestrup, C., Nielsen, M., and Olson, C. E. (1980): Urinary and brain β-carboline-3-carboxylates as potent inhibitors of brain benzodiazepine receptors. *Proc. Natl. Acad. Sci. USA*, 77: 2288–2292.
5. Braestrup, C., Nielsen, M., Skovbjerg, H., and Gredal, O. (1981): β-Carboline-3-carboxylates and benzodiazepine receptors. In: *GABA and Benzodiazepine Receptors*, edited by E. Costa, G. DiChiara, and G. L. Gessa, pp. 147–155. Raven Press, New York.
6. Braestrup, C., and Squires, R. F. (1977): Specific benzodiazepine receptors in rat brain characterized by high-affinity [³H]diazepam binding. *Proc. Natl. Acad. Sci. USA*, 74:3805–3809.
7. Costa, T., Rodbard, D., and Pert, C. B. (1979): Is the benzodiazepine receptor coupled to a chloride anion channel? *Nature*, 277:315–317.
8. DeLean, A., Stadel, J. M., and Lefkowitz, R. J. (1980): A ternary complex model explains the agonist-specific binding properties of adenylate cyclase-coupled β-adrenergic receptor. *J. Biol. Chem.*, 255:7108–7117.
9. Ehlert, F. J., Roeske, W. R., Braestrup, C., Yamamura, S. H., and Yamamura, H. I. (1981): γ-Aminobutyric acid regulation of the benzodiazepine receptor: biochemical evidence of pharmacologically different effects of benzodiazepines and propyl-β-carboline-3-carboxylate. *Eur. J. Pharmacol.*, 70:593–596.
10. Ehlert, F. J., Roeske, W. R., and Yamamura, H. I. (1981): Multiple benzodiazepine receptors and their regulation by γ-aminobutyric acid. *Life Sci.*, 29:235–248.
11. Gavish, M., and Snyder, S. H. (1980): Properties of soluble and partially purified benzodiazepine and γ-aminobutyric acid (GABA) receptors. *Soc. Neurosci. Abstr.*, 6:636.
12. Klepner, C. A., Lippa, A. S., Benson, D. I., Sano, M. C., and Beer, B. (1979): Resolution of two biochemically and pharmacologically distinct benzodiazepine receptors. *Pharmacol. Biochem. Behav.*, 11:457–462.
13. Lippa, A. S., Coupet, J., Greenblatt, E. N., Klepner, C. A., and Beer, B. (1979): A synthetic non-benzodiazepine ligand for benzodiazepine receptors: a probe for investigating neuronal substrates of anxiety. *Pharmacol. Biochem. Behav.*, 11:99–106.
14. Lippa, A. S., Klepner, C. A., Benson, D. I., Critchett, J. J., Sano, M. C. and Beer, B. (1980): The role of GABA in mediating the anticonvulsive properties of benzodiazepines. *Brain Res.*, Bull. 5 Suppl. 2:861–865.
15. Mitchell, R., and Martin, I. (1980): Ethyl β-carboline-3-carboxylate antagonises the effect of diazepam on a functional GABA receptor. *Eur. J. Pharmacol.*, 68:513–514.
16. Mackerer, C. R., and Kockman R. L. (1978): Effects of cations and anions on the binding of [³H]diazepam to rat brain. *Proc. Soc. Exp. Biol. Med.*, 158:393–397.
17. Martin, I. L., and Candy, J. M. (1978): Facilitation of benzodiazepine binding by sodium chloride and GABA. *Neuropharmacology*, 17:993–998.
18. Martin, I. L., and Candy, J. M. (1980). Facilitation of specific benzodiazepine binding in rat brain membrane fragments by a number of anions. *Neuropharmacology*, 19:175–179.
19. Mohler, H., and Okada T. (1977): Benzodiazepine receptor: demonstration in the central nervous system. *Science*, 198:849–851.
20. Mohler, H., and Okada, T. (1977): Properties of [³H]diazepam binding to benzodiazepine receptors in rat cerebral cortex. *Life Sci.*, 20:2101–2110.
21. Morin, A. M., Tanaku, I. A., and Wasterlin, C. G. (1981): Norharmane inhibition of [³H]diazepam binding in mouse brain. *Life Sci.*, 28:2257–2263.
22. Nielsen, M., and Braestrup, C. (1980): Ethyl β-carboline-3-carboxylate shows differential benzodiazepine receptor interaction. *Nature*, 286:606–607.
23. Nielsen, M., Schou, H., and Braestrup, C. (1981): [³H]propyl-β-carboline-3-carboxylate binds specifically to brain benzodiazepine receptors. *J. Neurochem.* 36:276–285.
24. Oakley, N. R., and Jones, B. J. (1980): The proconvulsant and diazepam-reversing effects of ethyl-β-carboline-3-carboxylate. *Eur. J. Pharmacol.*, 68:381–382.
25. Regan, J. W., Roeske, W. R., Malick, J. B., Yamamura, S. H., and Yamamura, H. I. (1981): GABA enhancement of CL 218,872 affinity and evidence of benzodiazepine receptor heterogeneity. *Mol. Pharmacol.*, 20:477–483.
26. Regan, J. W., Roeske, W. R., and Yamamura, H. I. (1980): [³H]Flunitrazepam binding to bovine retina and the effect of GABA thereon. *Neuropharmacology*, 19:413–414.

27. Rommelspacher, H., Nanz, C., Borbe, H. O., Fehske, K. J. Muller, W. E., and Wolert, U. (1980): 1-Methyl-β-carboline (harmane), a potent endogenous inhibitor of benzodiazepine receptor binding. *N-S Arch. Pharmacol.*, 314:97–100.
28. Seighart, W., and Karobath, M. (1980): Molecular heterogeneity of benzodiazepine receptors. *Nature*, 286:285–287.
29. Squires, R., Benson, D. I., Braestrup, C., Coupet, J., Klepner, C. A., Meyers, V., and Beer, B. (1979): Some properties of brain specific benzodiazepine receptors: new evidence for multiple receptors. *Pharmacol. Biochem. Behav.*, 10:825–830.
30. Squires, R. F., and Braestrup, C. (1977): Benzodiazepine receptors in rat brain. *Nature (Lond.)*, 266:732–734.
31. Supavilai, P., and Karobath, M. (1980): The effect of temperature and chloride ions on the stimulation of [$^3$H]flunitrazepam binding by the muscimol analogues THIP and piperidine-4-sulfonic acid. *Neuro. Sci. Lett.*, 19:337–341.
32. Tallman, J. F., Paul, S. M., Skolnick, P., and Gallager, D. W. (1980): Receptors for the age of anxiety: pharmacology of the benzodiazepines. *Science*, 207:274–281.
33. Tallman, J. F., Thomas, J. W., and Gallager, D. W. (1978): GABAergic modulation of benzodiazepine binding sensitivity. *Nature (Lond.)*, 274:383–385.
34. Tenen, S. S., and Hirsch, J. D. (1980): β-Carboline-3-carboxylate acid ethyl ester antagonizes diazepam activity. *Nature (Lond.)*, 288:609–610.

# Endogenous Modulating Mechanism of Cerebral Benzodiazepine Receptor: Roles of Membrane Phospholipids

Kinya Kuriyama and Eiko Ueno

*Department of Pharmacology, Kyoto Prefectural University of Medicine, Kyoto 602, Japan*

It has been well documented that a high-affinity binding site for benzodiazepines is present in the central nervous system (2,3,22,23,27,28,33). Since this binding is stereospecific and a close parallelism exists between the pharmacological potency of various benzodiazepines and their affinity to the binding site (22,28), it has been considered that this high-affinity site may be a pharmacologically relevant receptor for benzodiazepines. Furthermore, various biochemical (4,5,9,14,20,30) and electrophysiological (7) studies have suggested that the function of the benzodiazepine receptor is closely correlated with synaptic actions of GABA. In addition, recently it has been reported by several workers (1,8,13a) that benzodiazepine and GABA receptors are co-purified and these receptors are considered to reside on the same macromolecule. In our laboratory, Ito and Kuriyama (13a) have revealed that the binding of [$^3$H]-muscimol to solubilized GABA receptor is increased significantly as compared with that found in the membrane fraction, while the binding of [$^3$H]diazepam to solubilized benzodiazepine receptor is decreased considerably as compared with that found in the membrane. From these studies, we have suggested that the solubilization of GABA receptor from synaptic membrane with various detergents followed by ammonium sulfate fractionation removes endogenous inhibitor(s) on the GABA receptor binding. In contrast, it is not known whether or not a particular modulating mechanism on the benzodiazepine receptor binding may exist as in the case of GABA receptor binding. On the other hand, the state of membrane lipids has been considered to be an important factor for regulating neurotransmitter receptor binding at synapses. Hirata and Axelrod (11) have reported that enzymatic methylation of membrane phospholipids plays an important role in the biological signal transmission after the binding of ligand to their specific receptor sites. In addition, Hirata et al. (12,29) have reported that β-adrenergic receptor binding is affected by lipid fluidity in rat reticulocytes. Similarly, a modulatory role of lipid fluidity has been demonstrated in the binding of serotonin to its physiologically relevant receptor (10,25).

In the present study, we have observed that benzodiazepine receptor binding was altered significantly by treatment with phospholipase C and phospholipase $A_2$, and suggest that this phenomenon may be caused by the alteration of the state of membrane phospholipids.

## MATERIALS AND METHODS

### Preparation of Synaptic Membrane and Its Solubilized Fraction

Male Wistar rats weighing 180 to 200 g were decapitated and the brain was removed. The crude synaptic membrane was prepared according to the method of Enna and Synder (6). The prepared membrane was washed three times with 50 mM Tris-HCl buffer (pH 7.4) and stored at $-20°C$ for at least 12 hr. The frozen membrane was thawed, resuspended in 50 mM Tris-HCl (pH 7.4), and centrifuged at 48,000 $\times$ $g$ for 20 min. The resultant pellet was resuspended with 50 mM Tris-HCl buffer (pH 7.4) and used for the binding assay.

The solubilized fraction from cerebral synaptic membrane was obtained by treating the synaptic membrane fraction with 50 mM Tris-citrate buffer (pH 7.1) containing 1% Nonidet P-40 followed by the centrifugation at 100,00 $\times$ $g$ for 60 min. The supernatant thus obtained was dialyzed against 50 mM Tris-citrate buffer (pH 7.1) containing 0.1% Nonidet P-40 for 2 hr at 2°C, and subjected to ammonium sulfate precipitation (40% saturation). The resultant precipitate was resuspended with 50 mM Tris-citrate buffer (pH 7.1) containing 0.1% Nonidet P-40, and centrifuged at 100,000 $\times$ $g$ for 30 min. The supernatant was redialyzed against 50 mM Tris-citrate buffer (pH 7.1) containing 0.1% Nonidet P-40 at 2°C for 12 hr and this fraction was subjected to the binding assay.

### Assay of Benzodiazepine Binding

For the measurement of benzodiazepine binding to synaptic membrane, membrane preparations (containing 0.2-0.3 mg protein) were incubated with 0.5 nM [$^3$H]diazepam ([N-methyl-$^3$H]-diazepam, Spec. Act.: 76.8 Ci/mmol, The Radiochemical Center, Amersham) or [$^3$H]flunitrazepam ([N-methyl-$^3$H]-flunitrazepam, Spec. Act.: 75 Ci/mmol. The Radiochemical Center, Amersham) at 4°C for 20 or 60 min, respectively. In the case of solubilized fraction, the same experimental procedure as membrane fraction was employed except polyethylene glycol was added to the reaction mixture in a final concentration of 15 (wt/vol)%. Each incubation was terminated by filtrating under vacuum through Whatmann GF/B filter and then the filter was rinsed twice with 3 ml ice-cold 50 mM Tris-HCl buffer (pH 7.4). Radioactivity trapped on the filter was measured liquid-scintillation spectrometrically using toluene-Triton X-100 scintillation cocktail. The specific binding was calculated by subtracting the amount of nonspecific binding, found in the presence of $10^{-5}$ M diazepam (for [$^3$H]diazepam binding) or clonazepam (for [$^3$H]flunitrazepam binding) from the total binding. The GABA-induced stimulation of benzodiazepine receptor binding was determined in the presence of $10^{-5}$ M GABA.

## Procedure for Treatments with Various Enzymes and Drugs

Treatments with various enzymes were performed by preincubating the membrane and solubilized fractions at 37°C for 30 min before subjecting to the binding assay. In the case of treatments with phospholipase C, phospholipase $A_2$, and phospholipase D, 1 mM $CaCl_2$ was added to the preincubation medium. On the other hand, treatments with digitonin (0.05%), nystatin (0.5 mM), and polymixin B (0.5 mM) were carried out by incubating the membrane at 37°C for 30 min.

## Addition of Various Phospholipids to Phospholipase C- and Phospholipase $A_2$-Treated Membranes or to Solubilized Fraction

For examining the effect of addition of various phospholipids, each phospholipid was sonicated for 2 min with phospholipase C-treated and phospholipase $A_2$-treated membranes or solubilized fraction. After preincubating at 37°C for 30 min, 0.1 ml aliquot of the resultant suspension (containing 500 μg/ml each phospholipid) was used for the binding assay.

## Procedure for Photoaffinity Labeling of Benzodiazepine Receptor

Membrane preparations were incubated with 10 nM [$^3$H]flunitrazepam at 4°C for 90 min, and the samples were then irradiated with UV light for 5 min according to the method of Sieghart and Karobath (26). After the irradiation, the samples were further incubated at 4°C for 90 min in the presence of $10^{-5}$ M clonazepam and then filtered through Whatmann GF/B filter under vacuum. In the case of SDS-polyacrylamide gel electrophoresis (SDS-PAGE), the irradiated samples were centrifuged at 48,000 × $g$ for 20 min and the pellet thus obtained was resuspended in a small amount of $H_2O$. After adding the stop solution (containing 10 (wt/vol)% SDS, 100 mM Tris-HCl (pH 7.4), 5 mM β-mercaptoethanol, 0.2 g/ml sucrose, and 0.02 mg/ml bromophenol blue tracking dye) to this suspension, the sample was heated in a boiling water bath and then subjected to SDS-PAGE according to the method of Laemmli (16).

## Measurement of Protein

Protein content was measured by the method of Lowry et al. (18).

## RESULTS AND DISCUSSION

### Characteristics of Benzodiazepine Receptor Binding to the Membrane Fraction of Rat Brain

[$^3$H]Diazepam and [$^3$H]flunitrazepam bindings to the cerebral synaptic membrane were saturable and consisted of one component with a high affinity. The Scatchard analysis of [$^3$H]diazepam and [$^3$H]flunitrazepam bindings using variable concentrations (0.5–40.5 nM) of these drugs provided the apparent dissociation constants

($K_D$) of 6.36 ± 0.75 nM and 1.50 ± 0.08 nM, and the maximal number of the binding sites ($B_{max}$) of 0.94 ± 0.11 pmoles/mg protein and 1.12 ± 0.06 pmoles/mg protein, respectively. These results indicate that the affinity of flunitrazepam to benzodiazepine receptor is higher than that of diazepam, as reported previously by several sources (2,22,24,27,28). Moreover, both [$^3$H]diazepam and [$^3$H]flunitrazepam bindings were significantly enhanced by the addition of $10^{-5}$ M GABA and this enhancement was antagonized by $10^{-4}$ M bicuculline, a specific antagonist for GABA receptor. These data support the assumption, proposed by many workers, that GABA-induced stimulation of benzodiazepine receptor binding may be mediated through GABA receptor.

To examine some characteristics of the receptor site, synaptic membrane was pretreated with various enzymes at 37°C for 30 min before subjecting to the binding assay. The [$^3$H]diazepam binding was significantly reduced by pretreatment of the membrane with proteolytic enzymes such as trypsin and pronase, whereas that with neuraminidase, β-galactosidase, lipoxygenase, and phospholipase D had no significant effect on the binding. On the other hand, the treatment with phospholipase C and phospholipase $A_2$ significantly increased [$^3$H]diazepam binding, and these phenomena were also seen in the binding study using [$^3$H]flunitrazepam as a radioligand. Furthermore, the addition of $10^{-4}$ M bicuculline did not affect the increase induced by pretreatment with phospholipase C or phospholipase $A_2$, suggesting that these increases were not due to endogenous GABA newly released. These results also suggest that the benzodiazepine receptor site may be protein and the receptor binding may be modulated by membrane lipids. Accordingly, we have attempted to examine possible involvement of the membrane cholesterol in the modulation of the receptor binding. However, the pretreatment of membrane preparations with drugs that are known to interact with cholesterol, such as digitonin, nystatin, and polymixin B (15,32), had no effect on the binding. These results suggest that the membrane phospholipids which are susceptible to phospholipase C and phospholipase $A_2$ treatments may participate in the modulation of the benzodiazepine receptor binding, but cholesterol may not be involved in such a modulation mechanism.

**Properties of the Benzodiazepine Receptor in Solubilized Fraction**

We have attempted to solubilize benzodiazepine and GABA receptors from synaptic membrane preparations using Nonidet P-40, and have found that both receptor sites are solubilized, but are not separable from each other following ammonium sulfate precipitation as well as gel filtration on Sephadex G-200 of the supernatant (Fig. 1). In addition, it has also been found that the binding of [$^3$H]muscimol to GABA receptor increases following ammonium sulfate fractionation and gel filtration on Sephadex G-200, whereas that of [$^3$H]flunitrazepam is significantly reduced following the application of these procedures (Fig. 1). The former phenomenon is considered to be due to the removal of enodgenous inhibitor(s) for GABA receptor binding (13a), whereas the latter phenomenon is thought to be due to the removal of membrane lipids which may play a modulatory role for benzodiazepine receptor binding as described in the previous section.

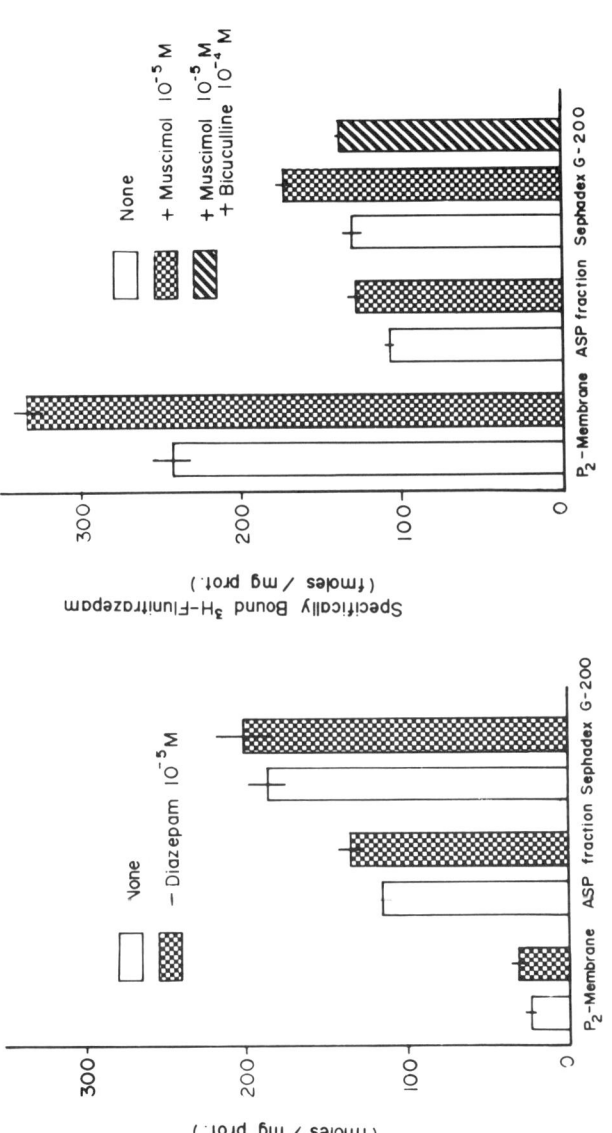

**FIG. 1.** Functional association of specific bindings of [3H]muscimol and [3H]flunitrazepam in synaptic (P$_2$) membrane, and solubilized ammonium sulfate precipitated (ASP) fraction and its eluate from Sephadex G-200 gel filtration. *Left:* Effect of diazepam on [3H]muscimol binding to various fractions indicated. Each fraction was incubated with 1 nM [3H]muscimol in the presence or absence of 10$^{-5}$ M diazepam. *Right:* Effect of muscimol and bicuculline on [3H]flunitrazepam binding to various fractions. Each fraction was incubated with 0.5 nM [3H]flunitrazepam in the presence or absence of 10$^{-5}$ M muscimol. Each value represents the mean ± SEM obtained from three separate experiments done in triplicate.

The Scatchard analysis of [$^3$H]flunitrazepam binding to the solubilized fraction revealed to $K_D$ of 4.7 nM and the $B_{max}$ of 1.42 pmoles/mg protein, respectively. The addition of $10^{-5}$ M GABA or muscimol increased the affinity without altering the $B_{max}$ value as shown in the case of membrane fraction. Furthermore, the enhancement of this binding was blocked by the addition of $10^{-4}$ M bicuculline (Fig. 1). The $K_D$ value for the binding to solubilized fraction was, however, lower than that found in the membrane fraction.

## Modulation of Benzodiazepine Receptor Binding by Phospholipids

Since the treatment of synaptic membrane preparations with phospholipase C and phospholipase $A_2$ induced an increase in [$^3$H]diazepam binding, kinetic studies on the binding were performed. The Scatchard analysis on the binding to the phospholipase C- and phospholipase $A_2$-treated membranes in the absence of GABA showed that phospholipase C treatment induced a significant increase (approximately 30%) of the $B_{max}$ without changing the $K_D$ value, whereas phospholipase $A_2$ treatment decreased the $K_D$ by approximately 30% without affecting on the $B_{max}$ (Table 1). On the other hand, [$^3$H]diazepam binding to the membrane treated with phospholipase C or phospholipase $A_2$ was also enhanced by $10^{-5}$ M GABA as found in untreated membrane. However, in the case of phospholipase $A_2$-treated membrane, the $K_D$ value in the presence of $10^{-5}$ M GABA tended to be higher than that for untreated or phospholipase C-treated membrane. On the other hand, the extent of the maximal stimulation induced by $10^{-4}$ M GABA found in the phospholipase $A_2$-treated membrane was significantly lower than that found in untreated as well as in phospholipase C-treated membrane. These results suggest that membrane lipids may have modulating roles on the affinity as well as on the number of binding sites for benzodiazepine receptor.

Since above data suggest that membrane phospholipids may play important roles in the modulation of the receptor binding, we have also examined whether or not the treatments with phospholipase C and phospholipase $A_2$ on the solubilized re-

TABLE 1. *Scatchard analysis of [$^3$H]diazepam binding to cerebral synaptic membrane treated with phospholipase C and phospholipase $A_2$*

| Treatment | $K_D$ (nM) | | $B_{max}$ (pmoles/mg prot.) | |
|---|---|---|---|---|
| | −GABA | +GABA($10^{-5}$ M) | −GABA | +GABA($10^{-5}$ M) |
| None | 6.48 ± 0.25 | 2.81 ± 0.14 | 1.03 ± 0.15 | 1.01 ± 0.24 |
| Phospholipase C[a] | 6.23 ± 0.33 | 2.36 | 1.34 ± 0.09[b] | 1.20 |
| Phospholipase $A_2$[a] | 4.59 ± 0.32[c] | 3.24 ± 0.04 | 0.97 ± 0.08 | 1.05 ± 0.16 |

[a] Cerebral synaptic membrane was preincubated with each enzyme (0.5 unit/mg of membraneous protein) in the presence of 1 mM $CaCl_2$ at 37°C for 30 min, and centrifuged at 48,000 × g for 20 min. The resultant pellet was resuspended with 50 mM Tris-HCL buffer (pH 7.4) and used for the assay of [$^3$H]diazepam binding as described in Materials and Methods. The data represent the mean ± SEM from three to seven separate experiments.
[b] $p < 0.05$, compared with each non-treated value.
[c] $p < 0.02$, compared with each non-treated value.

ceptor fraction affect the benzodiazepine receptor binding. The increase of the binding in membrane fraction induced by phospholipase C and phospholipase $A_2$ treatments disappeared following the solubilization of the membrane. These results indicate that the increased binding induced by the treatments with these lipolytic enzymes appears only at the membrane level, and also suggest that the solubilization of $P_2$ membrane removes phospholipids related to the modulation of the receptor binding and/or may dissociate the phospholipid-benzodiazepine receptor interaction which plays an important modulating role on the function of benzodiazepine receptor in the membrane.

It is well known that phospholipase C and phospholipase $A_2$ hydrolyze various glycerophospholipids at the position of $C_2$ ether (19) and $C_3$ ester bond (31), respectively. Therefore, there are two possibile causes for the increase of the receptor binding induced by these two lipolytic enzymes: Particular phospholipids in the membrane involved in the modulation of the receptor binding are removed by these enzymatic treatments, or the reaction products induce an increase of the binding. The addition of phosphatidylserine and phosphatidic acid eliminated the increase in the binding induced by both phospholipase C and phospholipase $A_2$ treatments. As shown in Fig. 2, the addition of phosphatidic acid to phospholipase $A_2$-treated membrane altered the $K_D$ without affecting the $B_{max}$. Although molecular mecha-

|  | $K_D$ (nM) | $B_{max}$ (pmoles/mg prot.) |
|---|---|---|
| Control | 6.5 | 0.98 |
| Phospholipase $A_2$ | 5.2 | 0.95 |
| Phospholipase $A_2$ + Phosphatidic Acid | 9.1 | 0.98 |

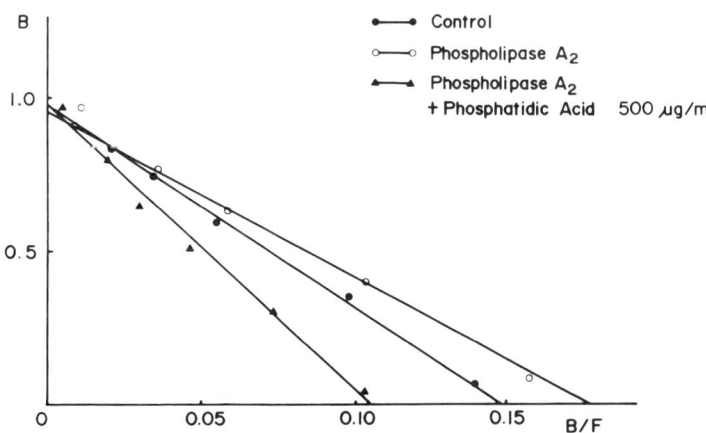

FIG. 2. Effect of addition of phosphatidic acid on [³H]diazepam binding to cerebral synaptic membrane treated with phospholipase $A_2$. Following the treatment of synaptic membrane with phospholipase $A_2$, phosphatidic acid was added, and its effect on the [³H]diazepam binding was examined.

nisms underlying the modulation of the function of benzodiazepine receptor by membrane phospholipids remain to be clarified, these results suggest that the removal of a certain type of phospholipid from synaptic membranes may be involved in the increase of the binding found in phospholipase C- and phospholipase $A_2$-treated membranes. The phenomena similar to this result have also been reported in GABA receptor under certain conditions (17). Considering the lipophilic property of benzodiazepines, it seems reasonable to assume that the state of membrane lipids located near the receptor site may modulate the binding of benzodiazepine to its receptor.

### Analysis of the Increase of [³H]Flunitrazepam Binding Induced by Phospholipase C and Phospholipase $A_2$ by Photoaffinity Labeling and SDS-PAGE

It has been reported that flunitrazepam irreversibly binds to the receptor site when irradiated with UV light (13,21,26). The incorporation of [³H]flunitrazepam has been reported to be inhibited by other benzodiazepines with the potency corresponding to their affinity to the receptor. As shown in Table 2B, this irreversible binding was enhanced by the addition of GABA. Furthermore, it was abolished by the treatment with trypsin but not by boiling at 100°C for 5 min (Table 2A). Since we have observed that the benzodiazepine receptor binding is increased by the treatment of the membrane with phospholipase C and phospholipase $A_2$ as described previously, we have determined whether or not these phenomena are also detected in the photolabeling system. The irreversible [³H]flunitrazepam binding to the membrane was also increased to a similar extent by phospholipase C treatment as found in the case of reversible [³H]flunitrazepam binding (Table 2B). The results obtained by SDS-PAGE on the irreversible binding indicated that the molecular weight of

TABLE 2. *Effect of various treatments on irreversible [³H]flunitrazepam binding to cerebral synaptic membrane*

| A. Treatment[a] | Irreversible binding of [³H]flunitrazepam (fmoles/mg prot.) |
|---|---|
| None | $602 \pm 49$ ($N = 4$) |
| Boiling (100°C, 5 min) | 415 |
| Trypsin (100 µg/ml) | 0 |
| B. Pretreatment[b] | |
| None | $602 \pm 49$ ($N = 4$) |
| Phospholipase C | $931 \pm 36$ ($N = 3$) |
| Phospholipase $A_2$[c] | $683 \pm 18$ ($N = 3$) |
| GABA $10^{-5}$ M added | 781 |

[a] After the photolabeling, the samples were treated in each condition as indicated.
[b] Before subjecting to the photolabeling, pretreatments were performed.
[c] $p < 0.01$, compared with "None."

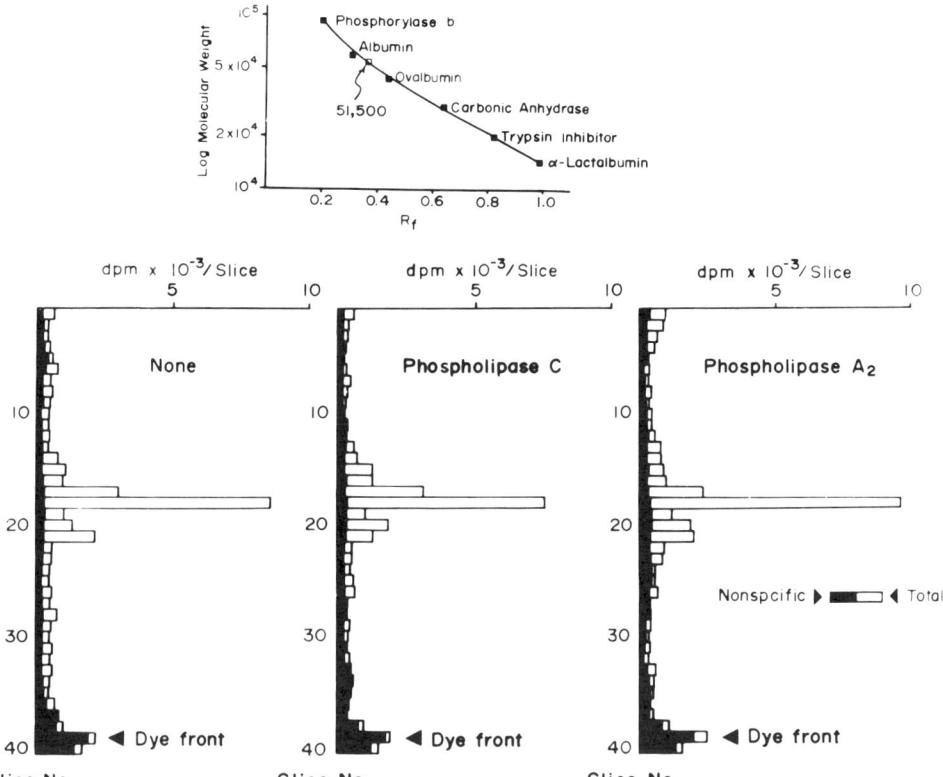

**FIG. 3.** SDS-PAGE pattern of irreversible binding of [$^3$H]flunitrazepam to synaptic membrane. Membrane preparations were pretreated with phospholipase C and phospholipase $A_2$ at 37°C for 30 min, and subjected to the photoaffinity labeling as described in Materials and Methods. SDS-PAGE was performed using the irradiated samples from untreated, phospholipase C-treated, and phospholipase $A_2$-treated membranes. The protein concentration applied is varied in each sample.

photolabeled receptor component was approximately 51,500. This value is identical to those reported by several workers (21,26). Furthermore, we have observed that the increase of radioactivity found in phospholipase C-treated membrane appears in the same band as that in the control (Fig. 3). These results clearly indicate that phospholipase C and phospholipase $A_2$ treatments do not induce transfer of the binding protein, and also support our previous assumption that phospholipids being susceptible to phospholipase C (or phospholipase $A_2$) treatment may participate in the modulation of the receptor function.

## CONCLUSION

The results obtained in this study strongly suggest that the binding of benzodiazepine to its synaptic receptor may be modulated by synaptic membrane lipids.

In addition, it has been found that benzodiazepine and GABA receptors co-solubilized and co-purified, at least a certain extent, and are not separable from each other under the experimental conditions employed in this study.

Further studies should be directed to clarify the physiological significance and exact molecular mechanisms underlying the modulatory actions of membrane lipids on the benzodiazepine receptor binding, and to analyze the functional and molecular links present in both GABA and benzodiazepine receptor sites in the brain.

## ACKNOWLEDGMENT

This work supported, in part, by a Grant-in-Aid for Scientific Research (56480104, 1981 and 1982) from The Ministry of Science and Culture, Japan.

## REFERENCES

1. Asano, T., and Ogasawara, N. (1980): Solubilization of γ-aminobutyric acid receptor from rat brain. *Life Sci.*, 26:1131–1137.
2. Braestrup, C., Albrechtsen, R., and Squires, R. F. (1977): High densities of benzodiazepine receptors in human cortical areas. *Nature*, 269:702–704.
3. Braestrup, C., and Squires, R. F. (1977): Specific benzodiazepine receptors in rat brain characterized by high affinity [³H]diazepam binding. *Proc. Natl. Acad. Sci. USA*, 74:3805–3809.
4. Brilely, M. S., and Langer, S. Z. (1978): Influence of GABA receptor agonists and antagonists on the binding of [³H]diazepam to the benzodiazepine receptor. *Eur. J. Pharmacol.*, 52:129–132.
5. Costa, E., Guidotti, A., Mao, C. C., and Suria, A. (1975): New concepts on the mechanism of action of benzodiazepines. *Life Sci.*, 17:167–186.
6. Enna, S. J., and Snyder, S. H. (1976): Influences of ions, enzymes and detergents on γ-aminobutyric acid receptor binding in synaptic membranes of rat brain. *Mol. Pharmacol.*, 13:442–453.
7. Gallager, D. W. (1978): Benzodiazepines: potentiation of a GABA inhibitory response on the dorsal raphe nucleus. *Eur. J. Pharmacol.*, 49:133–143.
8. Gavish, M., and Snyder, S. H. (1981): γ-Aminobutyric acid and benzodiazepine receptors: copurification and characterization. *Proc. Natl. Acad. Sci. USA*, 78:1939–1942.
9. Haefely, W. K., Kulcsar, A., Möhler, H., Pieli, L., Polc, P., and Schaffner, R. (1975): Possible involvement of GABA in the central actions of benzodiazepines. *Adv. Biochem. Psychopharmacol.*, 12:131–151.
10. Heron, D. S., Shinitzky, M., Hershkowitz, M., and Samuel, D. (1980): Lipid fluidity markedly modulates the binding of serotonin to mouse brain membranes. *Proc. Natl. Acad. Sci. USA*, 77:7463–7467.
11. Hirata, F., and Axelrod, J. (1980): Phospholipid methylation and biological signal transmission. *Science*, 209:1082–1090.
12. Hirata, F., Strittmatter, W. J., and Axelrod, J. (1979): β-Adrenergic receptor agonists increase phospholipid methylation, membrane fluidity, and β-adrenergic-adenylate cyclase coupling. *Proc. Natl. Acad. Sci. USA*, 76:368–372.
13. Johnson, R. W., and Yamamura, H. I. (1979): Photoaffinity labeling of the benzodiazepine receptor in bovine cerebral cortex. *Life Sci.*, 25:1613–1620.
13a. Ito, Y., and Kuriyama, K. (1982): Some properties of solubilized GABA receptor. *Brain Res.*, 236:351–363.
14. Karobath, M., and Sperk, G. (1979): Stimulation of benzodiazepine receptor binding by γ-aminobutyric acid. *Proc. Natl. Acad. Sci. USA*, 76:1004–1006.
15. Kinsky, S. C., Luse, S. A., and van Deenen, L. L. M. (1966): Interaction of polyene antibiotics with natural and artificial membrane systems. *Fed. Proc.*, 25:1503–1510.
16. Laemmli, U. K. (1970): Cleavage of structural proteins during the assembly of the head of bacteriophage T4. *Nature*, 227:680–685.
17. Lloyd, K. G., and Davidson, L. (1979): [³H]GABA binding in brains from Huntington's chorea patients: altered regulation by phospholipids? *Science*, 205:1147–1149.

18. Lowry, O. H., Rosebrough, N. J. Farr, A. L., and Randall, R. J. (1951): Protein measurement with the Follin phenol reagent. *J. Biol. Chem.*, 193:265–275.
19. Macfarlane, M. G., and Knight, B. C. J. G. (1941): The biochemistry of bacterial toxins I.: the lecithinase activity of CL. Wellchii toxins. *J. Biochem.*, 35:884–902.
20. Martin, I. L., and Candy, J. M. (1978): Facilitation of benzodiazepine binding by sodium chloride and GABA. *Neuropharmacology*, 17:993–998.
21. Möhler, H., Battersby, M. K., and Richards, J. G. (1980): Benzodiazepine receptor protein identified and visualized in brain tissue by a photoaffinity label. *Proc. Natl. Acad. Sci. USA*, 77:1666–1670.
22. Möhler, H., and Okada, T. (1977): Benzodiazepine receptors: demonstration in the central nervous system. *Science*, 198:849–851.
23. Möhler, H., and Okada, T. (1977): Properties of [$^3$H]diazepam binding to benzodiazepine receptors in rat cerebral cortex. *Life Sci.*, 20:2101–2110.
24. Möhler, H., and Okada, T. (1978): Biochemical identification of the site of action of benzodiazepines in human brain by [$^3$H]-diazepam binding. *Life Sci.*, 22:985–996.
25. Papaphilis, A., and Deliconstantinos, G. (1980): Modulation of serotonergic receptors by exogenous cholesterol in the dog synaptosomal plasma membrane. *Biochem. Pharmacol.*, 29:3325–3327.
26. Sieghart, W., and Karobath, M. (1980): Molecular heterogenity of benzodiazepine receptors. *Nature*, 286:285–287.
27. Speth, R. C., Wastek, G. J., Johnson, P. C., and Yamamura, H. I. (1978): Benzodiazepine binding in human brain: characterization using [$^3$H]-flunitrazepam. *Life Sci.*, 22:859–866.
28. Squires, R. F., and Braestrup, C. (1977): Benzodiazepine receptors in rat brain. *Nature*, 266:732–734.
29. Strittmatter, W. J., Hirata, F., and Axelrod, J. (1979): Phospholipid methylation unmasks cryptic β-adrenergic receptors in rat reticulocytes. *Science*, 204:1205–1207.
30. Tallmann, J. F., Thomas, J. W., and Gallager, D. W. (1978): GABA-ergic modulation of benzodiazepine binding site sensitivity. *Nature*, 274:383–385.
31. Van den Bosch, H., Postema, N. M., de Hass, G. H., and van Deenen, L. L. M. (1965): On the positional specificty of phospholipase A from pancreas. *Biochim. Biophys. Acta*, 98:657–659.
32. Weissmann, G., and Sessa, G. (1967): The action of polyene antibiotics on phospholipid–cholesterol structures. *J. Biol. Chem.*, 242:616–625.
33. Williamson, M., Paul, S. M., and Skolnick, P. (1978): Demonstration of [$^3$H]-diazepam binding to benzodiazepine receptors in vivo. *Life Sci.*, 23:1935–1940.

# Glycine Receptors in the Human Brain: Characterization of ³H-Strychnine Binding and Status in Pathological Conditions

K. G. Lloyd, G. De Montis, *F. Javoy-Agid, K. Beaumont, **A. Lowenthal, †J. Constantinidis, and *Y. Agid

*Neuropharmacology Unit, Synthelabo LERS, 92220, Bagneux, France;*
*\*Hôpital Pitié-Salpêtrière, Paris, France;*
*\*\*University of Antwerp, Antwerp, Belgium; and †Clinique Psychiatrique Bel-Air, Geneva, Switzerland*

Glycine is a likely neurotransmitter in many inhibitory synapses in the spinal cord (3,4,11,15). Attempts have been made to measure glycine receptors *in vitro* using ³H-glycine as the ligand (5); but it seems that ³H-glycine is not ideal as a ligand, since in addition to its binding to glycine receptors, it will also identify high-affinity glycine-uptake sites (5). An alternative approach to radiolabeling glycine receptors is to use ³H-strychnine (22), a specific antagonist of glycine-mediated inhibition (3,4,7,8). However, it appears that it is not the glycine recognition site of the receptor complex that binds ³H-strychnine, but rather another integral portion of the receptor macromolecule, perhaps more closely related to the glycine-regulated chloride ionophore (22,24).

In addition to a role at the level of the spinal cord neurons, glycinergic synapses have also been proposed to regulate motor function via inhibition of the nigrostriatal dopamine neurons. Thus, intranigral injection of glycine depresses single cell activity in both the pars compacta and pars reticulata (7), decreases striatal dopamine release (2), and induces ipsilateral rotations (12). However, results inconsistent with this hypothesis also have been reported (1,14).

In order to further understand the regulation of nigrostriatal dopamine neurons, we have studied the status of specific, glycine-sensitive ³H-strychnine binding in the human substantia nigra, pars compacta, and pars reticulata. Possible alterations in ³H-strychnine binding in nigrostriatal dysfunction (Parkinson's disease, Huntington's chorea) have also been investigated.

---

Present address of Dr. De Montis: 2nd Institute of Pharmacology, University of Cagliari, Cagliari, Italy.
Present address of Dr. Beaumont: Department of Medicine, University of California–San Diego, La Jolla, California 92093.

## MATERIALS AND METHODS

Human brains were obtained postmortem, frozen, and dissected as previously described (13,17). The presence of a clinically evident neurological disease (Parkinson's disease, Huntington's disease) was confirmed postmortem by neuroanatomical abnormalities. The control patients did not have any evident neurological or psychiatric abnormalities and were matched with respect to age and postmortem time with the neurological disorders.

Male albino rats weighing 180 to 220 g (CD-COBS strain from Charles River, France) were used. Bovine spinal cords were obtained from a local slaughterhouse within 12 hr after removal from the animal. $^3$H-Strychnine (13 Ci/mmole) was obtained from the Radiochemical Center, Amersham, U. K.

Rat spinal cord membranes were prepared according to Young and Snyder (23). Membranes were prepared from frozen tissue (rat, cow, human) by homogenizing

TABLE 1. $^3$H-Strychnine binding in different regions of brains from control patients

| Region | Data from Scatchard plots | | | | Binding at 10 nM $^3$H-strychnine (fmol/mg prot.) |
|---|---|---|---|---|---|
| | Affinity (nM) | | Binding sites (fmol/mg protein) | | |
| | $K_{D_1}$ | $K_{D_2}$ | $B_{max}1$ | $B_{max}2$ | |
| Spinal cord | 7.8 ± 2.3 (5) | 117 ± 19 (3) | 151 ± 60 (5) | 421 ± 25 (3) | 107 ± 43 (5) |
| Inferior olive | — | — | — | — | 55 ± 4 (8) |
| Substantia nigra compacta | 2.7; 4.6 (2) | 58 (1) | 90; 150 (2) | 790 (1) | 127 ± 10 (13) |
| Substantia nigra reticulata | 3.5; 3.6 (2) | — | 53; 60 (2) | — | 60 ± 12 (13) |

Results presented as mean ± SEM. Saturation curves were performed as described in the text, with the following concentration ranges of $^3$H-strychnine: spinal cord, 1 to 200 nM (8 points); substantia nigra compacta, 0.5 to 50 nM (6 points); substantia nigra reticulata, 1 to 10 nM (3 points). The number of different brains examined is indicated in parentheses.

TABLE 2. $^3$H-Strychnine binding to rat, bovine, and human spinal cord material

| Binding sites | Rat | Cow | Human |
|---|---|---|---|
| High-affinity site | | | |
| $K_D$ (nM) | 8.4 ± 1.0 (8) | 2.9; 4.3 (2) | 7.8 ± 2.3 (5) |
| $B_{max}$ (fmol/mg prot.) | 2,767 ± 773 (8) | 97; 149 (2) | 151 ± 60 (5) |
| Low-affinity site | ND | | |
| $K_D$ (nM) | — | 49.8; 66.2 (2) | 117 ± 19 (3) |
| $B_{max}$ (fmol/mg prot.) | — | 1,142; 905 (2) | 421 ± 25 (3) |

Results expressed as the mean ± SEM. The number of spinal cords examined is indicated in parentheses. ND, not detectable. When $N = 2$, the individual data are given. Saturation curves were performed with the following concentrations of $^3$H-strychnine: rat spinal cord, 0.5 to 24 nM (7 points); bovine spinal cord, 0.5 to 100 nM (8 points); human spinal cord, 1 to 200 nM (8 points).

(Polytron, setting 5) in 50 volumes of ice-cold distilled water for 30 sec. The suspension was centrifuged for 20 min (48,000 × g) and the pellet was rinsed three times.

Specific $^3$H-strychnine binding was performed as previously described (23,25). In brief, aliquots of resuspended pellets were incubated at 4°C for 10 min in 2.0 ml of sodium-potassium phosphate buffer (0.05 M, pH 7.1) containing 200 nM sodium chloride and the desired concentration of $^3$H-strychnine. Tubes containing 1 mM glycine plus all other components were used to account for nonspecific binding of $^3$H-strychnine. After centrifugation (10 min, 48,000 × g), the supernatant was discarded and the pellets were rinsed twice with ice-cold distilled water. The membranes were solubilized with Soluene-350, 4 ml of Demilune were added, and the radioactivity present assayed in a Nuclear Chicago Mark III scintillation spectrometer. The protein concentration of the resuspended membrane preparation was determined by the method of Lowry et al. (20). Statistical analysis was performed using the Student's $t$-test.

## RESULTS

Specific high-affinity $^3$H-strychnine binding was present in human spinal cord and substantia nigra, pars reticulata, and pars compacta (Table 1). The high affinity sites found in the spinal cord and the different regions of the substantia nigra exhibited a similar $K_D$ (2–8 nM). The $B_{max}$ of this high affinity site was similar for the pars compacta and spinal cord, but was considerably lower in the pars reticulata. A low-affinity site ($K_D$ = 117 nM) was observed in the spinal cord and pars compacta ($K_D$ = 58 nM), although this site could not be consistently demonstrated in all membrane preparations. When the $^3$H-strychnine specifically bound at 10 nM was assessed, the spinal cord and pars compacta exhibited binding capacities similar to the $B_{max}$ of the high-affinity site. At this concentration of $^3$H-strychnine, membranes from the pars reticulata and the inferior olivary nucleus exhibited approximately one-half the specific binding of the spinal cord or pars compacta.

$^3$H-Strychnine binding to rat and bovine spinal cord membranes was compared with the data found from the human material. For the rat spinal cord a single $K_D$ was observed, whereas bovine and human spinal cord tissue exhibited two binding sites (Table 2). The high-affinity sites of the human and rat spinal cords were very similar in terms of $K_D$ (8–10 nM), but the binding capacity of the rat spinal cord was about 10- to 15-fold that of the human; for the bovine tissue, the affinity of the high-affinity site was about twice that of the rat or human whereas the binding capacity was very similar to that of human spinal cord membranes. In terms of lower affinity sites, the bovine material had a lower $K_D$ and a greater $B_{max}$.

$^3$H-Strychnine binding was assessed in the substantia nigra and inferior olivary nucleus of patients who died with Parkinson's disease and in the substantia nigra from Huntington's disease (Table 3). In comparison with the material from control patients, the glycine displaceable $^3$H-strychnine binding was significantly lower in substantia nigra from parkinsonian patients both in the pars compacta and pars

TABLE 3. $^3$H-Strychnine binding (at 10 nM $^3$H-strychnine) to brain regions from patients with Parkinson's disease or Huntington's disease

|  | Substantia nigra pars compacta | Substantia nigra pars reticulata | Inferior olive |
|---|---|---|---|
| Controls |  |  |  |
| Mean (fmol/mg prot.) | 127 | 60 | 55 |
| ± SEM *(N)* | ± 10 (13) | ± 12 (13) | ± 4 (8) |
| Parkinson's disease |  |  |  |
| % Control | 67 ± 7 | 50 ± 10 | 113 ± 15 |
| *(N)* | (7) | (7) | (8) |
| Significance vs. control | $p < 0.05$ | $p < 0.05$ | NS |
| Huntington's disease |  |  |  |
| % Control | 149 ± 32 | 158 ± 37 | — |
| *(N)* | (4) | (4) |  |
| Significance vs. control | NS | NS | — |

Results are expressed as the mean ± SEM. The number of different brains examined is shown in parentheses. NS, not significant.

reticulata. In contrast, $^3$H-strychnine binding in the inferior olivary nucleus was similar in control and Parkinson material. $^3$H-Strychnine binding was about 50% greater than controls in both the pars compacta and pars reticulata for Huntington's disease patients but this did not reach a level of statistical significance.

## DISCUSSION

The $K_D$ for the $^3$H-strychnine high-affinity binding site in the human material (7.8 nM for the spinal cord, 3.5 nM for the substantia nigra) is very similar to that of the rat (8.4 nM for the spinal cord) or cow (3.4 nM for the spinal cord). These values for the rat spinal cord are in agreement with the literature (2–10 nM) (10,23,25). In contrast to the rat material, two binding sites are often observed in the human and bovine tissue preparations. This difference may be related to the more limited concentration ranges of $^3$H-strychnine used in the rat, due to the small amount of tissue available (see also legends to Tables 1 and 2).

The present binding capacity of the rat spinal cord is similar to that reported by Young and Snyder (24). The rat showed a much greater binding capacity ($B_{max}$ or binding at 10 nM $^3$H-strychnine) than either bovine or human material. Of the human brain regions currently examined, $^3$H-strychnine binding was similar for the spinal cord and substantia nigra, pars compacta, but was much lower (approximately half) in the inferior olive and pars reticulata. This is in agreement with strychinine binding in the rat brain (22). The greater binding capacity for $^3$H-strychnine of the rat membrane as compared with the human material may indicate that in the human there are fewer glycine receptor units. A similar difference between monkey and rat had been previously observed (13).

The presence of a $^3$H-strychnine binding site in the substantia nigra, together with the observations that: (a) glycine exerts a strychnine-sensitive depression of dopamine neurone activity (6,7); (b) there is a high-affinity glycine uptake system in the substantia nigra (14); and (c) local application of glycine is inhibitory to nigral dopamine neuron function (2,12,16) presents a strong argument for inhibitory glycinergic control of nigral dopamine neuron activity. However, the global glycine-dopamine interaction within the extrapyramidal system differs from the GABA-mediated inhibition of dopamine neurons, as blockade of the glycine receptor unit by strychnine does not reverse haloperidol catalepsy, whereas blockade of GABA receptor function by bicuculline or picrotoxinin results in a marked reduction (19).

The hypothesis of glycine receptors on dopamine cell bodies is supported by the distribution of $^3$H-strychnine binding in the human substantia nigra, the pars compacta having twice the capacity of the pars reticulata. Stronger evidence comes from the observation that in Parkinson's disease $^3$H-strychnine binding sites are low in the substantia nigra, but not in the inferior olive. This is consistent with the association of $^3$H-strychnine binding sites on dopamine cell bodies and/or dendrites, the loss of which is the major anatomical and neurochemical pathology of Parkinson's disease (9,17). The present observations, plus the previous reports of a loss of GABA receptors in the parkinsonian substantia nigra (18,21), indicate that normally dopamine cells receive both GABAergic and glycinergic inhibitory inputs.

The lower capacity for $^3$H-strychnine binding in the substantia nigra of parkinsonian patients does not appear to be due to nonspecific causes such as general cerebral atrophy or as a consequence of severe neurological disease. Thus, there is not any decrease in $^3$H-strychnine binding in the substantia nigra from Huntington's chorea patients (Table 3) and in 2 cases of senile dementia $^3$H-strychnine binding is well within the normal range (Lloyd et al., *unpublished data*).

## CONCLUSIONS

Glycine receptor units, as identified by $^3$H-strychnine binding, are present in the human spinal cord, pars compacta, and pars reticulata of the substantia nigra. The affinity constant of the high-affinity binding site is similar to that seen for the rat or bovine material, but the binding capacity is lower for the human. The decrease of $^3$H-strychnine binding in the substantia nigra in Parkinson's disease, together with previous observations from the literature, indicates the presence of glycine receptors on nigral dopamine cell bodies and/or dendrites.

## REFERENCES

1. Arnt, J., and Scheel-Kruger, J. (1979): GABAergic and glycinergic mechanisms within the substantia nigra: Pharmacological specificity of dopamine-independent contralateral turning behaviour and interaction with other neurotransmitters. *Psychopharmacology*, 62:267–277.
2. Cheramy, A., Nieoullon A., and Glowinski, J. (1978): Inhibition of dopamine release in the cat caudate nucleus by nigral application of glycine. *Eur. J. Pharmacol.*, 47:141–147.
3. Curtis, D. R., Duggan, A. W., and Johnston, G. A. R. (1971): The specificity of strychnine as a glycine antagonist in the mammalian spinal cord. *Exp. Brain Res.*, 12:547–565.
4. Curtis, D. R., Hösli, L., and Johnston, G. A. R. (1968): A pharmacological study of the depression of spinal neurons by glycine and related amino-acids. *Exp. Brain Res.*, 6:11–18.
5. DeFeudis, F. V. (1978): Central glycine receptors. *Gen. Pharmacol.*, 9:139–144.

6. Dray, A., and Gonye, T. J. (1975): Effects of caudate stimulation and microiontophoretically applied substances on neurones in the rat substantia nigra. *J. Physiol. (Lond.)*, 246:88P–89P.
7. Dray, A., and Straughan, D. W. (1976): Synaptic mechanisms in the substantia nigra. *J. Pharm. Pharmacol.*, 28:400–405.
8. Felpel, L. P. (1972): Effects of strychnine, bicuculline and picrotoxin on labyrinthine-evoked inhibition in neck motoneurons of the cat. *Exp. Brain Res.*, 14:494–502.
9. Hornykiewicz, O. (1966): Dopamine (3-hydroxytyramine) and brain function. *Pharmacol. Rev.*, 18:925–964.
10. Hunt, P., and Raynaud, J. P. (1977): Benzodiazepine activity: Is interaction with the glycine receptor, as evidenced by displacement of strychnine binding, a useful criterion? *J. Pharm. Pharmacol.*, 29:442–444.
11. Iversen, L. L., and Bloom, F. E. (1972): Studies of the uptake of ($^3$H)-GABA and ($^3$H)-glycine in slices and homogenates of rat brain and spinal cord by electron microscopic autoradiography. *Brain Res.*, 41:131–143.
12. James, T. A., and Starr, M. S. (1979): Is glycine an inhibitory synaptic transmitter in the substantia nigra? *Eur. J. Pharmacol.*, 57:115–125.
13. Javoy-Agid, F., and Agid, Y. (1980): Is the mesocortical dopaminergic system involved in Parkinson's disease? *Neurology*, 30:1326–1330.
14. Kerwin, R. W., and Pycock, C. J. (1979): Specific stimulating effect of glycine on $^3$H-dopamine efflux from substantia nigra slices of the rat. *Eur. J. Pharmacol.*, 54:93–98.
15. Krnjevic, K. (1974): Chemical nature of synaptic transmission in vertebrates. *Physiol. Rev.*, 54:418–540.
16. LeViel, V. Cheramy, A., Nieoullon, A., and Glowinski, J. (1979): Symmetric bilateral changes in dopamine release from the caudate nuclei of the cat induced by unilateral nigral application of glycine and GABA-related compounds. *Brain Res.*, 175:259–270.
17. Lloyd, K. G. Davidson, L., and Hornykiewicz, O. (1975): The neurochemistry of Parkinson's disease: Effect of L-DOPA therapy. *J. Pharmacol. Exp. Therap.*, 195:453–464.
18. Lloyd, K. G. Shemen, L. and Hornykiewicz, O. (1977): Distribution of high affinity sodium-independent ($^3$H)-gamma-aminobutyric acid ($^3$H-GABA) binding in the human brain: Alterations in Parkinson's disease. *Brain Res.*, 127:269–278.
19. Lloyd, K. G., and Worms, P. (1979): GABA-mediated regulation of dopaminergic neurons. In: *Catecholamines: Basic and Clinical Frontiers*, edited by E. Usdin, I. J. Kopin, and J. Barchas, pp. 1068–1070. Pergamon Press, New York.
20. Lowry, O. H., Rosebrough, N. J., Farr, A. L., and Randall, R. J. (1951): Protein measurement with the Folin phenol reagent. *J. Biol. Chem.*, 193:265–275.
21. Rinne, U. K., Koskinen, V., Laaksonen, H., Lönneberg, P., and Sonninen, V. (1978): GABA receptor binding in the Parkinsonian brain. *Life Sci.*, 22:2225–2228.
22. Snyder, S. H. (1975): The glycine receptor in the mammalian central nervous system. *Br. J. Pharmacol.*, 53:473–484.
23. Young, A. B., and Snyder, S. H. (1973): Strychnine binding associated with glycine receptors of the central nervous system. *Proc. Natl. Acad. Sci. USA*, 70:2832–2836.
24. Young, A. B., and Snyder, S. H. (1974): Strychnine binding in rat spinal cord membranes associated with the synaptic glycine receptor: Cooperativity of glycine interactions. *Mol. Pharmacol.*, 10:790–809.
25. Young, A. B., Zukin, S. R., and Snyder, S. H. (1974): Interactions of benzodiazepines with central nervous system glycine receptors: possible mechanism of action. *Proc. Natl. Acad. Sci. USA*, 71:2246–2250.

# Specific Binding of Cysteine Sulfinic Acid to Synaptic Membrane Fractions

Heitaroh Iwata and Akemichi Baba

*Department of Pharmacology, Faculty of Pharmaceutical Sciences, Osaka University, Osaka, Japan*

Cysteine sulfinic acid (CSA), a metabolic precursor of taurine, is known to have a strong excitation action on the central neurons when applied iontophoretically (4). It also may be responsible for the excitation neurotoxic effects observed after injection of L-cysteine (9). Moreover, CSA caused a greater increase than glutamate in the level of cyclic adenosine monophosphate (AMP) in guinea pig cerebral cortex (11). These findings indicate that CSA could have functional roles in the central nervous system. In previous studies, we demonstrated the distribution of CSA in rat brain (2), the $Na^+$-dependent high-affinity transport of CSA in the synaptosomes, and its $Ca^{2+}$-dependent release by depolarizing condition (1). Application of CSA to the lateral ventricle of rat brain induced EEG seizures, which were significantly suppressed by stimultaneous injection of taurine (6).

Excitatory amino acids, such as glutamate, aspartate, and CSA, stimulated the formation of cyclic AMP in cerebral cortical slices—possibly via an amino acid receptor (11). However, our separate study (Baba et al., *unpublished data*), showing a specific antagonism by taurine of CSA-induced increase of cyclic AMP in hippocampal slices of guinea pig, indicated that the mechanism of action of CSA was different from that of glutamate or aspartate. Among the excitatory amino acids, the $Na^+$-independent specific binding of L-glutamate by synaptic membranes has been studied extensively (5,10). It is therefore of interest to examine the possibility that synaptic membranes have a specific binding site for CSA that differs from that for glutamate. In the present study, we used [$^{35}S$]cysteic acid (CA), an analog of CSA, as a ligand for binding assay, since it has a similar excitation effect to CSA (4) and is more stable.

## MATERIALS AND METHODS

### Chemicals

L-[$^{35}S$]Cystine (370 Ci/mmole) was obtained from New England Nuclear. L-[$^3H$]Glutamate (35 Ci/mmole) was from the Radiochemical Centre, Amersham. D-Cysteic acid of more than 94% purity was prepared from D-cystine (7). L-[$^{35}S$]CA was synthesized from L-[$^{35}$S]cystine according to the HgCl$_2$ oxidation method (7). The purity of [$^{35}$S]CA was determined by paper chromatography or high voltage thin layer chromatography. More than 94% of the radioactivity was recovered in CA (17.5 Ci/mmole).

## Preparation of Crude Synaptic Membranes

Male Sprague-Dawley rats, weighing approximately 200 g, were used throughout. Crude synaptic membranes of the cerebral cortex were prepared as described by Simon et al. (13). The membrane fraction was stored at $-20°C$ for 16 hr. Before binding assay, frozen or fresh membranes were resuspended in deionized distilled water and incubated at 25°C for 40 min to eliminate possible endogenous ligands. Then the mixture was centrifuged and the pellet was suspended in 50 mM Tris-HCl (pH 7.4) and used for binding assay.

## Assay of [$^{35}$S]CA Binding and [$^3$H]Glutamate Binding

In the standard procedure for [$^{35}$S]CA binding assay, aliquots of the membrane suspension were incubated in triplicate at 37°C for 20 min in 1 ml of 50 mM Tris-HCl (pH 7.4) containing 140 mM [$^{35}$S]CA (4 × 10$^5$ cpm) alone, in the presence of 1 mM unlabeled L-CA, or other indicated reagents. [$^3$H]Glutamate binding assay was performed in the same way, except that 140 nM [$^3$H]glutamate and 1 mM unlabeled glutamate were used.

The incubation was stopped by rapid filtration of the mixture through a Whatman GF/B glass fiber filter, and the membranes on the filter were washed four times with 5 ml Tris-HCl buffer within 15 sec. The filter was then dried and its radioactivity was counted in a liquid scintillation spectrometer. Specific [$^{35}$S]CA binding was calculated by subtracting the amount of radioactivity not displaced by 1 mM L-CA from the total bound radioactivity. The amount of radioactivity retained by the filters in the absence of membranes was approximately 0.05% of the total [$^{35}$S]CA and was subtracted from each value. Specific [$^3$H]glutamate binding was calculated in the same manner.

## RESULTS

The specific binding of [$^{35}$S]CA to fresh synaptic membranes was approximately 70 times higher in the presence of Na$^+$ than in its absence. When the membranes were stored at $-20°C$, the specific binding in the presence of Na$^+$ was reduced to 10%, but in the absence of Na$^+$ did not change (*data not shown*).

Na$^+$-independent binding of [$^{35}$S]CA was also observed in the membranes of peripheral tissues (Fig. 1). Results showed a high localization of the binding in the membrane fractions of adrenal gland and skeletal muscle. On the other hand, the specific binding was negligible in the liver. The time course of Na$^+$-independent specific binding of [$^{35}$S]CA to cortical synaptic membranes was examined: It attained complete equilibrium after 20 min of incubation. Na$^+$-independent specific binding

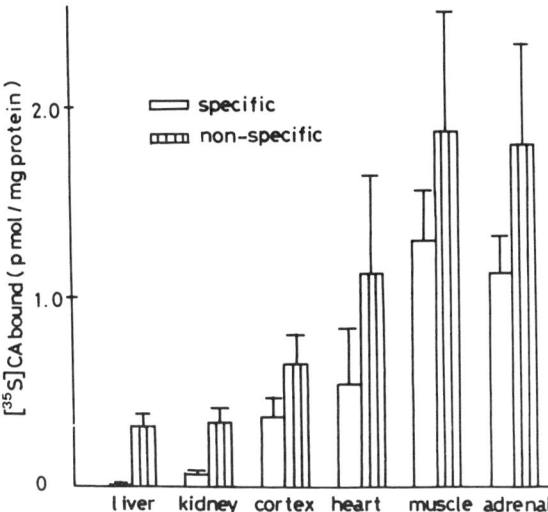

**FIG. 1.** Na+-independent binding of [35S]CA to crude membrane fractions of various tissues. Crude membrane fractions of each tissue were prepared as follows. Tissues were homogenized with 20 volumes 0.32 M sucrose, and the homogenates were centrifuged at 1,000 × $g$, for 10 min. Resulting supernatant was pelleted at 100,000 × $g$, for 60 min, and the pellet was used for the binding assay.

of CA was saturable; the nonspecific binding increased linearly with an increase in CA concentration and was not saturable over the concentration range up to 700 nM. Kinetics of Na+-independent specific binding of [35S]CA and [3H]glutamate was examined by Scatchard analysis. Results are shown in Table 1.

Na+-independent specific binding of [35S]CA was maximal at pH 7.4 and 37°C. To obtain information on whether the specific binding site of [35S]CA is involved in the binding site of CSA, we tested the abilities of various structural analogs to displace specifically bound CA (Table 2). Among the excitatory amino acids tested, L-CSA was the most effective displacer, being approximately 70 times more effective than L-CA. L-Glutamate and L-aspartate, respectively, were 11 and 95 times less effective than L-CSA. The specific binding of CA exhibited stereospecificity,

TABLE 1. *Kinetics of NA+-independent specific binding of [35S]CA and [3H]glutamate to the synaptic membranes*

|  | $K_D$ (nM) | $B_{max}$ (pmole/mg prot.) |
|---|---|---|
| [35S]CA | 474 | 3.29 |
| [3H]Glutamate | 363 | 13.10 |

The saturation of specific [35S]CA and [3H]glutamate binding was determined using increasing amounts of radioligands up to 700 nM. $K_D$ and $B_{max}$ values of the binding were calculated from the Scatchard analysis.

TABLE 2. *Displacement of Na$^+$- independent specific binding of [$^{35}$S]CA in crude synaptic membranes*

| Compound | IC$_{50}$ | (nM) |
|---|---|---|
| L-Cysteine sulfinate | 9.6 | |
| L-Glutamate | 107.4 | |
| DL-Homocysteate | 298.5 | |
| DL-Homocysteine | 545.6 | |
| L-Cysteate | 704.3 | |
| L-Aspartate | 912.0 | |
| D-Cysteate | 11.7 | µM |
| Kainate | 20 | µM |
| Taurine | > 1 | mM |
| Hypotaurine | > 1 | mM |
| Taurocyamine | > 1 | mM |

TABLE 3. *Displacement of NA$^+$- independent specific binding of [$^3$H]glutamate in crude synaptic membranes*

| Compound | IC$_{50}$ | (µM) |
|---|---|---|
| L-Glutamate | 0.24 | |
| L-Cysteine sulfinate | 5.75 | |
| DL-Homocysteine | 27.2 | |
| L-Cysteate | 64.2 | |
| Taurine | > 1 | mM |
| Hypotaurine | > 1 | mM |
| Taurocyamine | > 1 | mM |

since D-CA bound much less than the L-isomer. In addition, L-CSA competitively inhibited the Na$^+$-independent specific binding of CA, whereas L-glutamate inhibited it noncompetitively *(data not shown)*. IC$_{50}$ values of the related compounds for the [$^3$H]glutamate binding are shown in Table 3. L-Glutamate was the most effective, being 24 times more effective than L-CSA. L-CA had no significant effect.

## DISCUSSION

In the present study, we demonstrated the Na$^+$-independent specific binding of [$^{35}$S]CA to crude synaptic membranes. Radioligand binding studies have indicated multiplicity of binding sites for excitatory amino acids. Assuming a postsynaptic location of the CA binding sites, the question arises of whether these binding sites are identical with those of glutamate, since Na$^+$-independent specific binding of glutamate has been shown (5,8,10,12). L-CSA was the most potent displacer of the specific binding of [$^{35}$S]CA and it inhibited CA binding competitively. On the contrary, the inhibition by L-glutamate, which was 11 times less than that by L-

CSA, was noncompetitive. Unlabeled L-CA had only 1/70 of the affinity of L-CSA. In addition, the most potent displacer for the glutamate binding was L-glutamate: L-CSA was 24 times less effective than L-glutamate. In a recent study with hippocampal membranes, L-CSA was approximately six times weaker than L-glutamate in displacing [$^3$H]glutamate binding (3). As shown in Table 2, L-CSA has a very low IC$_{50}$ value for the CA binding. Although we did not examine this binding site using L-CSA as a ligand, it seems reasonable that it has very high affinity for L-CSA.

The present study suggests that L-CSA may be an endogenous ligand for the Na$^+$-independent specific binding sites of CA in synaptic membranes, which seems to differ from that of glutamate. There is increasing neurochemical evidence that both glutamate and aspartate function as excitatory synaptic transmitters in the mammalian central nervous system. CSA has also been characterized as an excitatory amino acid (4). Our previous and present studies support the idea that CSA is an excitatory synaptic transmitter in the central nervous system.

## REFERENCES

1. Baba, A., Yamagami, S., and Iwata, H. (1979): Uptake, release and metabolism of cysteine and cysteine sulfinic acid in the synaptosomal fraction of rat brain. *Sulfur-Containing Amino Acids*, 2:39–46.
2. Baba, A., Yamagami, S., Mizuo, H., and Iwata, H. (1980): Microassay of cysteine sulfinic acid by an enzymatic cycling method. *Anal. Biochem.*, 101:288–293.
3. Baudry, M., and Lynch, G. (1980): Characterization of two [$^3$H]glutamate binding sites in rat hippocampal membranes. *J. Neurochem.*, 36:811–820.
4. Curtis, S. R., and Watkins, J. C. (1960): The excitation and depression of spinal neurones by structurally related amino acids. *J. Neurochem.*, 6:117–141.
5. Foster, A. C., and Roberts, P. J. (1978): High affinity L-[$^3$H] glutamate binding to postsynaptic receptor sites on rat cerebellar membranes. *J. Neurochem.*, 31:1467–1477.
6. Iwata, H., Yamagami, S., Mizuo, H., and Baba, A. (1980): Inhibitory effects of taurine and GABA on cysteine sulfinic acid-induced seizures. *Sulfur-Containing Amino Acids*, 3:25–28.
7. Lavine, J. F. (1936): The action of mercuric sulfate and chloride on cystine, cysteine sulfinic acid (R-SO$_2$H), and cysteic acid with reference to the dismutation of cystine. *J. Biol. Chem.*, 147:309–313.
8. Michaelis, F. K., Michaelis M. L., and Boyarsky, L. L. (1974): High-affinity glutamic acid binding to brain synaptic membranes. *Biochim. Biophys. Acta*, 367:338–348.
9. Olney, J. W., Ho, O. L., and Rhee, V. (1971): Cytotoxic effects of acidic and sulphur containing amino acids on the infant mouse central nervous system. *Exp. Brain Res.*, 14:61–76.
10. Roberts, P. J. (1974): Glutamate receptor in the rat central nervous system. *Nature*, 252:399–401.
11. Shimizu, H., Ichishita, H., Tateishi, M., and Umeda, I. (1974): Characteristics of the amino acid receptor site mediating formation of cyclic adenosine 3′, 5′-monophosphate in mammalian brains. *Mol. Pharmacol.*, 11:223–231.
12. Sharif, N. A., and Roberts, P. J. (1980): Effects of protein- and membrane-modifying agents on the binding of L-[$^3$H]glutamate to cerebellar synaptic membranes. *Brain Res.*, 194:594–597.
13. Simon, J. R., Contrera, J. F., and Kuhar, M. J. (1976): Binding of [$^3$H]kainic acid, an analogue of L-glutamate, to brain membranes. *J. Neurochem.*, 26:141–147.

Molecular Pharmacology of Neurotransmitter
Receptors, edited by T. Segawa et al.
Raven Press, New York © 1983.

# Morphological Study of Neurotransmitter Receptors in the Rat Brain

Shozo Kito, Eiko Itoga, Takenobu Kishida, and Masanori Togo

*Third Department of Internal Medicine, Hiroshima University School of Medicine, Hiroshima 734, Japan*

In recent years, receptor-binding experiments of neurotransmitters with use of minutely fractionated brain materials have been acquiring increasing popularity. Multiple subtypes of receptors have been described pharmacologically, whereas only a few morphological studies on neurotransmitter receptors have been published. This is especially true of electron microscopic observations of the receptors, for which the only method is autoradiography. Autoradiography of a diffusible ligand is commonly applied *in vivo*. However, *in vitro* labeling procedures of autoradiography have been performed by several scientists at the light microscopic level (1,3,4,11). This method has several advantages compared with studies employing *in vivo* labeling, although it has a limitation of ligands. We can wash specimens sufficiently to minimize nonspecific binding whereas washing is impossible in the *in vivo* labeling procedure. We can use ligands that do not pass through the blood-brain barrier and we can use autopsy human materials.

In this chapter, we describe the autoradiographic distribution of receptor sites of the lightly fixed rat brain, which were observed using $^3$H-muscimol and $^3$H-D-alanine-methionine-amide-enkephalin (DAMA) at light and electron microscopic levels.

## MATERIALS AND METHODS

### Tissue Preparation

Wistar strain male rats weighing 180 to 200 g were used for the experiments. Sampling for light microscopic autoradiography was performed as follows. The animals were anesthetized with pentobarbital (subcutaneous injection of 0.3 ml/100 g body weight) and perfusion-fixed with 500 ml of 0.1% paraformaldehyde in 0.1 ml phosphate buffer, pH 7.2, intracardially. The brains were removed, sagitally sliced in four to five pieces by a sharp razor blade, and the pieces were immersed into the above-mentioned fixative. The immersed tissue pieces were taken out of the fixative after 30 min and left in 7% phosphate dextrose buffer for several hours at 4°C. After embedded in OCT compound and frozen in acetone with dry ice, the specimens were stored at $-30°C$ and used for the next step within 2 weeks. The frozen specimens were cut in sections of 8 or 12 μM thickness with a Sakura cryostat and then thaw-mounted onto clean acid-washed slides coated with 0.5% gelatine solution.

### Receptor Binding with Cryostat Sections

Slides with mounted 12-μm thick tissue sections were brought to room temperature and preincubated with buffer solution. The slides were then transferred to an incubation medium containing the tritiated ligand. After incubation with the ligand, the slides were rinsed in the buffer solution and the tissue sections were scraped by Whatman GF/B filter paper and placed in scintillation vials. After dissolving the tissue in 1 ml of soluene, 10 ml of the scintillation fluid was added for measurement of radioactivity.

For $^3$H-muscimol binding, 0.31 M Tris-HCl buffer was used and the displacer was GABA. In $^3$H-DAMA binding experiments, 0.17 M Tris-HCl buffer was used and nonradioactive met-enkephalin was utilized to obtain blank values.

### Autoradiography

The 8-μm frozen sections were brought to room temperature and preincubated with the same buffer as used in the biochemical binding experiments. After preincubation, the sections were incubated with 5 nM radiolabeled ligands dissolved in the buffer for 40 min at 25°C. The slides were rinsed with the same buffer without radioactivity and postfixated with 95% ethanol. After the tissues were dried, the sections were coated either with Ilford L-4 or with Sakura NTR-M2 as nuclear track emulsion by dipping and stored at 4°C for 4 to 8 weeks. After exposure, the slides were developed by Konidol X, and stained with toluidine blue. Excess unlabeled GABA at 0.2 mM for $^3$H-muscimol binding and 1 μM unlabeled met-enkephalin for $^3$H-DAMA were utilized as displacers. One-minute washing was selected for muscimol binding and 10-min washing for $^3$H-DAMA binding.

For electron microscopic observations, the brains of rats were perfusion-fixated with modified Zamboni's solution (0.2% picric acid 1% paraformaldehyde in phosphate buffer). Then, 80-μm Vibratome sections were incubated with 5 nM $^3$H-muscimol for 60 min at 25°C. The sections were then postfixed with mixture of 2% glutaraldehyde and 2% $OsO_4$. We processed the ultrathin sections of electron microscopic autoradiography by the "touch method," using Sakura NR-H2 and elon ascorbic acid (EAA) developer. The EAA developer was needed to develop silver grains into finer ones. Through this method, the diameters of developed silver grains were as small as 20–80 nm.

## RESULTS

### Receptor Binding with Cryostat Sections

The preliminary experiments consisted of receptor binding experiments on slides with mounted tissue sections. Figure 1 shows a saturation curve of $^3$H-muscimol

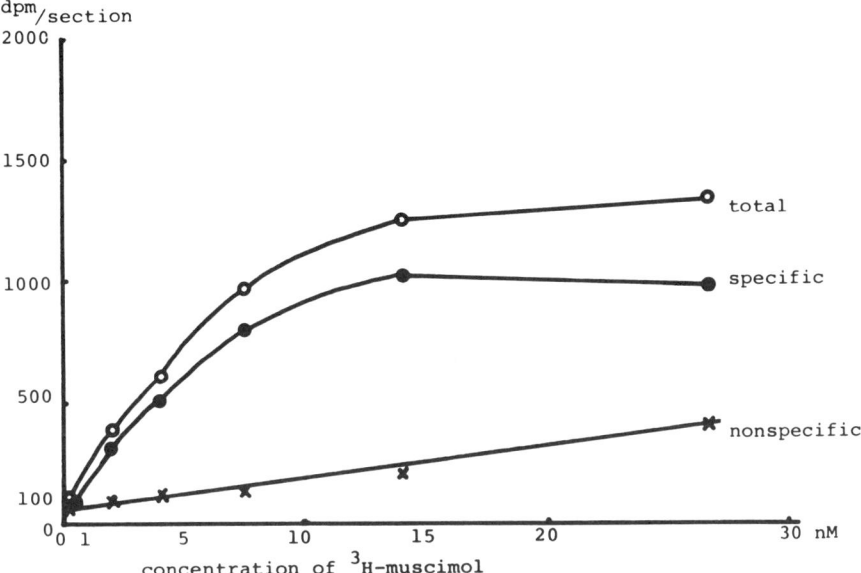

**FIG. 1.** The saturation of ³H-muscimol binding in the rat cerebellum. The specific binding curve *(closed circles)* was obtained by subtracting nonspecific *(crosses)* from total *(open circles)* binding.

binding of cryostat sections of the rat cerebellum which was fixed slightly with 0.1% paraformaldehyde. The results of these studies were compared with those of binding experiments that used nonperfused materials which were obtained as follows. Wistar strain rats were decapitated and the brains were removed rapidly. The tissues were embedded in OCT, frozen and sectioned by a cryostat in 12 μm thickness. Scatchard plots of saturation data of these two experiments are shown in Fig. 2. The $K_D$ value was 8.41 nM and the $B_{max}$ was 184.2 fmole per two sections in the lightly fixed material. The ligand binding of the tissues that were not perfused with fixative revealed a slightly lower $K_D$ value (5.99 nM). In the unfixed cerebellum, the $B_{max}$ was 207.8 fmole per two sections and there was no significant difference from that of the fixed material. We subsequently examined the effects of pentobarbital anesthesia on these studies. Table 1 shows the comparison of specific binding of ³H-muscimol to cryostat sections of various regions of the rat brain among (a) the unfixed materials from unanesthetized animals, (b) unfixed materials from pentobarbital-anesthetized animals, and (c) fixed materials. The effect of pentobarbital anesthesia on muscimol binding was negligible except in the section of the striatum.

Figure 3 shows the saturation plot of ³H-DAMA binding using cryostat sections of the lightly fixed rat hypothalamus. The binding was saturable and the $K_D$ value was 1.67 nM and the $B_{max}$ was 20 fmole per two sections (Fig. 4). The specific binding of ³H-DAMA to cryostat sections of various regions of the rat brain was highest in the hypothalamus and striatum (697 dpm/section and 693 dpm/section).

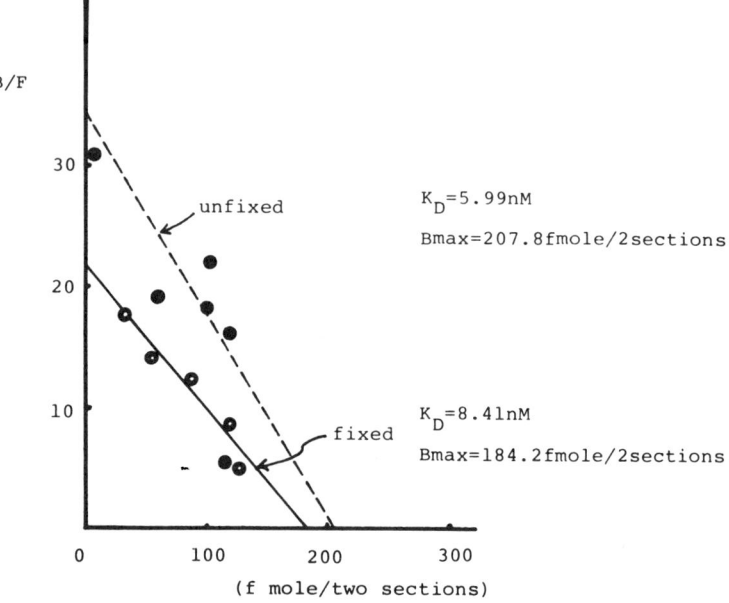

**FIG. 2.** Scatchard plots of saturation data of $^3$H-muscimol binding experiments. The results of studies on fixed materials *(open circles)* are compared with those on unfixed materials *(closed circles)*.

TABLE 1. *The effect of fixation and pentobarbital anesthesia on $^3$H-muscimol binding to a cryostat section*

| Brain regions | $^3$H-Muscimol bound (dpm/section) | | |
|---|---|---|---|
| | Unfixed materials | Materials from anesthetized animals | Pentobarbital anesthesia followed by fixation |
| Cerebellum | 1101 (100)[a] | 1154 (114) | 460 (45) |
| Hypothalamus | 246 (100) | 296 (120) | 187 (76) |
| Striatum | 448 (100) | 264 (59) | 139 (31) |
| Midbrain | 200 (100) | 190 (95) | 108 (54) |

[a] % of binding.

Unfixed materials were obtained, as described in the text, by decapitation. Unfixed materials from anesthetized animals were obtained as follows: pentobarbital (0.3 ml/100 g body wt) was injected s.c. to the animals. After 15 min decapitation was done, the brains were removed, and 12-μm cryostat sections were made. Incubations with 5 nM $^3$H-muscimol for 30 min at 25°C followed preincubation with 0.31 M Tris citrate buffer for 20 min at 4°C. The sections were then washed for 1 min at 4°C in the same buffered solution and scraped by Whatman GF/B filter paper and dissolved in 1 ml soluene. Examined rats were almost of the same body weight and brain size. Comparisons were made among the sections cut through the same level of the brain. All the figures in the table are the means of the results obtained from four tissue sections.

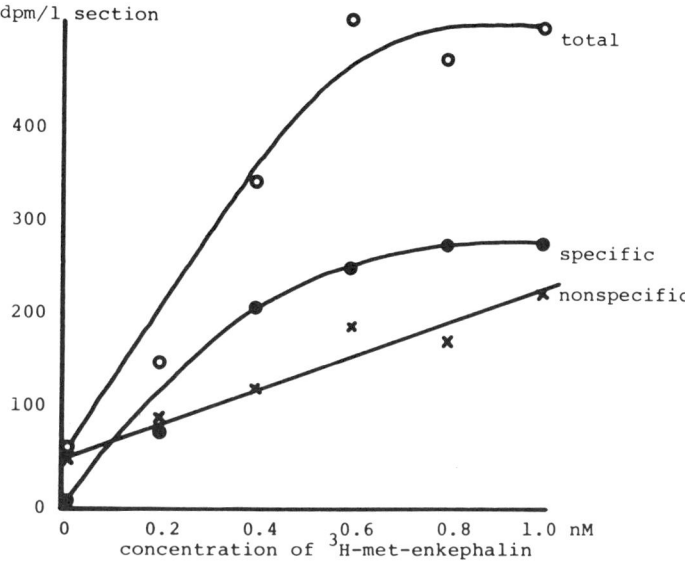

**FIG. 3.** The saturation of ³H-DAMA binding in cryostat sectioned tissue of the rat hypothalamus.

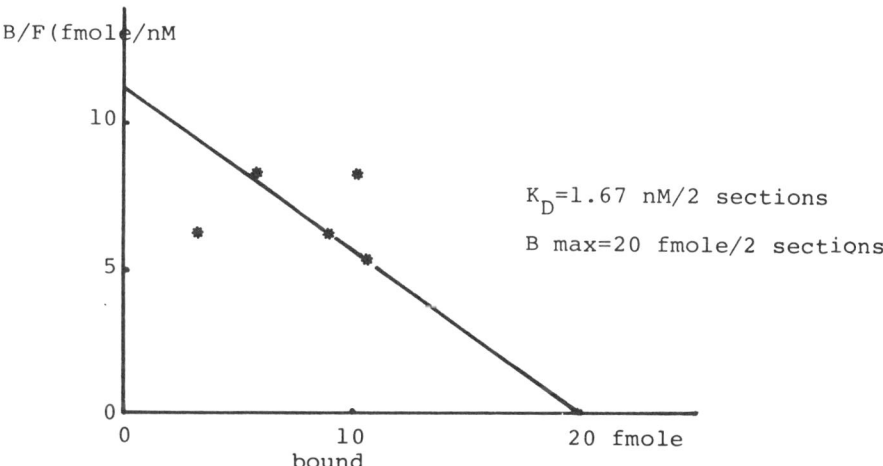

**FIG. 4.** Scatchard analysis for the specific binding of ³H-DAMA to cryostat sections of the rat brain.

In the midbrain it was 421 dpm/section, and met-enkephalin receptor density was lowest in the cerebellum (33 dpm/section).

## Autoradiography

$^3$H-Muscimol binding sites were widely distributed in the central nervous system. In the cerebellar cortex, they formed a laminar distribution. The highest density of the silver grains was observed in the granular layer (17.8 ± SD 2.7/6.25 μm$^2$; $N$ = 5 areas), followed by the molecular layer (11.6 ± 2.1/6.25 μm$^2$; $N$ = 5 areas); background levels were found in the white matter (6.8 ± 1.8/6.25 μm$^2$; $N$ = 5 areas) (Fig. 5).. In higher magnification, silver grains were observed surrounding the cell bodies of the Purkinje cells, stellate cells, and Basket cells (Fig. 6).

In electron microscopic autoradiography of the cerebellar molecular layer, the GABA receptor site labeled by EAA developed silver grains on the axodendritic synaptic membrane surface (Fig. 7). Synaptic vesicles can be observed in the figure as can be a synapse of inhibitory nature in which the pre-and postsynaptic membranes are unequal in thickness. In addition, numerous $^3$H-muscimol binding sites can be

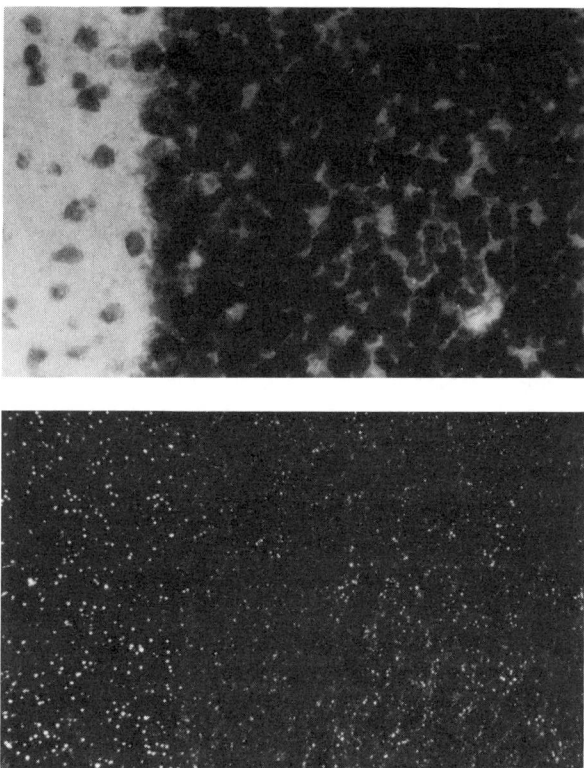

**FIG. 5.** Darkfield **(top)** and brightfield **(bottom)** photomicrographs of the rat cerebellum. High density of GABA receptors can be seen in the granular cell layer, and receptors are less dense in the molecular layer. Silver grains are observed surrounding the stellate and basket cells. ×200.

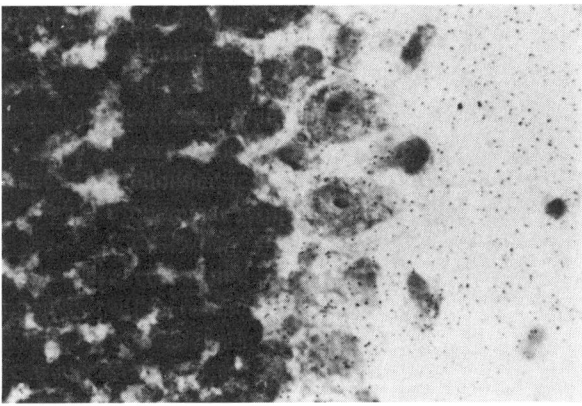

FIG. 6. Brightfield photomicrograph of the rat cerebellum in higher magnification. ×400.

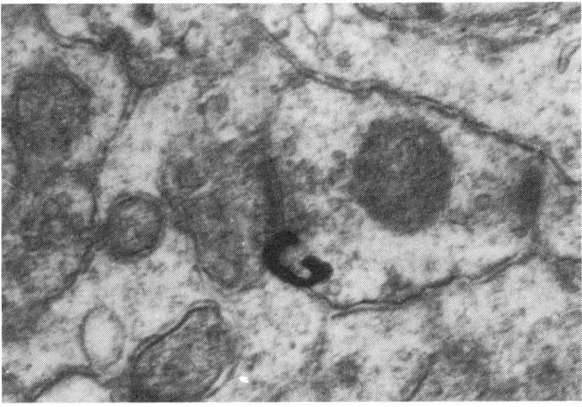

FIG. 7. An electron microscopic autoradiograph of the molecular cell layer of the cerebellum incubated with ³H-muscimol. Developed silver grains are observed on axodendritic synapses. The section was developed with EAA developer (18°C, 8 min) preceded by gold latensification (18°C, 10 sec).

seen on the plasma membranes of both dendrites and axons, but not necessarily in the synaptic sites (Fig. 8).

Generally, the shorter the development time, the less the silver grains spread. In a short development time, the specific grains are observed in a more specifically localized pattern on the neuronal plasma membrane. Figure 9 shows small silver grains precisely localized on the dendritic membranes.

Figure 10 shows the neuropile of the substantia nigra in which silver grains of muscimol binding sites are scattered around the synaptic regions and the plasma membranes. In electron microscopic autoradiography, we sometimes cannot escape from the scatter of β-particles from the bound ³H-muscimol.

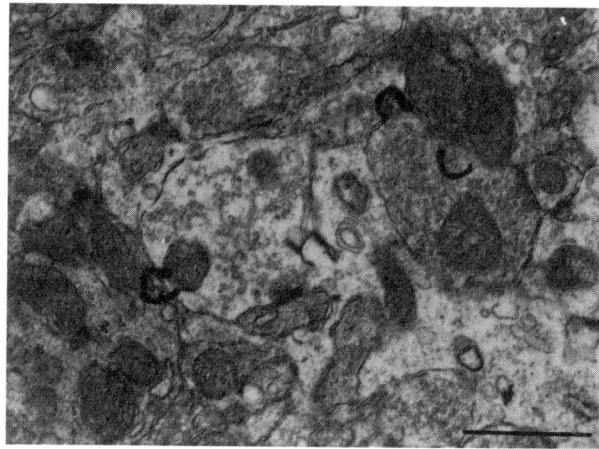

**FIG. 8.** A finding similar to that of Fig. 7. Silver grains are observed on the plasma membrane in the rat cerebellar molecular layer. Development time is 7 min with EAA developer. Bar = 1 µm.

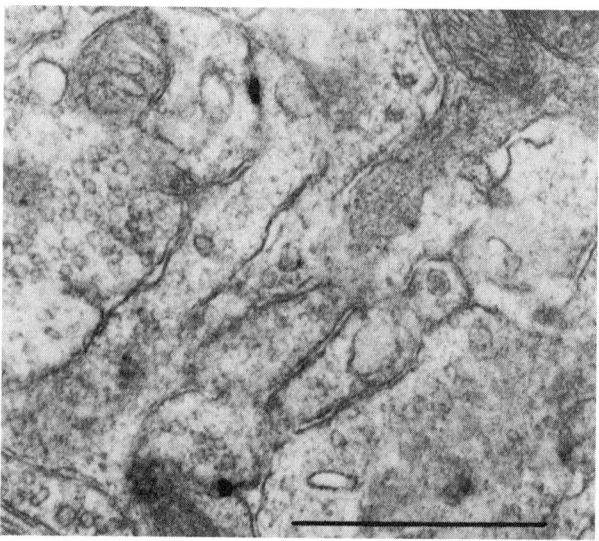

**FIG. 9.** An electron microscopic autoradiograph of the cerebellar molecular layer. The sections are developed with EAA developer for 5 min. Silver grains are smaller in size when compared with those in Figs. 7 and 8. Bar = 1 µm.

Figure 11 shows high magnification of the $^3$H-muscimol binding sites in the substantia nigra observed autoradiographically.

Much emphasis has recently been placed on the amygdaloid nucleus which is considered to play important roles in regulating neuroendocrinological functions. There is met-enkephalin-like immunoreactivity in the numerous nerve terminals

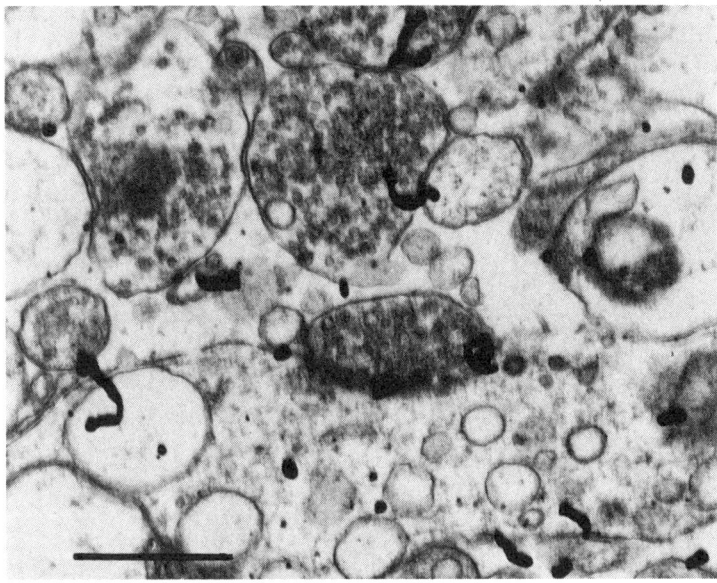

**FIG. 10.** An electron microscopic autoradiograph of the substantia nigra of a rat incubated with ³H-DAMA. Bar = 1 μm.

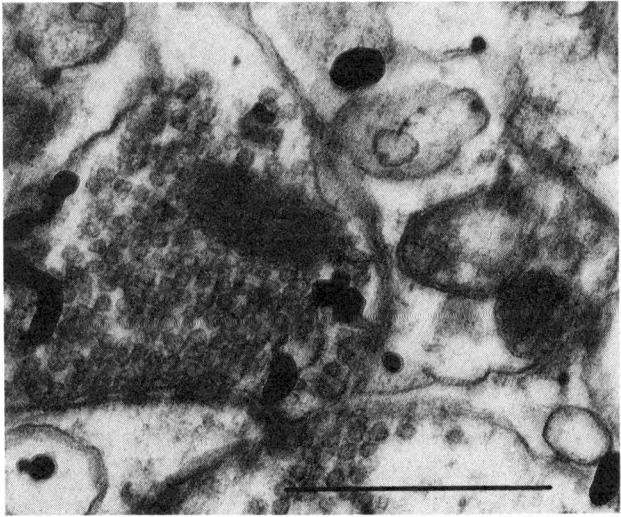

**FIG. 11.** Higher magnification of the same section as of Fig. 10.

and cell bodies of the amygdaloid nucleus (Fig. 12). From this viewpoint, we examined receptor sites of met-enkephalin at the electron microscopic level.

In the neuropile of the amygdaloid nucleus, we observed that met-enkephalin receptor sites labeled by EAA developed silver grains on the plasma membranes

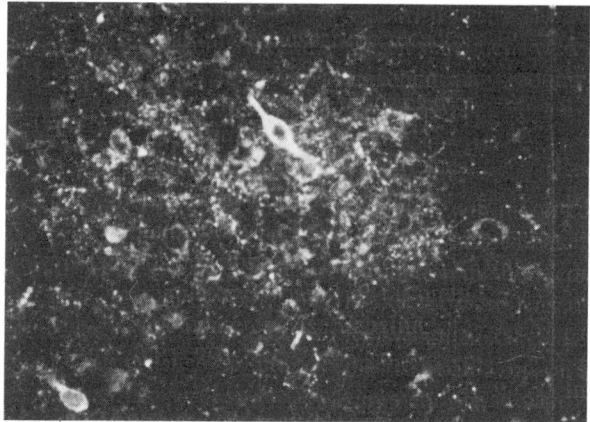

**FIG. 12.** Met-enkephalin-like immunoreactivity in the rat amygdaloid nucleus. Immunoreactive nerve terminals and cell bodies are observed. ×200.

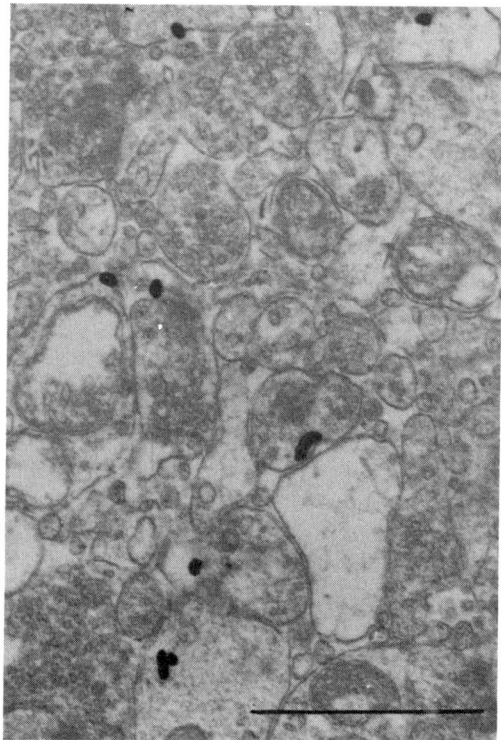

**FIG. 13.** $^3$H-DAMA binding sites of the amygdaloid nucleus. The section is developed with EAA developer for 5 min. Bar = 1 μm.

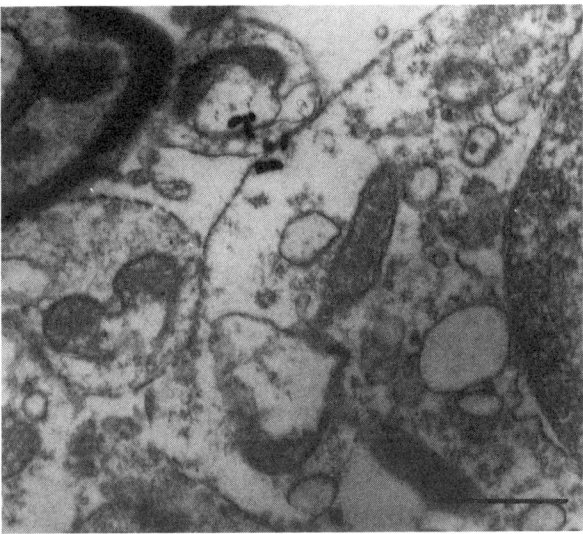

FIG. 14. An electron microscopic autoradiograph of the amygdaloid nucleus. Met-enkephalin binding receptor sites on the surface of the cytosome of a nerve cell in the amygdaloid nucleus are observed. Bar = 1 μm.

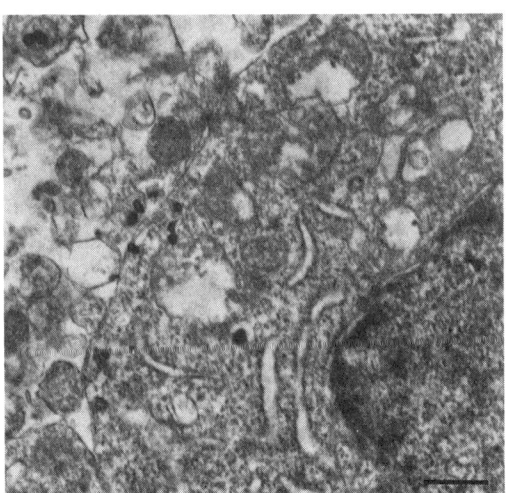

FIG. 15. 3H-DAMA binding sites of the caudate nucleus. Bar = 1 μm.

(Fig. 13). In Fig. 14, met-enkephalin receptor sites can be seen on the surface of the cytosome of the nerve cell in the amygdaloid nucleus. In the caudate nucleus, numerous met-enkephalin receptor sites are also observed in cytosome of a nerve cell and dendrites (Fig. 15).

## DISCUSSION

Our autoradiographic observations of ligand bindings to neurotransmitter receptors in the brain were performed with the use of $^3$H-muscimol and $^3$H-DAMA. Important points for those observations are, first, that binding affinity of the ligand should be high enough (the $K_D$ value should be less than $10^{-9}$–$10^{-10}$ M) and second, that the ligand should be held firmly and diffusion during preparation of a specimen should be minimum (2). Kuhar et al. (10,11) devised a method of light microscopic autoradiography of neurotransmitter receptors in which biochemical binding experiments on the lightly fixed tissue slices were previously performed to decide the optimal conditions for autoradiography. According to Chan-Palay and Palay (4,5), tritiated muscimol is a suitable ligand for autoradiography of GABA receptors since it has a free amino group that enables the substance, when it is bound to receptor sites in tissue constituents, to be covalently bound by aldehyde fixation. Chan-Palay performed autoradiographic observations on the distribution of GABA receptors of the cerebellar cortex and the hippocampus (3,4), then applied $^3$H-muscimol by means of three ways and compared them. These were direct application to a slice of the brain, microinjection into the localized region of the brain, and intravenous injection to animals. We adopted a method principally based on Kuhar's technique. The differences in our methods from Kuhar's are first, that tissues are fixed for longer time (30 min) in order to obtain better preservation of tissue structure histologically; second, that the sections are coated with emulsion by dipping method; and third, that the sections are coated with carbon to prevent diffusion of a radiolabeled ligand from the tissue.

As the result of longer fixation, we were able to get better histological specimens although the slightly lower $K_D$ value was inevitable.

Furthermore, we performed electron microscopic autoradiography of neurotransmitters in which development method was critical. In general, resolution power of electron microscopic autoradiography is poor when compared with that of electron microscopic immunohistochemistry. To overcome this difficulty, phenidon developer has been utilized in recent years (8). We used EAA developer which developed silver grains that were much smaller than the grains of silver bromide of undeveloped emulsion. Furthermore, in EAA development the growing speed of silver grains during the development process is so slow that we can easily select the development time adequate for our purpose (9). On the other hand, EAA development may fail to make grains of silver bromide visible. Therefore, it is necessary to set development time in various ways between 5 and 9 min and find the optimum development time.

In our study, we observed GABA-receptor sites labeled with silver grains not only on the synaptic membranes but also on the plasma membranes of the dendrites and the axons not corresponding to synaptic sites. They were also noticed on the plasma membranes of the glia cells. In the substantia nigra, GABA-receptor sites were also abundantly observed autoradiographically and some of them were not on the synaptic regions. The physiological significance of these binding sites that were not related to syanpses was left for further investigations.

We observed numerous binding sites of $^3$H-DAMA autoradiographically in the amygdaloid nucleus on the plasma membranes of dendrites and nerve cell somas where not only met-enkephalin but also other neuropeptides such as substance P and somatostatin were immunohistochemically identified in nerve terminals as well as in nerve cell bodies (6,7). In addition, the presence of met-enkephalin receptor sites was confirmed on the plasma membranes of both dendrites and cytosomas in the caudate nucleus where met-enkephalin positive nerve terminals were believed to be richly contained.

There are still problems to be solved in the autoradiographical observation of neurotransmitter receptors. Nevertheless, this technique is very important in observing the morphological relationship between transmitters and their receptor sites: It is known that the distribution of GABA receptors indicated by $^3$H-muscimol binding differs from that indicated by $^3$H-GABA uptake and by GABA synthesizing and degradative sites.

## SUMMARY AND CONCLUSION

1. We performed light and electron microscopic autoradiography of GABA and opiate receptors using $^3$H-muscimol and $^3$H-DAMA.

2. Selection of development method is important for electron microscopic autoradiography. The authors obtained silver grains in a pattern precisely localized to the cytoplasmic membrane, i.e., the receptor site by means of EAA development.

3. We observed $^3$H-muscimol binding site in the neuropiles of the cerebellar molecular layer and the substantia nigra ultrastructurally. Receptor sites labeled with silver grains are located not only on the synaptic regions but also on the plasma membranes of the dendrites and axons not corresponding to synaptic sites. $^3$H-DAMA binding sites in the caudate nucleus and the amygdaloid nucleus are noticed on the plasma membranes of the axons, dendrites, and nerve cell somas, some corresponding to synapses, others not.

There are still problems to be solved in the autoradiographical observation of neurotransmitter receptors. Nevertheless, this technique is very important in observing the morphological relationship between transmitters and their receptor sites.

## ACKNOWLEDGMENT

This study was supported in part by a Grant-in-aid for Science Research 56440040 and 56770411 from the Ministry of Education, Japan.

## REFERENCES

1. Arimatsu, Y., Seto, A., and Amano, T. (1978): Localization of α-bungarotoxin binding sites in mouse brain by light and electron microscopic autoradiography. *Brain Res.*, 147:165–169.
2. Barnard, E. A. (1979): Visualization and counting of receptors at the light and electron microscopic levels. In: *The Receptors. A Comprehensive Treatise, Vol. 1*, edited by R. D. O'Brien, pp. 247–293. Plenum Press, New York.

3. Chan-Palay, V. (1978): Autoradiographic localization of γ-aminobutyric acid receptors in the rat central nervous system by using ³H-muscimol. *Proc. Natl. Acad. Sci. USA*, 75:1024–1028.
4. Chan-Palay, V. (1978): Quantitative visualization of γ-aminobutyric acid receptors in hippocampus and area dentata demonstrated by ³H-muscimol autoradiography. *Proc. Natl. Acad. Sci. USA*, 75:2516–2520.
5. Chan-Palay, V., and Palay, S. L. (1978): Ultrastructural localization of γ-aminobutyric acid receptors in the mammalian central nervous system by means of ³H-muscimol binding. *Proc. Natl. Acad. Sci. USA*, 75:2977–2980.
6. Kishida, T., Kito, S., Itoga, E., Yanaihara, N., Ogawa, N., and Sito, S. (1980): Immunohistochemical distribution of neuropeptides in the rat central nervous system. *Acta Histochem. Cytochem.*, 13:463–485.
7. Kishida, T., Kito, S., Itoga, E., Yanaihara, N., Ogawa, N., and Wakabayashi (1979): Immunohistochemical studies on the distribution of biologically active oligopeptides in the rat central nervous system. *Acta Histochem. Cytochem.*, 12:301–324.
8. Lettre, H., and Paweletz, N. (1966): Probleme der elektroenmicroskopischen Autoradiographie. *Nature*, 53:268.
9. Mizuhira, V., and Futaesaku, Y. (1976): Limits of resolution in electron microscope autoradiography. In: *Recent Progress in Electron Microscopy of Cells and Tissues*, edited by E. Yamada, V. Mizuhira, K. Kurosumi, and T. Nagami, p. 147. Igakushoin, Tokyo; University Park Press, Baltimore, London.
10. Palacios, M., Young, W. S., and Kuhar, M. J. (1980): Autoradiographic localization of γ-aminobutyric acid (GABA) receptors in the rat cerebellum. *Proc. Natl. Acad. Sci. USA*, 77:670–674.
11. Young, W. S., and Kuhar, M. J. (1980): A new method for receptor autoradiography: ³H-opioid receptors in rat brain. *Brain Res.*, 180.

Molecular Pharmacology of Neurotransmitter Receptors, edited by T. Segawa et al.
Raven Press, New York © 1983.

# Involvement of Sulfhydryl Groups in the Functional Integrity of the Opiate Receptors of Neuroblastoma × Glioma Hybrid NG108-15

Arthur J. Blume, D. Mullikin-Kilpatrick, and N. E. Larsen

*Department of Physiological Chemistry and Pharmacology, Roche Institute of Molecular Biology, Nutley, New Jersey 07110*

The involvement of sulfhydryl (SH) groups in the maintenance of the structure and function of many membrane bound receptors has been observed. Included among these are the acetylcholine (7), insulin (6), and β-adrenergic (11,18) receptors. The interaction of opiate ligands with their specific receptors in the brain has likewise been shown to be regulated by SH groups (13,17). As postulated at present, there is supposed to be an SH site closely associated with the ligand binding site on these opiate receptors (17). It is also possible that another SH group exists which is selectively involved in the formation of high affinity opiate agonist receptor complexes. This supposition arises from the observation that a wide variety of SH reagents can cause preferential losses in agonist ligand binding and increased sensitivity of agonist binding to regulation by monovalent cations (13,17).

Therefore, we felt that it would be worthwhile to examine the effects of SH-modifying reagents on ligand binding to the opiate receptors in the mouse neuroblastoma × rat glioma hybrid cell NG108-15 (8). These cells have a single population of stereospecific opiate receptors (8) which have high affinity for many of the opioid enkephalin peptides (1). In addition, it is known that agonist ligands, through these receptors, can regulate the activity of the cells' adenylate cyclase (16). The coupling of these receptors with the catalytic moiety of adenylate cyclase as well as ligand binding to these receptors has been shown to be regulated by guanine nucleotides and cations (2,3,10).

This chapter summarizes our recent studies using SH reagents to gain information concerning the mechanism by which opiates regulate adenylate cyclase. The cells used here, NG108-15, have been described along with their method of growth, harvest, and the preparation of intact cells and nuclei-free membranes (8,9). The

---

Present address of Dr. Larsen: Evans Building, Room 501, Hematology Research, 75 E. Newton Street, Boston, Massachusetts 02118.

methods used for determining the affinity and number of opiate binding sites using $^3$H-naloxone, $^3$H-naltrexone, $^3$H-etorphine, and $^3$H-Dala$^2$met$^5$enkephalinamide as well as the affinity of nonradiolabeled ligands based on their competition with $^3$H-naloxone have been as previously detailed (2,3,9,10). Treatment of membranes with thiol reagents was done as previously reported (9).

Incubating NG108-15 membrane preparations with either of the thiol reagents NEM or PCMB alters the binding of both $^3$H-opiate agonists and $^3$H-opiate antagonists (Fig. 1). The magnitude of the change observed with either reagent is clearly dependent upon the concentration of the compound used when the incubation period is fixed. Iodoacetamide, even at concentrations of up to 10 mM, does not produce any such observable alterations. Interestingly, the binding of the opioid peptide agonist $^3$H-Dala$^2$met$^5$enkephalinamide is more sensitive to NEM (i.e., exhibits a lower IC$_{50}$ value of NEM) than for $^3$H-naltrexone binding. This is not the case with PCMB, as under identical conditions PCMB affects equally the binding of $^3$H-agonist and $^3$H-antagonist. The differential effectiveness of NEM is also seen with membranes incubated with a fixed concentration of NEM for increasing periods of time (9). These experiments show a much faster loss in the binding of subsaturating concentrations of the agonist $^3$H-Dala$^2$met$^5$amide than either of the two classical opiate antagonists $^3$H-naltrexone and $^3$H-naloxone (see Fig. 3A and B). Furthermore, the binding of the stable enkephalin analog and the two antagonists disappears in a pseudo first-order manner. However, the rate constant is almost nine times slower for loss in $^3$H-antagonist binding than for the enkephalin. Upon similar treatment

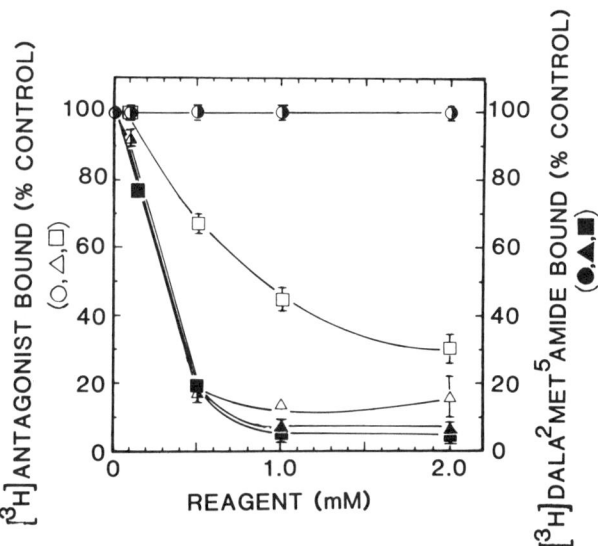

**FIG. 1.** Reactivity of NG108-15 opiate receptors with different SH reagents. NG108-15 membranes incubated with NEM *(squares)*, PCMB *(triangles)*, or iodoacetamide *(circles)* for 60 min at 32°C. The specific binding, assayed after termination of above reactions with DTT, was done using $^3$H-Dala$^2$met$^5$amide *(closed symbols)*, or $^3$H-naltrexone, or $^3$H-naloxone *(open symbols)*. (Data from ref. 12.)

with NEM the binding of another opiate agonist, etorphine, also decays in a pseudo first-order manner, which is also faster than that for naloxone. Based on these effects of NEM and PCMB, at least four different aspects of SH-group involvement in NG108-15 opiate receptor function become evident: (a) modification of an SH group(s) must either decrease the number or affinity of these binding sites, (b) since the decay in binding is pseudo first-order, only one SH may need be altered so as to change ligand binding, (c) as washing the membranes free of NEM does not reverse these alterations, the effects of NEM are considered irreversible and, (d) the binding of an opiate agonist is more sensitive than the binding of opiate antagonists to such NEM treatments.

An analysis of the resulting saturation binding isotherms after treatment with a fixed concentration of NEM for up to 80 min indicates that with increasing time of incubation with NEM, there is an increasingly larger loss in the number of binding sites for naloxone and/or naltrexone (Fig. 2). These effects of NEM on receptor number are also described by a single pseudo first-order rate constant. Furthermore, no loss in antagonist affinity is seen to accompany these NEM treatments! In fact, with NEM treatments of ~20 min, there appears to be an increase (up to 100%) in the affinity of naloxone (9). This increase in binding affinity for antagonists, post-NEM treatment, can readily account for the fact that the apparent decay rate for the binding of subsaturating concentrations of naloxone is slower ($t\frac{1}{2} \sim 50$ min) than is the rate of loss of antagonist binding sites ($t\frac{1}{2} \sim 30$ min).

Before NEM treatment, the number of opiate agonist and antagonist binding sites are equal (1,8,9). Furthermore, we have assumed that both agonist and antagonist can bind to the same receptors, but only one at a time as any opiate antagonist blocks totally all specific $^3$H-agonist binding and vice versa. Losses in antagonist sites, therefore, should be accompanied by identical losses in agonist binding sites. This appears to be the case for NG108-15 membranes treated with NEM (2 mM)

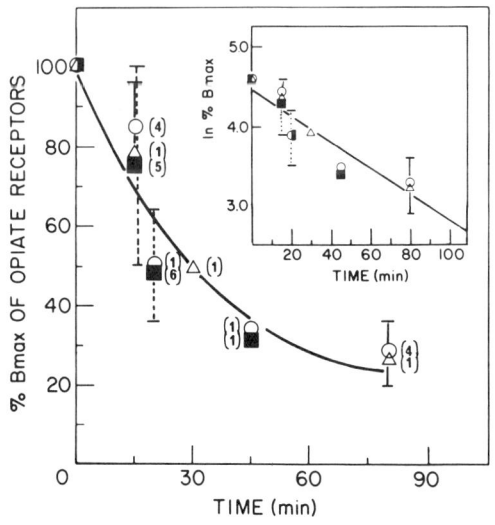

FIG. 2. Loss in receptor number produced by NEM. Membranes and appropriate controls reacted with 2 mM NEM for up to 80 min. Afterwards, the number of receptor sites/mg protein for $^3$H-naltrexone *(triangles)*, $^3$H-naloxone *(circles)*, and $^3$H-Dala$^2$met$^5$amide *(squares)* were determined. These values are given as a % of the receptors in controls. Number of experiments given in parentheses. (Data from refs. 9 and 12.)

for 20 min as the reduction in the number of binding sites is quantitatively the same whether judged by $^3$H-agonist or $^3$H-antagonist binding (9,12). From many such experiments conducted after different times of incubation with NEM, the number of sites for opiate agonists is observed to decrease in a pseudo first-order fashion, which is not significantly different from that seen for the antagonist binding sites. We concluded that (a) there is a single, essential SH group within the opiate receptor which, when modified by NEM (or presumably PCMB), prevents the binding of either agonist or antagonist ligands and, (b) that some other additional site must be responsible for the apparent increased sensitivity of Dala$^2$met$^5$amide binding to NEM inactivation.

As indicated above, the rate of loss in binding sites is not fast enough to account for the much more rapid loss ($t^{1/2} \sim 8$ min) in $^3$H-enkephalin binding observed with subsaturating concentrations of $^3$H-ligand. An explanation of this rapid loss is provided by a comparison of the actual binding isotherms for $^3$H-enkephalin to NG108-15 membranes before and after a short treatment (i.e., $\sim 20$ min) with 2 mM NEM. One finds that although the number of binding sites has been reduced somewhat (i.e., $\sim 30\%$), the affinity of $^3$H-Dala$^2$met$^5$amide to the surviving receptor sites has also gotten much poorer after such NEM treatment: before NEM, nM $K_D = 5.5 \pm 1.8$ ($N = 7$) whereas post-NEM, nM $K_D = 37.2 \pm 7.6$ ($N = 7$) (9). This effect of NEM on affinity is apparently irreversible, as washing away the free NEM does not return control agonist affinity. Therefore, a modification by NEM of another SH group, which is not the one described above as being at the ligand-binding domain of the receptor, produces a significant loss in affinity at the modified receptor. These losses in affinity for this enkephalin analog as well as other types of opiate agonists have been substantiated in experiments in which affinity is determined from competition by the nonradiolabeled ligand of $^3$H-naloxone binding (9). In these cases, a five- to sevenfold shift in $K_I$ for Dala$^2$met$^5$amide is found after these NEM treatments. Using this method, we find that NEM decreases the NG108-15 opiate receptor's affinity for (a) enkephalin peptides, (b) two purported "μ" receptor selective agonists, normorphine and dihydromorphine, (c) the "δ" selective agonist Dala$^2$D-leu-enkephalin and, (d) etorphine, an agonist which has high affinity at most known opiate receptors, but not for the antagonist naltrexone (Table 1). We, therefore, propose that there is a second SH group which is essential for the formation of the high-affinity agonist-opiate receptor complex observed in NG108-15. This group is not the one involved in the general ligand-binding domain of these opiate receptors.

In order to support the individuality of these two different SH groups postulated above, we investigated the ability of ligands to protect against the actions of NEM. In these experiments, protection against the action of NEM on the SH groups controlling the ligand binding site can be selectively monitored by determining the survival of binding of subsaturating concentrations of $^3$H-naloxone after removal of NEM and the "protecting" ligand. On the other hand, preferential alteration by NEM of agonist receptor affinities can be monitored by following the rapid losses in binding of subsaturating concentrations of $^3$H-Dala$^2$met$^5$amide also after removal

TABLE 1. *Summary of the selective loss in opiate agonist affinity induced by NEM treatment*

| | Apparent $K_D$ (nM) | | $K_D$ ratios Post-NEM |
|---|---|---|---|
| Opiate | Control | Post-NEM | Control |
| Naltrexone | 14.4 | 12.9 | 0.9 |
| Cyclazocine | 7.7 | 6.1 | 0.8 |
| Pentazocine | 176 | 339 | 1.9 |
| β-Endorphine | 26.5 | 39.7 | 1.5 |
| Dala$^2$D-leu$^5$enkephalin | 5.8 | 26.4 | 4.5 |
| Dala$^2$met$^5$amide | 10.9 | 75.3 | 6.9 |
| Etorphine | 3.4 | 7.5 | 2.2 |
| Dihydromorphine | 131 | 353 | 2.7 |
| Normorphine | 631 | 2,983 | 4.7 |

The affinity of various ligands for the opiate receptor as judged from their ability to compete for the specific binding of $^3$H-naloxone (6–8 nM) using 150–250 μg membrane protein/rx. The apparent $K_D$ were determined from the equation $K_D$ = IC$_{50}$ ÷ (1 + conc. $^3$H-naloxone/$K_D$ $^3$H-naloxone). The $K_D$ of $^3$H-naloxone in control and NEM-treated membranes was taken as 40 and 20 nM, respectively. Data from ref. 9.

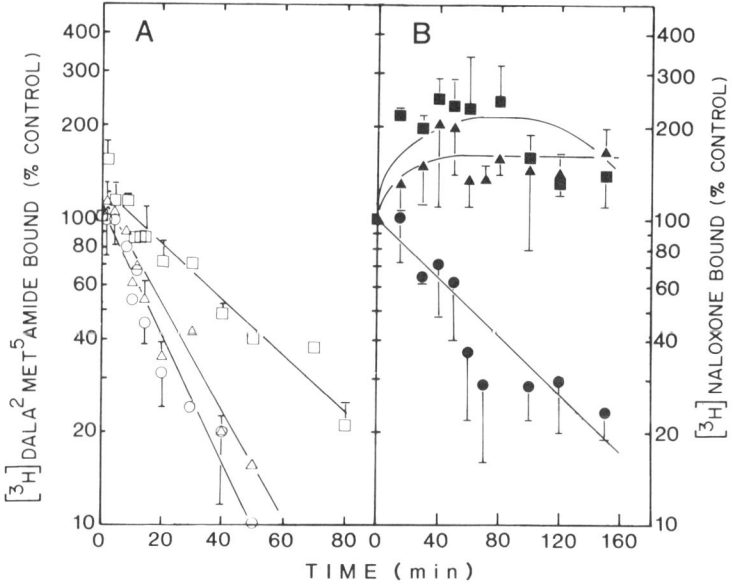

**FIG. 3.** Protection by ligands of losses in $^3$H-ligand binding induced by NEM. Membranes incubated at 32°C without *(circles)* or with 50 nM Dala$^2$met$^5$amide *(squares)* or with 150 nM naltrexone *(triangles)* and 2 mM NEM; the reactions were stopped with DTT, and the membranes then washed. The specific binding assayed subsequently with $^3$H-naloxone *(closed symbols)* or $^3$H-Dala$^2$met$^5$amide *(open symbols)*. (Data from ref. 12.)

of NEM and the "protecting" ligand(s). The results (Fig. 3) indicate that naltrexone or Dala$^2$met$^5$amide (at ~10 times their $K_D$ values) provide excellent protection against the loss of $^3$H-naloxone binding for periods up to 80 min. As proposed above, losses in subsaturating $^3$H-antagonist binding should reflect losses in numbers of binding sites. Protection against such losses, therefore, should be indicative of protection in the number of sites surviving the NEM treatment. This is actually what is observed when the binding isotherm for $^3$H-naloxone is investigated in membranes which have been incubated with naltrexone or Dala$^2$met$^5$amide during their NEM treatments (Fig. 4). It appears that the occupation of the ligand's binding site by either an opiate agonist or antagonist provides significant protection of the general ligand binding sites from interaction with NEM.

However, the degree of protection afforded by opiate agonists and antagonists of $^3$H-enkephalin binding from NEM inactivation is very different. Judged from losses in $^3$H-Dala$^2$met$^5$amide binding (using subsaturating concentrations of $^3$H-ligand) (see Fig. 3), the presence of naltrexone (at 10 times its $K_D$ value) affords little, if any, protection. Although the $t^{1/2}$ of the loss of $^3$H-Dala$^2$met$^5$amide binding increases by about 50%, the variability is too large to allow any significance to be given to this change. The presence of Dala$^2$met$^5$amide (also at 10 times its $K_D$ value) affords significant protection against losses in $^3$H-enkephalin binding an almost sixfold reduction in the decay rate being noted. This is still, however, less protection than seen for $^3$H-antagonist binding. In a separate series of experiments, we assessed the ability of other opiates and opiate antagonists to provide protection against losses in binding of subsaturating concentrations of $^3$H-enkephalin that occur during a 20-min treatment with 2 mM NEM. The results (12) indicate that some protection can be provided by many different ligands when tested at 10 times their $K_D$ values. Included among these is the larger endogenous peptide, β-endorphin, as well as two nonpeptide opiates, normorphine and etorphine. In addition, some

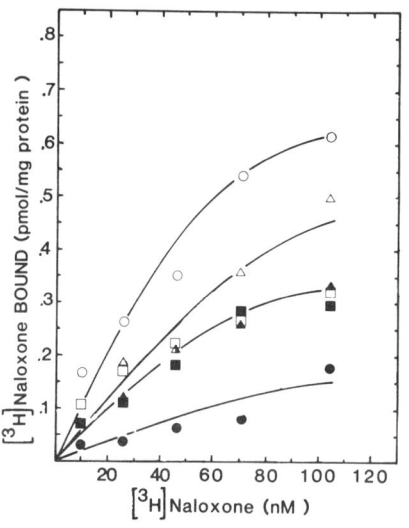

FIG. 4. $^3$H-Antagonist binding to membranes treated with NEM with or without "protecting" ligands. Membranes incubated at 32°C with 2 mM NEM for 80 min alone (closed circles), with 50 nM Dala$^2$met$^5$amide (closed squares), or 8,000 nM naltrexone (closed triangles); non-NEM treated control membranes (open symbols). $^3$H-Naloxone binding assessed after washing. The receptor $B_{max}$ (fmol/mg protein) in control plus nothing (877), plus amide (370), plus naltrexone (575); $B_{max}$ post-NEM plus nothing (117), plus amide (457), and plus naltrexone (417). (Data taken from ref. 12.)

protection is provided by ligands having mixed agonist-antagonist activities such as cyclazocine and pentazocine and even the pure antagonist naloxone (when tested at 20 times its $K_D$ value). In no case, however, was the protection complete.

When the binding isotherm for the $^3$H-enkephalinamide was investigated after NEM treatments carried out in the presence of "protecting" ligands, we found variable results, but always that (a) the inclusion of protecting ligands leads to increases in the number of surviving binding sites, and (b) whereas antagonists never protect against the loss in agonist affinity, agonists sometimes partially protect and sometimes they do not. The reason for the degree of variability found in these results is not yet fully evident and, at the present time, we do not have any statistically significant evidence for agonist protection against the NEM inactivation of high-affinity opiate agonist form of binding.

Nevertheless, we remained interested in the loss in high-affinity agonist binding. We had demonstrated previously that both monovalent cations and guanine nucleotides can regulate the opiate receptors in NG108-15 (1). Both of these regulators act to decrease the binding of opiate agonists and no inhibitory action of monovalent cations could be detected on opiate antagonist binding. The question arose as to what happens to cation and nucleotide regulation after receptor modification by NEM. For some β-adrenergic receptors, NEM modification prevents its normal association with a coupling factor (termed G/F or N) and without this association, nucleotides do not decrease agonist binding and there is also a loss in the high-affinity form of β-agonist binding (5,11,18). Our studies (9,12) on the ability of Dala$^2$met$^5$amide to compete for $^3$H-naltrexone binding as well as the ability of $^3$H-enkephalinamide to bind to membranes treated for $\sim$20 min with 2 mM NEM showed the following: (a) that Na$^+$ is still capable of selectively decreasing agonist affinity up to 100-fold, (b) the effects of Na$^+$ are still dose-dependent and exhibit an IC$_{50}$ value of 7 mM, (c) the rank order of potency of cations to produce such effects is Na$^+$ ≥ Li$^+$ >> K$^+$ ≥ choline$^+$, and (d) guanosine triphosphate (GTP) no longer has any significant effect on $^3$H-enkephalinamide affinity (Fig. 5).

When contrasted to the picture of regulation in control membranes, these facts indicate that the NEM-induced loss in high opiate-agonist affinity binding is accompanied by a loss in sensitivity to guanine nucleotides and an increase in sensitivity to monovalent cations. Control membranes are effected by monovalent cations, with the same rank order, but Na$^+$ has an IC$_{50}$ value of $\sim$100 mM (9)!

Since Na$^+$ and GTP normally play key roles in NG108-15 opiate receptor function (1,2,9,10), we also tested if either regulator could act as a protector against either of the two different actions of NEM. In these experiments, Na$^+$ was used at 400 mM and GTP at 200 μM and, after the incubations, the membranes were washed free of these agents (12). With regard to protection against losses in the binding of subsaturating concentrations of $^3$H-naloxone, GTP offers no protection, whereas NaCl provides almost complete protection. Furthermore, a definite order is found in the ability of various monovalent cations to protect $^3$H-opiate antagonist binding (i.e., Na$^+$ ≥ Li$^+$ >> K$^+$ ≥ choline$^+$). This is the same order of potency observed for cation modulation of opiate agonist binding to control as well as to NEM-treated

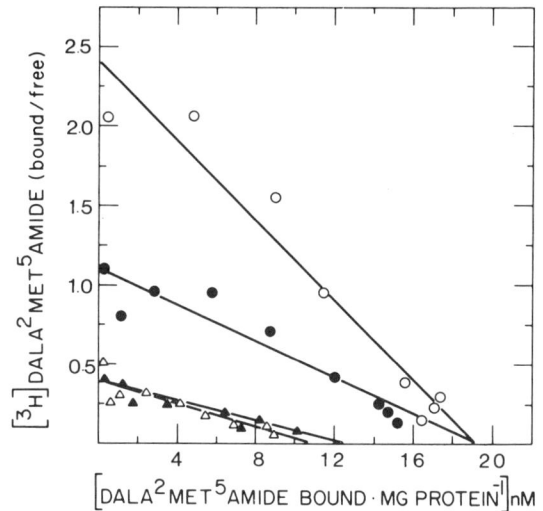

**FIG. 5.** Effects of NEM on $^3$H-Dala$^2$met$^5$amide binding. Membranes treated with 2 mM NEM at 32°C for 15 min *(triangles)*, control membranes *(circles)*. Specific $^3$H-enkephalinamide binding tested over the range 0.3–115 nM in buffer alone *(open symbols)* or plus 200 µM GTP *(closed symbols)*. (Data from ref. 9.)

NG108-15 membranes. With regard to protecting the binding of subsaturating concentrations of $^3$H-enkephalinamide from NEM action, we find that GTP again offers no protection (if anything, sensitivity to NEM may be slightly increased). In addition, NaCl now has only a minimal protecting effect (i.e., the rate of loss in $^3$H-agonist binding being decreased by ~50%). A lack of protection by Na$^+$ of the high-affinity form of agonist binding was confirmed in separate experiments on the binding isotherm for $^3$H-enkephalinamide and the ability of nonradioactive enkephalinamide to compete for $^3$H-naloxone binding after NEM treatment (12).

In summary, our results are consistent with the following model of the opiate receptors in these NG108-15 cells. An NEM sensitive site exists (probably an SH group) that is closely associated with the opiate receptor's ligand-binding domain. This site is essential for both opiate agonist and antagonist binding; its modification by NEM (or PCMB) results in a total inability to bind ligands. There is one such site per opiate ligand-binding site as evidenced by the pseudo first-order decay in binding sites observed during these NEM treatments. Binding of opiate agonists and antagonists protects this site from NEM, most simply, by covering the sensitive SH group. The known action of monovalent cations to decrease agonist affinity appears to correlate with its modification of the receptors, which makes this SH group less accessible to NEM alkylation. Since Na$^+$ can alter the dissociation rates of $^3$H-opiate agonists from these NG108-15 receptors (1), its effect on the ligand binding site is considered allosteric. Our findings on monovalent cation protection of opiate binding sites from NEM inactivation is consistent with such an allosteric effect of cations. An absolutely conclusive location of the actual site of action of Na$^+$ would require more information.

Second, there exists another NEM sensitive site (probably an SH group) which is uniquely involved in the formation of high-affinity agonist-receptor complexes. Furthermore, it is this complex which is the site of action of guanine nucleotides responsible for regulating opiate binding. Modification of this SH group by NEM prevents formation of such a complex thereby eliminating nucleotide effects without changing the number of opiate binding sites. This SH group is apparently not involved in opiate antagonist binding nor required for the formation of an "$Na^+$-sensitive" state of ligand binding and can be considered to be distal to the receptor's general ligand-binding domain. This high-affinity form of binding is most likely required for regulation of adenylate cyclase. Protection of this site from NEM action is not afforded by $Na^+$ or guanine nucleotides or opiate antagonists (at least under our present conditions of treatment). We have no evidence at the present time that opiate agonists protect at this site. A priori, this SH group could be located on the receptor or on some independent membrane component such as the guanine nucleotide regulatory unit, which binds nucleotides and is known to modulate many receptor-mediated regulations of adenylate cyclase activity (4,14,15).

## REFERENCES

1. Blume, A. J. (1978): Opiate binding to membrane preparations of neuroblastoma × glioma hybrid cells NG108-15: Effects of ions and nucleotides. *Life Sci.*, 22:1843–1852.
2. Blume, A. J.: Opiate receptor mediated regulation of the activity of adenylate cyclase in the mouse neuroblastoma × rat glioma hybrid cell NG108-15. In: *Psychopharmacology and Biochemistry of Neurotransmitter Receptors*, edited by H. I. Yamamura, R. W. Olsen, and E. Usdin., Elsevier/North-Holland, New York.
3. Blume, A. J., Boone, G., and Lichshtein, D. (1979): Regulation of the neuroblastoma × glioma hybird opiate receptors by $Na^+$ and guanine nucleotides. In: *Modulators, Mediators and Specifiers in Brain Function*, edited by Y. H. Ehrlich, J. Volavka, L. G. Davis, and E. G. Brunngraber, pp. 163–174. Plenum Press, New York.
4. Citri, Y., and Schramm. M. (1980): Resolution, reconstitution, and kinetics of the primary action of a hormone receptor. *Nature*, 287:297–300.
5. DeLean, A., Stadel, J. M., and Lefkowitz, R. J. (1980): A ternary complex model explains the agonist-specific binding properties of the adenylate cyclase-coupled β-adrenergic receptor. *J. Biol. Chem.*, 255:7108–7117.
6. Jacob, S., Hazum, E., and Cuatrecasas, P. (1980). The subunit structure of rat liver insulin receptor. *J. Biol. Chem.*, 255:6937–6940.
7. Karlin, A., and Bartels, E. (1966): Effects of blocking sulfhydryl groups and of reducing disulfide bonds on the acetylcholine-activated permeability system of electroplax. *Biochim. Biophys. Acta*, 120:525–535.
8. Klee, W. A., and Nirenberg, M. (1974): A neuroblastoma × glioma hybrid cell line with morphine receptors. *Proc. Natl. Acad. Sci. USA*, 71:3474–3477.
9. Larsen, N. E., Mullikin-Kilpatrick, D., and Blume, A. J. (1981): Two different modifications of the neuroblastoma × glioma hybrid opiate receptors induced by N-ethylmaliemide. *Mol. Pharmacol.*, 20:255–262.
10. Lichshtein, D., Boone, G., and Blume, A. J. (1979): A physiological requirement of $Na^+$ for the regulation of cAMP levels in intact NG108-15 cells. *Life Sci.*, 25:985–992.
11. Mukherjee, C., and Lefkowitz, R. J. (1977): Regulation of β-adrenergic receptors in isolated frog erythrocytes plasma membranes. *Mol. Pharmacol.*, 13;291–303.
12. Mullikin-Kilpatrick, D., Larsen, N. E., and Blume, A. J. (1983): Protection of the opiate receptors in NG108-15 against modification by N-ethylmaliemide. *J. Neurosci. (in press)*.
13. Pasternak, G. W., Wilson, A., and Snyder, S. H. (1975): Differential effects of protein modifying reagents on receptor binding of opiate agonists and antagonists. *Mol. Pharmacol.*, 11:340–351.

14. Ross, E. M., and Gilman, A. G. (1977): Resolution of some components of adenylate cyclase necessary for catalytic activity. *J. Biol. Chem.*, 252:6966–6969.
15. Ross, E. M., Haga, T., Howlett, A. C., Schwarzmeir, J., Schleifer, L. S., and Gilman, A. G. (1978): Hormone-sensitive adenylate cyclase: Resolution and reconstitution of some components necessary for regulation of the enzyme. *Adv. Cyclic Nucleotide Res.*, 9:56–67.
16. Sharma, S. K., Nirenberg, M., and Klee, W. A. (1975): Morphine receptors as regulators of adenylate cyclase activity. *Proc. Natl. Acad. Sci. USA* 72:590–594.
17. Simon, E. J., and Groth, J. (1975): Kinetics of opiate receptor inactivation by sulfhydryl reagents: Evidence for conformational change in the presence of $Na^+$. *Proc. Natl. Acad. Sci. USA* 72:2404–2407.
18. Stadel, J. M., and Lefkowitz, R. J. (1979): Multiple reactive sulfhydryl groups modulate the function of adenylate cyclase coupled beta-adrenergic receptors. *Mol. Pharmacol.*, 16:709–718.

ated by T. Segawa et al.

# Structural Modifications of the Ergopeptine Molecule and Their Differential Influence on the Affinities to Different Receptor Binding Sites—A Structure Affinity Analysis

A. Closse, G. Bolliger, A. Dravid, W. Frick, D. Hauser,
P. Pfäffli, A. Sauter, and H. J. Tobler

*Preclinical Research, SANDOZ Ltd., CH 4002 Basle, Switzerland*

Ergot alkaloids are pharmacologically multipotent substances that show affinities to several neurotransmitter receptor systems in the mammalian central nervous system (2,6,7,11–13,26,32). Their $IC_{50}$ values for eight different binding sites were determined and their affinity profiles established. In this chapter it will be shown that structural modifications of ergopeptines change their affinities to the different binding sites differentially. From these results some conclusions concerning the properties of the different receptors will be drawn. Figure 1 shows the ligands used and their specificity. The methods used were those of refs. 3,6,9,21,29–31.

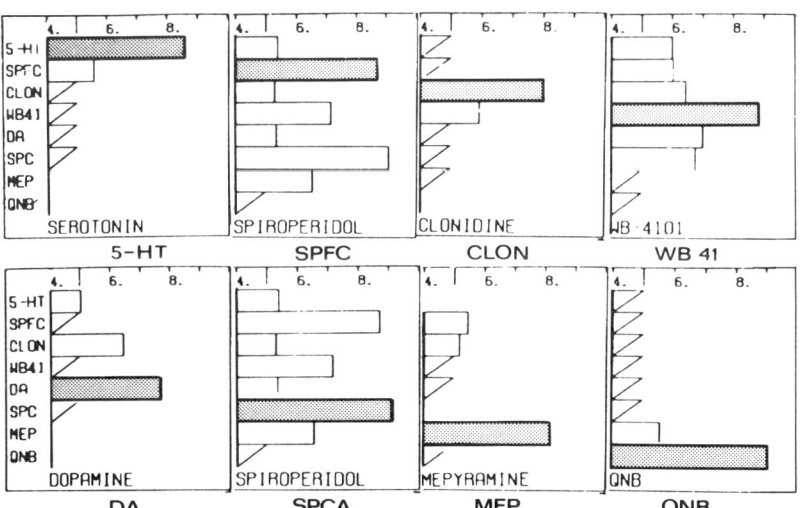

FIG. 1. Affinity profiles of the ligands used. The length of the bars is proportional to the negative logarithm of the corresponding $IC_{50}$ value ($pIC_{50}$) and therefore to the affinity. $IC_{50}$ values are means of 2 to 4 independent determinations (SEM ≤ 25%). SPFC = spiroperidol in frontal cortex (5-HT$_2$ receptors), SPC = spiroperidol in caudate (dopamine receptors.)

Dihydro-α-ergocryptine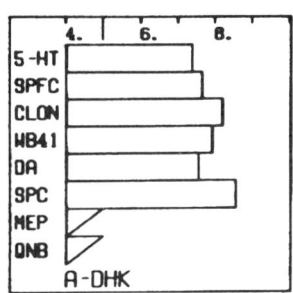

Affinity profile (pJC$_{50}$)

IC$_{50}$ (nM)

| 5-HT | SPFC | CLON | WB | DA | SPC | MEP | QNB |
|------|------|------|-----|-----|-----|--------|--------|
| 40 | 21 | 11 | 5,8 | 26 | 2,5 | >10000 | >10000 |

**FIG. 2.** Affinity profile of dihydro-α-ergocryptine. (Abbreviations as in Fig. 1.)

The commercially available ligand dihydro-α-ergocryptine consisting of a peptide moiety linked by an amide bond to the lysergic acid molecule is shown in Fig. 2. Dihydro-α-ergocryptine has high affinity to the binding sites of serotonin, spiroperidol, clonidine, WB 4101, and dopamine and no affinity to the muscarinic-cholinergic or the histamine H$_1$ receptor.

Common structures of neurotransmitters superimposed on the ergot structure are shown in Fig. 3 (2,4). It was proposed by Nichols (19) and by Bach et al. (1) that the five-membered ring in the ergot molecule should correspond to the aromatic ring of dopamine. The main argument in favor of this theory is that if the phenyl ring A of the ergot molecule would correspond to the phenyl ring of dopamine, the conformation of the dopamine skeleton within the ergot molecule (C$_5$) would be opposite to the conformation within the apomorphine molecule (C$_{6a}$), whereas the proposed structure 2b (Fig. 4) would correspond to the rigid dopamine structure in apomorphine. Whether the same would apply to the rigid conformation of noradrenaline, we do not know.

To obtain information about the influence of minor modifications of the ergot molecule upon the affinities to different receptors we evaluated the results of our binding studies by a simple SAR analysis (SAR = Structure Activity Relationship). For the simple SAR analysis the IC$_{50}$ values under consideration were divided to give a factor by which the affinity to a given receptor was augmented or diminished. For example, if the hydrogen in position 1 is substituted by a rather voluminous group, like pivaloyloxymethyl, which does not lead to delocalization of the free electron pair at the nitrogen atom, the affinities to serotonin and clonidine binding sites are much less influenced than those to WB and the spiroperidol sites (Fig. 5). A factor of 3 or 0.3 should be well off the limit of error.

Serotonin

Dopamine
and Noradrenalin

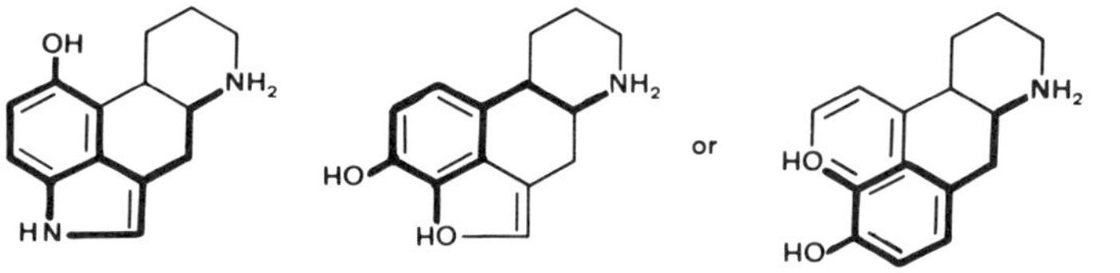

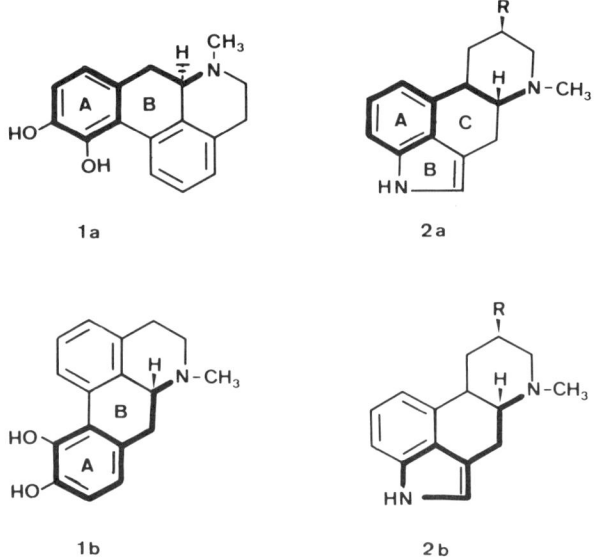

**FIG. 3.** Common structures of ergot alkaloids and neurotransmitters.

1a

2a

1b

2b

**FIG. 4.** Different possibilities of superimposing dopamine over ergot and apomorphine structures.

If the substituent at position 1 is not only voluminous but leads also to a delocalization of the electron pair at the nitrogen, for example $R_1$ = t-BOC, then all affinities are greatly diminished (Fig. 6).

Therefore we conclude that, for affinities to all binding sites an electron-rich aromatic system, at a certain distance from the basic nitrogen in position 6, is needed, whereas for binding to the serotonin and the clonidine binding site, the hydrogen position 1 is not obligatory; besides there seems to be enough space in this area to accommodate quite a voluminous residue, which does not seem to be available for the binding sites of spiroperidol and WB 4101. The affinity to the dopamine binding sites also seems to be influenced by this substitution, but clearly less so than the affinity to the spiroperidol-caudate binding site.

If the electron configuration of the pyrrol ring is disturbed by 2,3-dihydrogenation, the nitrogen in position 1 becomes basic. As a consequence, the affinities are

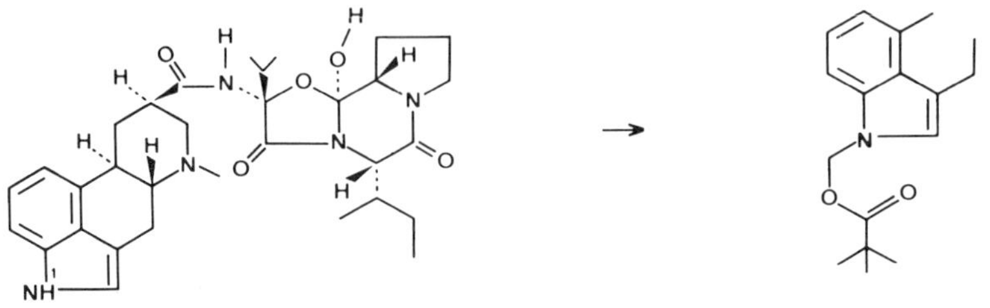

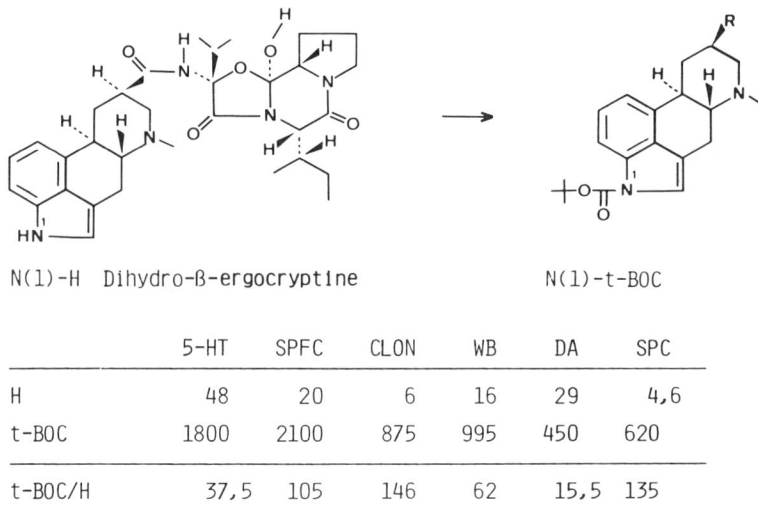

N(1)-H  Dihydro-β-ergocryptine                                N(1)-POM

|        | 5-HT | SPFC | CLON | WB  | DA  | SPC |
|--------|------|------|------|-----|-----|-----|
| H      | 48   | 20   | 6    | 16  | 29  | 4,6 |
| POM    | 130  | 185  | 17   | 405 | 125 | 125 |
| POM/H  | 2,7  | 9,3  | 2,8  | 25  | 4,3 | 27  |

**FIG. 5.** $IC_{50}$ values (nM) of dihydro-β-ergocryptine and its 1-pivaloyloxymethyl derivative and the factors by which the affinities of dihydro-β-ergocryptine are diminished after substitution of the hydrogen in position 1 by pivaloyloxymethyl (POM). (Abbreviations as in Fig. 1.)

N(1)-H  Dihydro-β-ergocryptine                                N(1)-t-BOC

|         | 5-HT | SPFC | CLON | WB  | DA   | SPC |
|---------|------|------|------|-----|------|-----|
| H       | 48   | 20   | 6    | 16  | 29   | 4,6 |
| t-BOC   | 1800 | 2100 | 875  | 995 | 450  | 620 |
| t-BOC/H | 37,5 | 105  | 146  | 62  | 15,5 | 135 |

**FIG. 6.** $IC_{50}$ values (nM) of dihydro-β-ergocryptine and 1-t-BOC derivative and factors showing the change in affinities after this substitution. (Abbreviations as in Fig. 1.)

diminished. Again, the affinity to the serotonin binding site is least affected. Here one can also distinguish quite well serotonin-1 from serotonin-2 receptor sites (Fig. 7).

Not only the lysergic acid part but also the peptide moiety contributes to the affinites of the ergopeptines: If the carbonyl group in position 6' is reduced, there is a loss of affinity to all receptors with the least effect on the dopamine binding

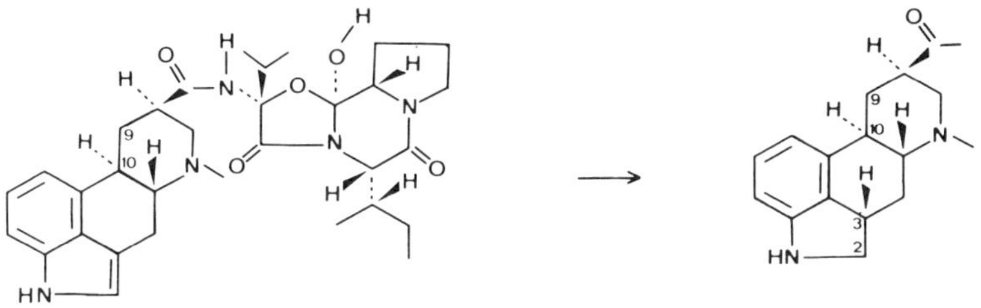

|            | 5-HT | SPFC | CLON | WB  | DA  | SPC |
|------------|------|------|------|-----|-----|-----|
| Dihydro    | 48   | 20   | 6    | 16  | 29  | 4,6 |
| Tetrahydro | 135  | 240  | 64   | 68  | 430 | 90  |
| Tetra/Di   | 2,9  | 12   | 11   | 4,3 | 15  | 20  |

**FIG. 7.** IC$_{50}$ values (nM) of 9,10-dihydro-β-ergocryptine and 2,3,9,10-tetrahydro-β-ergocryptine and factors showing affinity changes after hydrogenation. (Abbreviations as in Fig. 1.)

site (Fig. 8). Either the carbonyl group in position 6' may serve as a hydrogen acceptor from an accessory binding site or the basic pyramidal nitrogen of the reduced form may exert a repulsive effect.

If carbonyl group is introduced in position 8' of the reduced molecule, all affinities except one are restored (Fig. 9). Only in the case of the spiroperidol-caudate binding site is the affinity of the C8'-carbonyl compound about five times lower than that of the C6'-carbonyl compound. Therefore we suggest an acceptor function for the carbonyl group rather than the "basic nitrogen repulsion" theory, at least in the case of the spiroperidol-caudate binding site (Fig. 10). The dopamine binding site, on the contrary, seems to be much less influenced by the manipulations at 6' and 8' positions (Fig. 9).

The angle between the lysergic acid moiety and the peptide group, when the compound is bound to the receptors or to the accessory binding sites, is not known. It is clear, however, that the peptide part has to have a certain distance from the lysergic acid part: If a CH$_2$-group is inserted between the ergoline system and the C$_8'$ carbonyl group, and thus the distance between the two parts is increased, the affinities to all binding sites are significantly reduced (Fig. 11).

The configuration at position 8 of the lysergic acid moiety seems also to play an important role (Fig. 12): Of both naturally occurring ergot compounds, α-ergocryptin with the β-configuration at C8 is a much more active compound than the epimeric α-ergocryptinin.

There is also some evidence that the relative positions of the two parts of the ergopeptine molecule might not be the same for all the receptor sites. For example, the affinity to both serotonin receptors is higher if there is a methyl group in position 2' instead of an isopropyl group. For the spiroperidol binding site in the caudate the opposite is the case (Fig. 13). The bigger isopropyl group allows unhindered

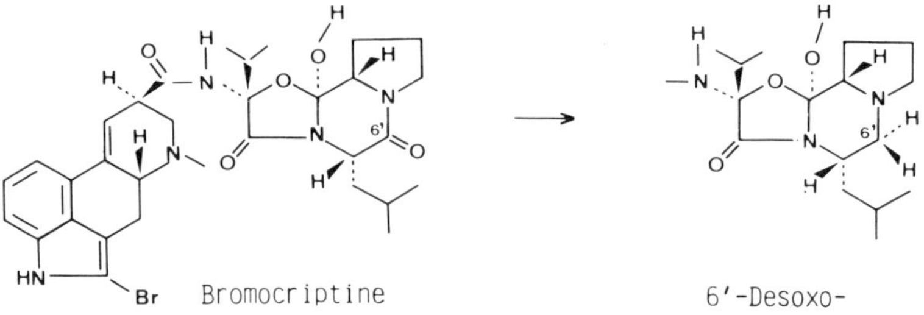

|              | 5-HT | SPFC | CLON | WB  | DA  | SPC |
|--------------|------|------|------|-----|-----|-----|
| Bromocriptine | 225  | 76   | 29   | 33  | 84  | 13  |
| 6'-Desoxo b.  | 1250 | 545  | 560  | 490 | 220 | 340 |
| 6'-Desoxo/Bromo | 5,6 | 7,2 | 19   | 15  | 2,6 | 26  |

**FIG. 8.** IC$_{50}$ values (nM) of bromocriptine and 6'-desoxobromocriptine and factors referring to affinity changes after reduction. (Abbreviations as in Fig. 1.)

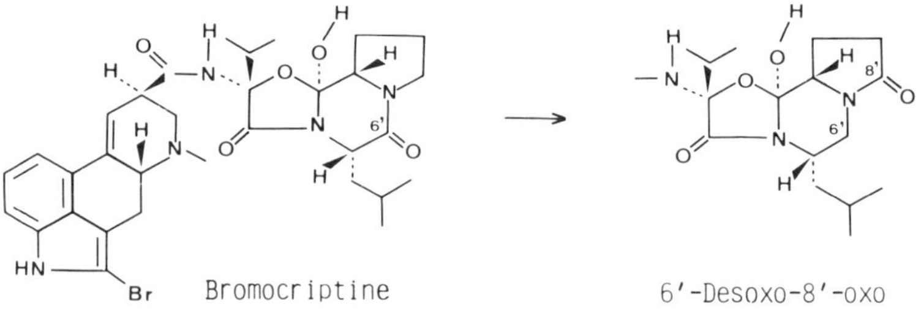

|                | 5-HT | SPFC | CLON | WB  | DA  | SPC |
|----------------|------|------|------|-----|-----|-----|
| Bromocriptine  | 225  | 76   | 29   | 33  | 84  | 13  |
| 6'-Desoxo-8'-Oxo | 360 | 180  | 16   | 70  | 54  | 65  |
| 8'-Oxo/6'-Oxo  | 1,6  | 2,4  | 0,55 | 2,1 | 0,64 | 5  |

**FIG. 9.** IC$_{50}$ values (nM) of bromocriptine, 6'-desoxo-, and 6'-desoxo-8'-oxobromocriptine and factors comparing the affinities of bromocriptine and 6'-desoxo-8'-oxobromocriptine. (Abbreviations defined in Fig.1.)

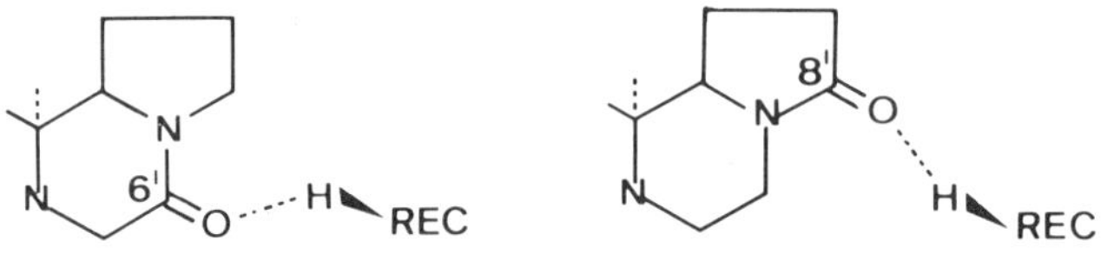

**FIG. 10.** Possible mode of attachment of the peptide moiety to the binding sites.

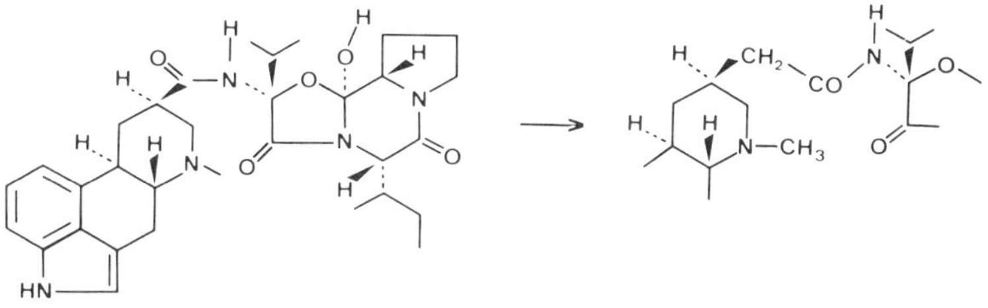

Dihydro-β-ergocryptine → 8-Homo-

|  | 5-HT | SPFC | CLON | WB | DA | SPC |
|---|---|---|---|---|---|---|
| Dihydro-β-ergocryptine | 48 | 20 | 6 | 16 | 29 | 4,6 |
| 8-Homo-... | 3900 | 1550 | 2000 | 365 | 610 | 430 |
| 8-Homo/Dihydro-β | 82 | 77 | 333 | 23 | 21 | 93 |

**FIG. 11.** $IC_{50}$ values (nM) of dihydro-β-ergocryptine and 8-homodihydro-β-ergocryptine and factors showing the affinity changes. (Abbreviations as in Fig. 1.)

α-Ergocryptine         α-Ergocryptinin

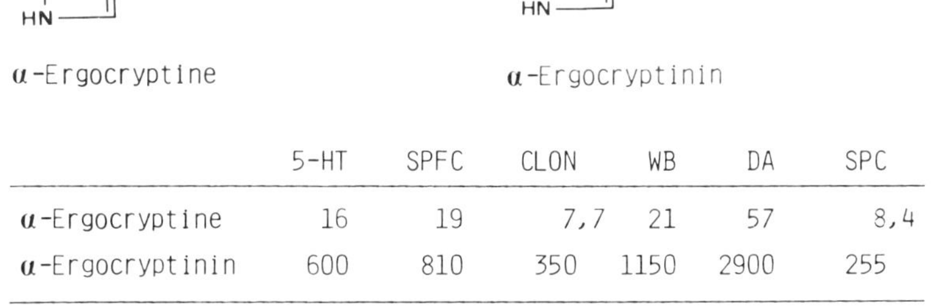

|  | 5-HT | SPFC | CLON | WB | DA | SPC |
|---|---|---|---|---|---|---|
| α-Ergocryptine | 16 | 19 | 7,7 | 21 | 57 | 8,4 |
| α-Ergocryptinin | 600 | 810 | 350 | 1150 | 2900 | 255 |
| "in"/"inin" | 37,5 | 43 | 45,5 | 55 | 51 | 30 |

**FIG. 12.** $IC_{50}$ values of α-ergocryptine and factors showing the affinity changes. (Abbreviations as in Fig. 1.)

rotation only around the bond between C8 and the carbonyl group. With a methyl group in position 2', peptide and lysergic acid moiety have additional rotational freedom around the bond between nitrogen and C2'. For the serotonin binding site the isopropyl group also might be too large for a perfect fit.

In conclusion, it can be said that, by minor structural modifications, one can change the affinity of the ergopeptine molecule to the serotonergic, α-adrenergic, or the dopaminergic receptors differentially. Furthermore, a differentiation between serotonin-1 and serotonin-2 receptors, $\alpha_1$ and $\alpha_2$ receptors, and between dopamine and spiroperidol binding sites can also be seen. This is not astonishing for the α-adrenergic system, since $\alpha_1$ and $\alpha_2$ receptors have been shown to be different and differently localized (15). The same might apply for serotonin-1 and serotonin-2 receptors (22).

For the dopaminergic system the situation is still controversial (8,10,20,24,25,27). In our studies most of the ergopeptines under investigation show normal displacement curves with Hill coefficients close to unity. As can be seen in Fig. 14 the ergot molecule can accommodate not only the natural transmitter structure but also part of the spiroperidol molecule. However, dopamine and spiroperidol displace each other from their respective binding sites with shallow displacement curves and Hill coefficients well below unity. Based on the observed displacement profiles the differential effects of ergot derivatives on spiroperidol and dopamine binding sites seem more likely due to the structural modifications (Fig. 15) rather than to changes in the lipophilicity (18,23) of ergot alkaloids since these compounds, in general, are known to be highly lipophilic.

These findings are in accordance with the concept of separate binding sites (5,10,14,16) for spiroperidol and dopamine. On the other hand, if spiroperidol and

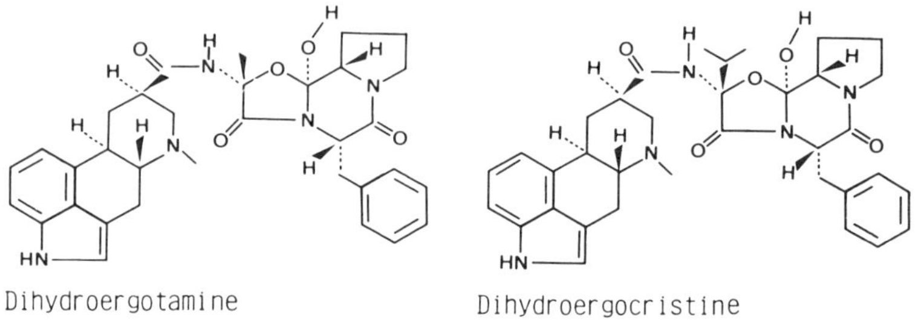

|  | 5-HT | SPFC | CLON | WB | DA | SPC |
|---|---|---|---|---|---|---|
| 2'-Methyl | 8 | 13,5 | 5,2 | 15 | 33 | 8,9 |
| 2'-Isopropyl | 35 | 27 | 8 | 12 | 55 | 3 |
| 2'-Methyl/ 2'-Isopropyl | 0,2 | 0,5 | 0,65 | 1,25 | 0,6 | 3 |

**FIG. 13.** $IC_{50}$ values (nM) of dihydroergotamine and dihydroergocristine and factors showing affinity differences between the two molecules. (Abbreviations as in Fig. 1.)

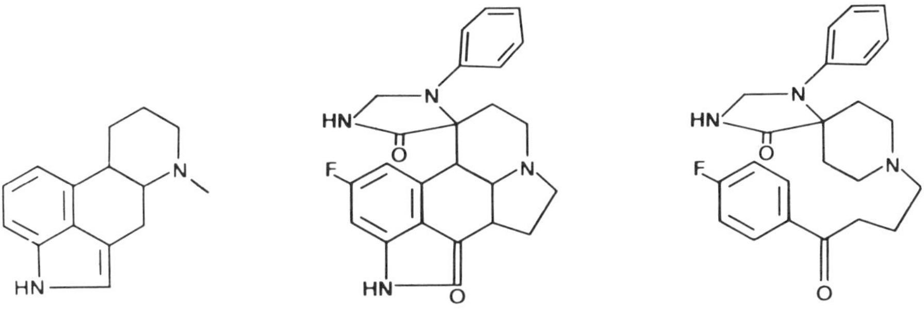

FIG. 14. Common structural conformation of ergot compounds and spiroperidol.

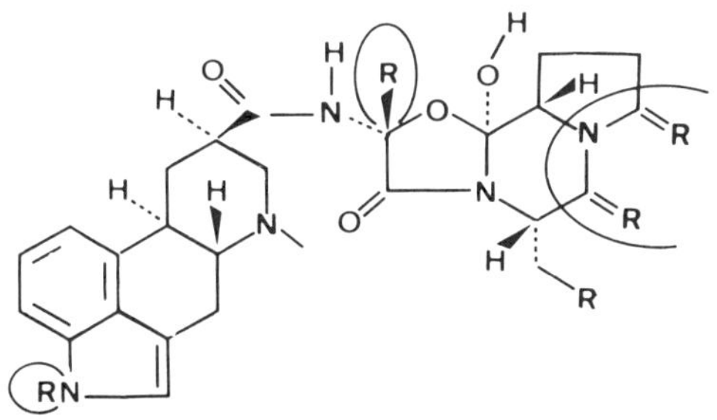

FIG. 15. Sites where structural variations influence the affinities to the binding sites of spiroperidol and dopamine different.

dopamine are considered to bind to the same site, some specific features of the receptor, like subunit (17) or accessory binding sites, will have to be postulated to account for the observed differences.

## ACKNOWLEDGMENTS

The skilled technical assistance of Mrs. E. Hehle, Th. Hotz, Mr. J. Jermann, D. Langenegger, M. Petignat, A. Wanner, Miss B. Wimmer, and Mr. C. Zwingelstein is gratefully acknowledged.

## REFERENCES

1. Bach, N. J., Kornfeld, E. C., Jones, N. D., Chaney, M. O., Dorman, D. E., Paschal, J. W., Clemens, J. A., and Smalstig, E. B. (1980): Bicyclic and tricyclic ergoline partial structures. Rigid 3-(2-aminoethyl)pyrroles and 3- and 4-(2-aminomethyl)pyrazoles as dopamine agonists. *J. Med. Chem.*, 23:481–491.
2. Berde, B., and Schild, H. O., editors (1978): *Ergot Alkaloids and Related Compounds*. Springer-Verlag, Berlin.
3. Burt, D. R., Creese, I., and Snyder, S. H. (1976): Properties of [$^3$H]haloperidol and [$^3$H]dopamine binding associated with dopamine receptors in calf brain membranes. *Mol. Pharmacol.*, 12:800–812.

4. Cannon, J. G., Demopoulos, B. J., Long, J. P., Flynn, J. R., and Sharabi, F. M. (1981): Proposed dopaminergic pharmacophore of lergotrile, pergolide and related ergot alkaloid derivatives. *J. Med. Chem.*, 24:238–240.
5. Clement-Cormier, Y., Meyerson, L. R., and McIsaak, A. (1980): Solubilization of multiple binding sites for the dopamine receptor from calf striatal membranes. *Biochem. Pharmacol.*, 29:2009–2016.
6. Closse, A., Frick, W., Hauser, D., and Sauter, A. (1980): Characterization of [$^3$H]bromocriptine binding to calf caudate membranes. In: *Psychopharmacology and Biochemistry of Neurotransmitter Receptors*, edited by H. I. Yamamura, R. W. Olsen, and E. Usdin, pp. 463–474.
7. Closse, A., and Hauser, D. (1976): Dihydroergotamine binding to rat brain membranes. *Life Sci.*, 19:1851–1864.
8. Costall, B., and Naylor, R. J. (1981): Minireview: The hypotheses of different dopamine receptor mechanisms. *Life Sci.*, 28:215–229.
9. Creese, I., Schneider, R., and Snyder, S. H. (1977): [$^3$H]Spiroperidol labels dopamine receptors in pituitary and brain. *Eur. J. Pharmacol.*, 46:377–381.
10. Creese, I., and Sibley, D. R. (1979): Radioligand binding studies: Evidence for multiple dopamine receptors. *Commun. Psychopharmacol.* 3:385–395.
11. Davis, D. N., Strittmatter, W. J., Hoyler, E., and Lefkowitz, R. J. (1977): Dihydroergocryptine binding in rat brain. *Brain Res.*, 132:327–336.
12. Goldstein, M., Lieberman, A., Calne, D. B. and Thorner, M. O., editors (1980): *Ergot Compounds and Brain Function, Vol. 23: Advances in Biochemical Pharmacology*. Raven Press, New York.
13. Greenberg, D. A., and Snyder, S. H. (1978): Pharmacological properties of [$^3$H]dihydroergocryptine binding sites associated with α-noradrenergic receptors in rat brain membranes. *Mol. Pharmacol.*, 14:38–49.
14. Hamblin, M., and Creese, I. (1980): Phenoxybenzamine discriminates multiple dopamine receptors. *Eur. J. Pharmacol.*, 65:119–121.
15. Langer, S. Z., Briley, M., and Dubocovich, M. L. (1980): Adrenergic receptor mechanisms in the central nervous system in relation to catecholamine neurons. In: *Central Adrenaline Neurons, Basic Aspects and their Role in Cardiovascular Functions*, edited by K. Fuxe, M. Goldstein, B. Hökfelt, and T. Hökfelt, pp. 199–211. Pergamon Press, New York.
16. Lew, J. Y., and Goldstein, M. (1979): Dopamine receptor binding for agonists and antagonists in thermal exposed membranes. *Eur. J. Pharmacol.*, 55:429–430.
17. Leysen, J. E. (1979): Unitary dopaminergic receptor composed of cooperatively linked agonist and antagonist sub-unit binding sites. *Commun. Psychopharmacol.* 3:397–410.
18. Leysen, J. E., and Gommeren, W. (1981): Optimal conditions for [$^3$H]apomorphine binding and anomalous equilibrium binding of [$^3$H]apomorphine and [$^3$H]spiperone to rat striatal membranes: Involvement of surface phenomena versus multiple binding sites. *J. Neurochem.* 36:201–219.
19. Nichols, D. E. (1976): Structural correlation between apomorphine and LSD: Involvement of dopamine as well as serotonin in the actions of hallucinogens. *J. Theor. Biol.*, 59:167–177.
20. Nishikori, K., Noshiro, O., Sano, K., and Maeno, H. (1980): Characterization, solubilization, and separation of two distinct dopamine receptors in canine caudate nucleus. *J. Biol. Chem.*, 255:10909–10915.
21. Peroutka, D. J., and Snyder, S. H. (1979): Multiple serotonin receptors: Differential binding of [$^3$H]5-hydroxytryptamine, [$^3$H]lysergic acid diethylamide and [$^3$H]spiroperiodol. *Mol. Pharmacol.*, 16:687–699.
22. Peroutka, S. J., and Snyder S. H. (1981): Two distinct serotonin receptors: Regional variations in receptor binding in mammalian brain. *Brain Res.*, 208:339–347.
23. Sibley, D. R., and Creese, I. (1980): Pseudo non-competitive interactions with dopamine receptors. *Eur. J. Pharmacol.*, 65:131–133.
24. Sokoloff, P., Martres, M., and Schwartz, J. C. (1980): Three classes of dopamine receptors (D-2, D-3, D-4) identified by binding studies with [$^3$H]-apomorphine and [$^3$H]domperidone. *Naunyn Schmiedebergs Arch. Pharmacol.*, 315:89–102.
25. Spano, P. F., Memo, M., Govoni, S., and Trabucchi, M. (1980): Similarities and dissimilarities between dopamine and neuroleptic receptors: Further evidence for type 1 and type 2 dopamine receptors in the CNS. *Adv. Biochem. Psychopharmacol.*, 24:113–121.
26. Thorner, M. O., Flückiger, E., and Calne, D. B., editors (1980): *Bromocriptine. A Clinical and Pharmacological Review*. Raven Press, New York.
27. Titeler, M., List, S., and Seeman, P. (1979): High affinity dopamine receptors ($D_3$) in rat brain. *Commun. Psychopharmac.*, 3:411–420.

28. Titeler, M., Weinrich, P., Sinclair, D., and Seeman, P. (1978): Multiple receptors for brain dopamine. *Proc. Natl. Acad. Sci USA*, 75:1153–1156.
29. Tran, V. T., Chang, R. S. L., and Snyder, S. H. (1978): Histamine-$H_1$ receptors identified in mammalian brain membranes with [$^3$H]mepyramine. *Proc. Natl. Acad. Sci USA*, 75:6290–6294.
30. U'Prichard, D. C., Greenberg, D. A., and Snyder, S. H. (1977): Binding characteristics of a radiolabelled agonist and antagonist at central nervous system alpha noradrenergic receptors. *Mol. Pharmacol.*, 13:454–473.
31. Wastek, G. J., and Yamamura, H. I. (1978): Biochemical characterization of the muscarinic cholinergic receptor in human brain: Alterations in Huntington's disease (slightly varied). *Mol. Pharmacol.*, 14:68.
32. Williams, L. T., and Lefkowitz, R. J. (1977): Molecular pharmacology of α-adrenergic receptors: Utilization of [$^3$H]dihydroergocryptine binding in the study of pharmacological receptor alterations. *Mol. Pharmacol.*, 13:304–313.

*Molecular Pharmacology of Neurotransmitter Receptors*, edited by T. Segawa et al.
Raven Press, New York © 1983.

# Labeling of a GTP-Binding Regulatory Protein of Rat Brain Adenylate Cyclase System by Cholera Toxin-Catalyzed ADP-Ribosylation

Keiichi Enomoto and Takeo Asakawa

*Department of Pharmacology, Saga Medical School, Saga 840-01, Japan*

The activity of adenylate cyclase is regulated through the binding of guanine nucleotides to a guanosine triphosphate (GTP)-binding regulatory protein (16). The regulatory protein is also believed to modulate the affinity of hormones and neurotransmitters to their receptors. It is therefore essential to detect and quantify the regulatory protein for the analysis of receptor-adenylate cyclase coupling. Preceding studies of the regulatory proteins of rat liver (3), fat cells (13), and reticulocytes and erythrocytes (12) have shown that a protein of 42,000 daltons was involved in the regulation of adenylate cyclase activity. The recent purification of the regulatory protein from rat liver plasma membranes has demonstrated that the purified protein contained the 42,000-dalton peptide and two other kinds of peptides (15). This finding suggests that the structure of the regulatory protein is more complex than has previously been considered.

In this chapter, we show that a protein which can be ADP-ribosylated by cholera toxin and has a molecular weight of 48,000 daltons is at least one of components of the regulatory protein in rat brain synaptic plasma membranes. The distribution of the 48,000-dalton protein and other ADP-ribosylated proteins in various brain membrane fractions are discussed as well.

## METHODS AND MATERIALS

### Cholera Toxin and Chemicals

Purified cholera toxin was a generous gift from Dr. Nobuya Ohtomo, the Chemo-Sero Therapeutic Research Institute, Kumamoto, Japan. [Adenylate-$^{32}$P]-NAD (10–50 Ci/mmol) was purchased from New England Nuclear.

### Buffer

Buffer A consisted of 0.13 M NaCl, 0.01% sodium azide, 2 kallikrein inactivator units/ml of aprotinin, 10 mM *N*-2-hydroxyethylpiperazine-*N'*-2-ethanesulfonic acid (HEPES) and NaOH to give pH 7.3.

## Brain Membrane Fractions

Synaptic plasma membranes were prepared from rat brains as described by Whittaker et al. (19). Myelin was purified according to the method of Uyemura et al. (18). Mitochondria fraction sedimented at the bottom of the tube during the centrifugation in a sucrose density gradient and was washed with 0.24 M sucrose three times. A membrane fraction floating between 0.35 and 0.6 M sucrose after the centrifugation of disrupted synaptosomes was collected as synaptic vesicle fraction.

## Cytosolic Protein Factor

The homogenate of rat brains or livers in 2 volumes of buffer A was centrifuged for 10 min at 9,500 × g and the resultant supernatant was further centrifuged at 105,000 × g for 60 min. The supernatant collected was partially purified by gel filtration. Some properties and further purification of the factor been reported (4–6).

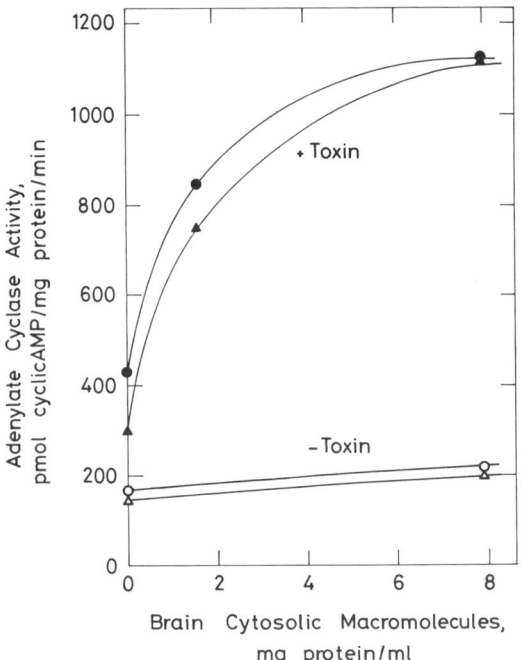

**FIG. 1.** Stimulation of cholera toxin-catalyzed activation of adenylate cyclase by the cytosolic protein factor. Adenylate cyclase in synaptic membranes was activated as described in Methods and Materials except that 4.3 mM NAD, 2.2 µg/ml of the toxin, and the cytosolic protein factor from brain were used. The incubation continued for 30 min in the presence (closed symbols) or absence (open symbols) of the toxin. Membranes were pre-washed with buffer A (triangles) before the ADP-ribosylation. Assay of the cyclase was conducted for 5 min at 30°C in the presence of 0.1 mM GTP.

## ADP-Ribosylation

ADP-ribosylation was usually conducted at 25°C for 60 min in the medium containing 100 μM NAD (0.5–2.5 Ci/mmol), 0.4 mM GTP, 5 mM ATP, 1 mM $MgCl_2$, 4 mg/ml bovine serum albumin, 15.5 mg protein/ml of cytosolic protein factor from rat liver, 8 mM nicotinamide, 8 mM thymidine, 20 μl of buffer A, 10 μg/ml of cholera toxin, and 70–100 μg protein of membranes in a final volume of 50 μl. Cholera toxin was pre-activated before use as described (6). Solubilized membranes were subjected to electrophoresis in 8–15% linear gradient polyacrylamide gel containing 0.1% SDS, and then the dried gel was exposed to a Kodak X-Omat R film as reported (6).

## Assay of Adenylate Cyclase

Adenylate cyclase was assayed as described before (6) in 100 μl of the medium at pH 7 containing 80 mM KCl, 12 mM $MgCl_2$, 3 mM EDTA, 13 mM phosphoenolpyruvate, 0.3 mM papaverine, 0.2 mM dithiothreitol, 0.01% sodium azide, 2 mM ATP, 25 units/ml of myokinase, and 15 units/ml of pyruvate kinase. The amount of cyclic AMP formed was determined by the cyclic AMP-binding protein assay (8). Assay continued for 5 min at 37°C unless mentioned.

## Enzyme Activities

5′-Nucleotidase and succinate dehydrogenase were assayed according to the methods of Aronson and Touster (1) and Kirshner et al. (10), respectively. The activity of 2′,3′-cyclic nucleotide 3′-phosphohydrolase was determined by the colorimetric method as reported (11).

## RESULTS AND DISCUSSION

Cholera toxin has been shown to activate adenylate cyclase by ADP-ribosylating the GTP-binding regulatory protein of adenylate cyclase (2,7). We could activate adenylate cyclase in brain synaptic plasma membranes by incubating membranes with toxin, NAD, GTP, and the cytosolic protein factor from brain or liver cytosols. Figure 1 shows that the activation by cholera toxin was remarkably stimulated by the endogenous cytosolic protein factor from brain. Pre-washing of the membranes reduced the activation by the toxin in the absence of the factor, probably by removing the factor which associated with the membranes.

To label the GTP-binding regulatory protein, we incubated synaptic membranes in the presence of cholera toxin and [$^{32}$P]-NAD. The solubilized membrane proteins were separated by SDS-polyacrylamide gel electrophoresis and ADP-ribosylated proteins were detected by autoradiography, as shown in Fig. 2. Several proteins were ADP-ribosylated dependently on the concentration of the toxin. Proteins of 66,000, 48,000, 25,000, and 18,000 daltons were labeled in every preparation of synaptic membranes used, but proteins of 110,000, 43,000, 38,000, and 23,000

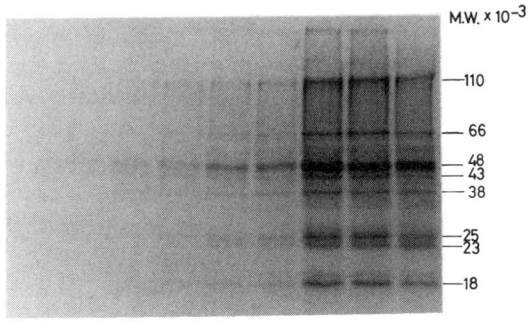

**FIG. 2.** Cholera toxin-catalyzed ADP-ribosylation of proteins in synaptic plasma membranes. ADP-ribosylation and autoradiography were carried out as described in Methods and Materials.

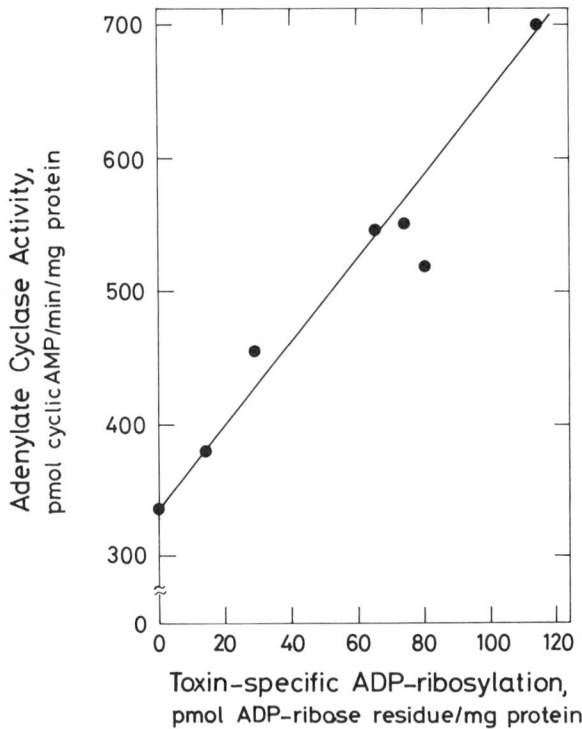

**FIG. 3.** Activation of adenylate cyclase by the toxin-catalyzed ADP-ribosylation. Synaptic membranes were treated with [$^{32}$P]-NAD and 0–10 µg/ml of cholera toxin. After washing of the membranes with buffer A, adenylate cyclase activity in the presence of 0.1 mM GTP and the radioactivity incorporated into the membranes were determined.

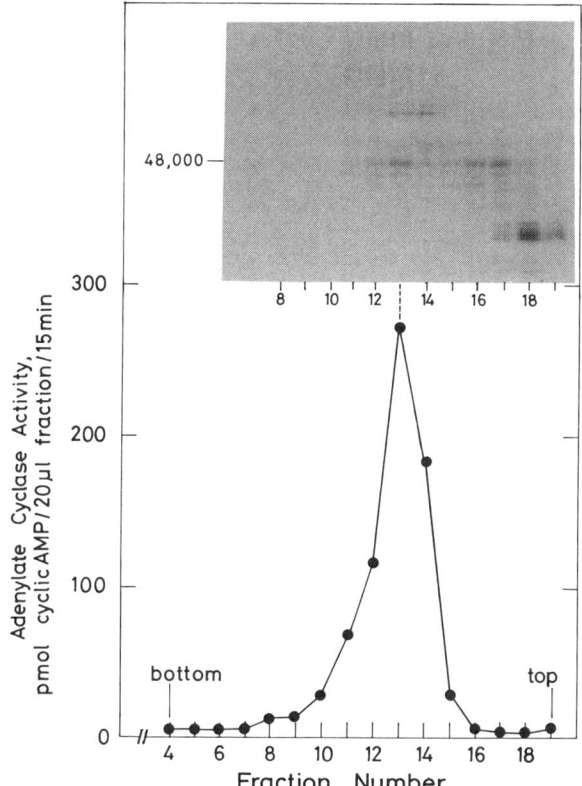

**FIG. 4.** Sucrose density gradient centrifugation of ADP-ribosylated proteins. Synaptic membranes (1.34 mg protein) were preincubated for 30 min at 30°C with 40 μM Gpp(NH)p and other necessary cofactors for ADP-ribosylation. The concentration of $Mg^{2+}$ during the preincubation was 4 mM, and no GTP and ATP was added. ADP-ribosylation was started by the addition of [$^{32}$P]-NAD and cholera toxin. Washed membranes were solubilized with Lubrol PX and centrifuged in a 5–20% sucrose density gradient as reported by Neer et al. (14). Adenylate cyclase was assayed for 15 min at 37°C in the presence of 10 μM Gpp(NH)p.

daltons were slightly or very faintly labeled in some membrane preparations. A 43,000-dalton protein, which had a molecular weight similar to that of the GTP-binding regulatory protein reported in some tissues, was slightly labeled particularly in fresh membrane preparations and did not associate with the regulatory protein activity in the gel filtration experiment to be described below. In all labeling experiments, a protein of 48,000 daltons (48K protein) was always the major product by the toxin-catalyzed ADP-ribosylation.

This ADP-ribosylation of membrane proteins was accompanied by the enhancement of the adenylate cyclase activity. As shown in Fig. 3, adenylate cyclase activity increased in parallel with the ADP-ribosylation of membrane proteins. In the presence of 100 μM NAD and 10 μg/ml of the toxin, approximately 120 pmoles of ADP-ribosyl residues were incorporated into 1 mg protein of the membranes. About 12.4% of the radioactivity in a polyacrylamide gel was incorporated into the 48K

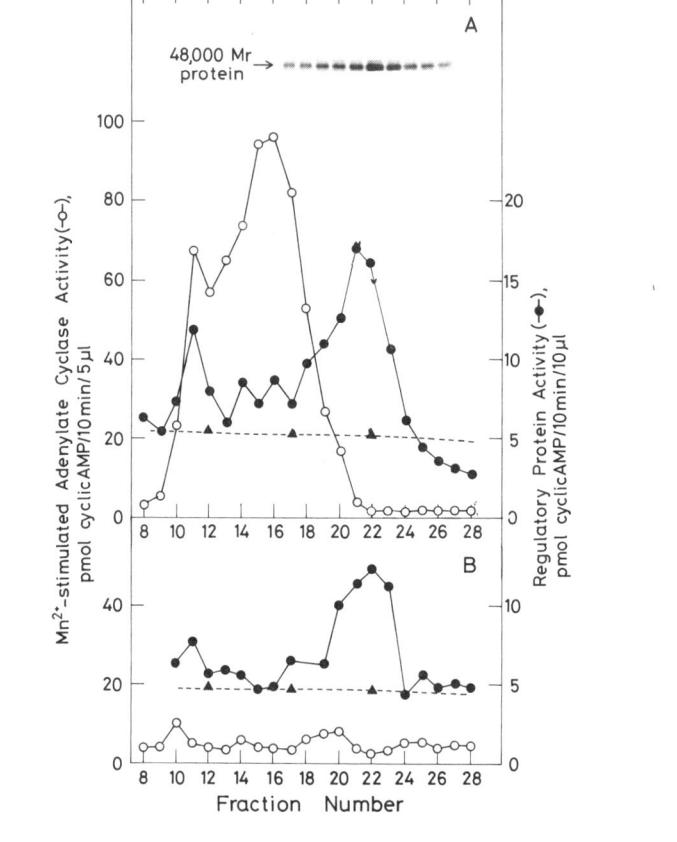
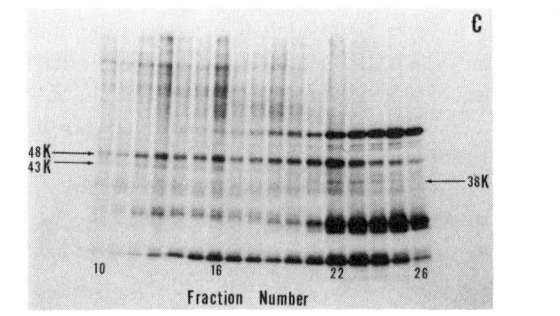

protein. Thus we can calculate the content of the 48K protein in the membranes as approximately 15 pmol/mg protein.

To determine which ADP-ribosylated protein has the activity of the regulatory protein, we carried out following experiments. Synaptic membranes were treated with cholera toxin and [$^{32}$P]-NAD in the presence of 5′-guanylylimidodiphosphate [Gpp(NH)p], which can activate adenylate cyclase through the formation of the stable complex of the catalytic component of adenylate cyclase and the regulatory protein that binds Gpp(NH)p. The treated membranes was solubilized with Lubrol PX and then subjected to centrifugation in a sucrose density gradient.

The distributions of adenylate cyclase activity and ADP-ribosylated proteins are shown in Fig. 4. A part of the 48K protein was present in fractions near the top, but a considerable amount of the protein co-sedimented with adenylate cyclase activity between fractions 12 and 14. This result suggests that the 48K protein can associate with the catalytic unit of adenylate cyclase. The presence of the 48K protein in fractions near the top may be the result of insufficient activation by Gpp(NH)p or the presence of the extra 48K protein.

Recently Strittmatter and Neer (17) succeeded in separating the regulatory protein activity from the catalytic unit of adenylate cyclase by gel filtration of solubilized brain membrane proteins. We conducted a similar experiment, using the ADP-ribosyl [$^{32}$P]-labeled synaptic membranes as the marker. As shown in Fig. 5A, the regulatory protein activity was separated from the activity of the catalytic unit of adenylate cyclase assayed in the presence of $Mn^{2+}$. The elution pattern of the 48K protein in the autoradiogram in Fig. 5A indicates that the 48K protein apparently co-eluted with the regulatory protein activity. Some of the 48K protein was detected in the fractions of the catalytic unit, as shown in the autoradiogram in Fig. 5C. The 43,000-dalton ADP-ribosylated protein was present in the catalytic unit fractions but absent in the regulatory protein fractions. Faintly labeled 38,000-dalton protein also eluted in the regulatory protein fractions. Other ADP-ribosylated proteins were mainly distributed in fractions 22–26 (66,000-dalton protein), 22–25 (25,000-dalton), and 22–24 (18,000-dalton).

**FIG. 5.** Gel filtration of the solubilized regulatory protein. Synaptic membranes (0.37 mg protein) were ADP-ribosylated as described in Methods and Materials except that 14.5 μM [$^{32}$P]-NAD (25 Ci/mmol) and 20 μg/ml cholera toxin were used. The ADP-ribosylated synaptic membranes mixed with 4.7 mg protein of untreated membranes were solubilized with cholate and ammonium sulfate and subjected to gel filtration according to the method of Strittmatter and Neer (17). Ultrogel AcA 34 column (1 × 24.5 cm) was used and 0.64 ml fractions were collected. Myelin (4.8 mg protein) was solubilized in the same way and applied to the same column. The activity of the catalytic unit of adenylate cyclase *(open circles)* was assayed in the presence of 5 mM $MnCl_2$. Assay of the regulatory protein activity *(closed circles)* was conducted as described by Strittmatter and Neer (17) by incubating 10 μl of each fraction with 60 μM Gpp(NH)p and 10 μl of catalytic unit of adenylate cyclase (1.8 mg protein/ml) separately prepared from rat brain. Adenylate cyclase was assayed for 10 min at 30°C. Basal adenylate cyclase activity due to the catalytic unit of the cyclase used for the reconstitution was assayed by the incubation of the catalytic unit with heated column fractions in the presence of Gpp(NH)p *(triangles)*. The elution patterns of the regulatory protein and the catalytic unit activities from solubilized synaptic membranes **(A)** and myelin fraction **(B)** are shown. ADP-ribosylated proteins from synaptic membranes eluted in each fraction were analyzed by autoradiography **(C)**.

From the evidence described above, it is likely that the 48K protein was the regulatory protein itself or at least a part of the regulatory protein in rat brain. The low regulatory protein activity in the catalytic unit fractions 13–16, in spite of the presence of the 48K protein, may be due to the lack of the second component of the regulatory protein that is necessary for the reconstitution. The 38,000-dalton protein may satisfy such a requirement.

We then examined the possibility of other brain membrane fractions contained the 48K protein as well. Figure 6 shows the specific activities of several enzymes in brain membrane fractions. It is apparent that mitochondria and synaptic vesicle

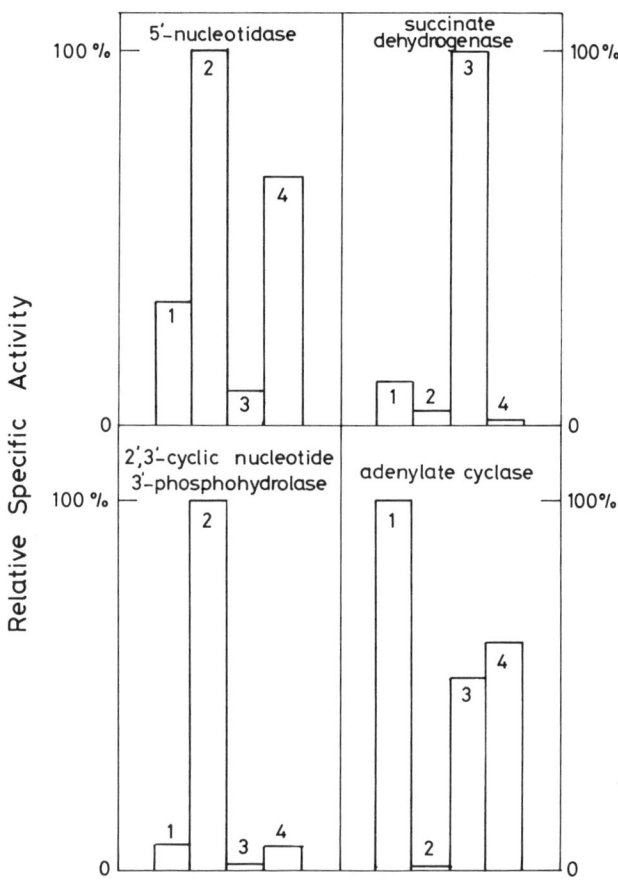

FIG. 6. Enzyme activities in brain membrane fractions. **1**: Synaptic plasma membranes; **2**: myelin fraction; **3**: mitochondria fraction; **4**: synaptic vesicle fraction. Maximum enzyme activities (100%) were 5.88 μmol Pi/hr/mg protein (5'-nucleotidase), 0.539 $\Delta OD_{500}$/hr/mg protein (succinate dehydrogenase), 28.2 μmol Pi/min/mg protein (2',3'-cyclic nucleotide 3'-phosphohydrolase) and 421 pmol cyclic AMP/min/mg protein (adenylate cyclase). Adenylate cyclase was assayed in the presence of 10 mM NaF. The distribution of total adenylate cyclase activity was 86% in synaptic plasma membranes, 5% in mitochondria fraction, and 9% in synaptic vesicle fraction. Less than 1% of the activity was found in myelin fraction.

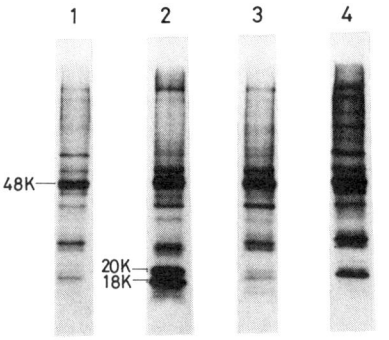

FIG. 7. ADP-ribosylated proteins in brain membrane fractions. Membrane fractions (83 μg protein) were treated with cholera toxin and [$^{32}$P]-NAD as described. **1:** Synaptic membranes; **2:** myelin fraction; **3:** mitochondria fraction; **4:** synaptic vesicle fraction.

fractions were not completely devoid of plasma membranes, as indicated by considerable activity of 5'-nucleotidase and adenylate cyclase. Myelin fraction, however, demonstrated little adenylate cyclase activity. ADP-ribosylated proteins by cholera toxin in membrane fractions are represented in an autoradiogram (Fig. 7). A protein which has a molecular weight of 48,000 was present in every membrane fraction as the major ADP-ribosylated protein. Mitochondria fraction and synaptic vesicle fraction showed similar patterns of ADP-ribosylated proteins to that of synaptic membranes. Myelin fraction contained two unique ADP-ribosylated proteins which have molecular weights of 20,000 and 18,000. These proteins were similar to myelin basic proteins in that they were easily solubilized with acid. Incubation of myelin membranes with 0.03 N HCl solubilized 43 and 62% of the 20,000- and 18,000-dalton proteins, respectively. There was no doubt that at least some of the 48,000-dalton protein present in mitochondria and synaptic vesicle fractions originated in plasma membranes in those fractions. However, the presence of the 48,000-dalton protein in myelin fraction could not be attributed to such contamination by plasma membranes because the specific activity of adenylate cyclase in myelin fraction was less than 2% of that in synaptic membranes. The observation, therefore, indicated that myelin had the 48,000-dalton protein which was very similar to the 48K protein in synaptic membranes.

As a natural result, this question has arisen: Whether or not the 48,000-dalton protein in myelin has the regulatory protein activity. To examine this, we subjected solubilized myelin to the gel filtration used for the separation of the regulatory protein. Figure 5B shows that the activity of the regulatory protein eluted at the same regulatory protein fractions as synaptic membranes. Although further study is required to verify that this activity is due to the 48,000-dalton protein in myelin, the results suggest the presence of the regulatory protein in the membranes which lack adenylate cyclase activity. This result is not very surprising, however, in view of the finding by Kaslow et al. (9) the regulatory protein in human erythrocyte membranes which also lack adenylate cyclase activity. The regulatory protein activity in myelin may have an unknown but physiologically important role in the membranes.

Proteins in brain cytosol were also ADP-ribosylated by cholera toxin. Major ADP-ribosylated protein has a molecular weight of 52,000. The ADP-ribosylation of cytosol proteins was strongly dependent on the presence of nucleotides such as ATP and GTP.

## SUMMARY

Cholera toxin ADP-ribosylated several proteins in synaptic plasma membranes of rat brains such as peptides of 66,000, 48,000, 38,000, 25,000, and 18,000 daltons. A 42,000-dalton protein reported to be the GTP-binding regulatory protein in several tissues was faintly labeled and its content varied from preparation to preparation. Adenylate cyclase activity was concomitantly enhanced by more than twice in proportion to the ADP-ribosylation. Accumulated evidence indicated that a protein of 48,000 daltons (48K protein) was a component which constituted the GTP-binding regulatory protein of adenylate cyclase system in rat brain. Among ADP-ribosylated proteins, the 48K protein was the major substrate for the ADP-ribosylation, and the content of this protein was estimated to be about 15 pmol/mg membrane protein. When synaptic membranes were solubilized and applied on a Ultrogel AcA34 gel filtration column to separate the regulatory protein from other components of adenylate cyclase, the 48K protein—but not other ADP-ribosylated proteins—co-eluted with the regulatory protein activity assayed by the reconstitution with catalytic unit of adenylate cyclase. The 48K protein was also detected in myelin fraction which lack adenylate cyclase activity. When solubilized proteins from myelin were subjected to the gel filtration in the AcA34 column, the regulatory protein activity eluted in the 48K protein fractions where the regulatory protein from synaptic membranes appeared.

Myelin contained basic protein-like peptides of 20,000 and 18,000 daltons ADP-ribosylated by cholera toxin. These peptides were solubilized from the membranes with acid. Soluble proteins in brain cytosol were ADP-ribosylated by cholera toxin, which was dependent on the presence of nucleotides.

## REFERENCES

1. Aronson, N. N., Jr., and Touster, O. (1974): Isolation of rat liver plasma membrane fragments in isotonic sucrose. In: *Methods in Enzymology, Vol. 31*, edited by S. Fleischer and L. Packer, pp. 90–102. Academic Press, New York.
2. Cassel, D., and Pfeuffer, T. (1978): Mechanism of cholera toxin action: Covalent modification of the guanyl nucleotide-binding protein of the adenylate cyclase system. *Proc. Natl. Acad. Sci. USA*, 75:2669–2673.
3. Doberska, C. A., MacPherson, A. J. S., and Martin, B. R. (1980): Requirement for guanosine triphosphate for cholera-toxin-catalysed incorporation of adenosine diphosphate ribose into rat liver plasma membranes and for activation of adenylate cyclase. *Biochem. J.*, 186:749–754.
4. Enomoto, K., and Asakawa, T. (1980): Effect of rat liver cytosol on the activation of adenylate cyclase by cholera toxin. *Proceedings of the 16th Joint Conference on Cholera*. U.S.-Japan Cooperative Medical Science Program *(in press)*.
5. Enomoto, K., and Gill, D. M. (1979): Requirement for guanosine triphosphate in the activation of adenylate cyclase by cholera toxin. *J. Supramol. Struc.*, 10:51–60.
6. Enomoto, K., and Gill, D. M. (1980): Cholera toxin activation of adenylate cyclase. *J. Biol. Chem.*, 255:1252–1258.
7. Gill, D. M., and Meren, R. (1978): ADP-ribosylation of membrane proteins catalysed by cholera toxin: Basis of the activation of adenylate cyclase. *Proc. Natl. Acad. Sci. USA*, 75:3050–3054.

8. Gilman, A. G., and Murad, F. (1974): Assay of cyclic nucleotides by receptor protein binding displacement. In: *Methods in Enzymology, Vol. 38*, edited by J. G. Hardman and W. O'Malley, pp. 49–61. Academic Press, New York.
9. Kaslow, H. R., Johnson, G. L., Brothers, V. M., and Bourne, H. R. (1980): A regulatory component of adenylate cyclase from human erythrocyte membranes. *J. Biol. Chem.*, 255:3736–3741.
10. Kirshner, N., Kirshner, A. G., and Kamin, D. L. (1966): Adenosine triphosphate activity of adrenal medulla catecholamine granules. *Biochim. Biophys. Acta*, 113:332–335.
11. Kurihara, T., and Takahashi, Y. (1973): Potentiometric and colorimetric methods for the assay of 2′,3′-cyclic nucleotide 3′-phosphohydrolase. *J. Neurochem.*, 20:719–727.
12. Limbird, L. E., Gill, D. M., Stadel, J. M., Hickey, A. R., and Lefkowitz, R. J. (1980): Loss of β-adrenergic receptor-guanine nucleotide regulatory protein interactions accompanies decline in catecholamine responsiveness of adenylate cyclase in maturing rat erythrocytes. *J. Biol. Chem.*, 255:1854–1861.
13. Malbon, C. C., and Gill, D. M. (1979): ADP-ribosylation of membrane proteins and activation of adenylate cyclase by cholera toxin in fat cell ghosts from euthyroid and hypothyroid rats. *Biochim. Biophys. Acta*, 586:518–527.
14. Neer, E. J., Echeverria, D., and Knox, S. (1980): Increase in the size of soluble brain adenylase cyclase with activation by guanosine 5′-(β,γ-imino)triphosphate. *J. Biol. Chem.*, 255:9782–9789.
15. Northup, J. K., Sternweis, P. C., Smigel, M. D., Schleifer, L. S., Ross, E. M., and Gilman, A. G. (1980): Purification of the regulatory component of adneylate cyclase. *Proc. Natl. Acad. Sci. USA*, 77:6516–6520.
16. Ross, E. M., and Gilman, A. G. (1980): Biochemical properties of hormone-sensitive adenylate cyclase. *Annu. Rev. Biochem.*, 49:533–564.
17. Strittmatter, S., and Neer, E. J. (1980): Properties of the separated catalytic and regulatory units of brain adenylate cyclase. *Proc. Natl. Acad. Sci. USA*, 77:6344–6348.
18. Uyemura, K., Tobari, C., Hirano, S., and Tsukada, Y. (1972): Comparative studies on the myelin proteins of bovine peripheral nerve and spinal cord. *J. Neurochem.*, 19:2607–2614.
19. Whittaker, V. P., Michaelson, I. A., and Kirkland, R. J. A. (1964): The separation of synaptic vesicles from nerve-ending particles ('synaptosomes'). *Biochem. J.*, 90:293–303

# Subject Index

# Subject Index

Acetylcholine, in substantia nigra, 92–93,95
Acetylcholine receptors, muscarinic, in smooth muscles, 31–40
Acetylcholinesterase, identification and isolation of, 7–10
Adenylate cyclase
 DA receptors and, in canine caudate nucleus, 175–182
 rat brain, labeling of GTP-binding regulatory protein of, 281–291
 receptor inversely coupled to, $\alpha_2$-adrenergic receptor as, 53–70
 VIP-sensitive, inhibition of, by DA, in rat anterior pituitary, 199–206
ADP-ribosylation, cholera toxin-catalyzed, labeling of GTP-binding regulatory protein of rat brain adenylate cyclase by, 281–291
Adrenergic-cholinergic interaction, in cardiac tissue, mechanisms of, 22–24
$\alpha_2$-adrenergic receptor, multiple affinity states and regulation of, 53–70
$\alpha_2$-adrenergic systems, changes in, during long-term desensitization, 32–35
$\beta$-adrenergic receptor subtypes, in rat brain, 73–80
$\beta$-adrenergic receptors
 6-OHDOPA, isoproterenol, DMI and, 84–86
 postsynaptic, in splenic tissue, 43–50
Affinity states, multiple, of $\alpha_2$-adrenergic receptor, 53–70
[$^3$H]agonist binding sites, in striatum, DA receptors as, 129–130
Agonists, dopaminergic, regulation of antagonist binding by, 24–25
Alkylation, phenoxybenzamine-selective, of [$^3$H]BUTY binding sites, 130–131
Antagonism of apomorphine-induced behavior, comparison of neuroleptics in, 167–171
Antagonist binding, regulation of, by dopaminergic agonists, 24–25
Anterior pituitary, rat, inhibition of VIP-sensitive adenylate cyclase by DA in, 199–206
Antidepressants, tricyclic, postsynaptic 5-HT receptor and, 120–121
Antipsychotics, two distinct classes of DA receptor mediating actions of, 163–171
Aorta, bovine, $\alpha_2$-adrenergic receptors in, 67–68
Apomorphine-induced behaviors, comparison of neuroleptics in antagonism of, 167–171
Apomorphine-induced stereotypy, in rats, inhibitory effects of 2-methoxybenzamide derivatives on, 177–179
Autonomic receptors, splenic, 43–50

Autoradiography, of morphology of neurotransmitter receptors, 250–255

Behavioral studies, of two distinct classes of DA receptor mediating actions of antipsychotics, 167–170
Behaviors, apomorphine-induced, comparison of neuroleptics in antagonism of, 167–171
Benzodiazepine receptor, 209–218
  cerebral, endogenous modulating mechanism of, 221–230
Binding
  antagonist, regulation of, by dopaminergic agonists, 24–25
  benzodiazepine receptor
    to membrane fraction of rat brain, properties of, 223–224
    modulation of
      by phospholipids, 226–228
      by GABA, 214–217
    of [$^3$H]propyl β-carboline-3-carboxylate, 211–214
  dopamine, to $D_1$ and $D_2$
    biochemical events subsequent to, 179–182
    inhibitory effects of 2-methoxy-benzamide derivatives on, 175–177
  [$^3$H]flunitrazepam, induced by phospholipase C and phospholipase $A_2$, 228–229
  muscarinic receptor, ionic effects on, 25–26
  radioligand, to dopamine receptors in pituitary, 126–127
  receptor, with cryostat sections, 246–249
  $^3$H-serotonin, spiperone inhibition of, in cat, 105–108
  specific, of cysteine sulfinic acid, to synaptic membrane fractions, 239–243
  stereospecific
    effects of lesions on, 149–153,157,159
    effects of proteolytic enzymes on, 153–161
  $^3$H-strychnine, characterization of, 233–237
Binding properties, heterogeneous, of benzodiazepine receptor, 209–211
Binding protein, curare, identification and isolation of, 11–13
Binding sites
  [$^3$H]agonist, in striatum, DA receptors as, 129–130
  [$^3$H]BUTY
    phenoxybenzamine-selective alkylation of, 130–131
    in striatum, DA receptors as, 127–129
  D-2 and D-4
    definition and comparison of, 164–167
    pharmacology of, 166–168
  $^3$H-serotonin, multiple
    discrimination of, by tryptamine analogues, 106,108–110
    pharmacological and species differences of, 103–112
  structural modifications of ergopeptine molecule and affinities to, 269–277
Binding studies, of two distinct classes of DA receptor mediating actions of antipsychotics, 164–168
Binding subunit, recognition, of $D_1$ DA receptor, identification and localization of, 135–143
Biochemical events, subsequent to dopamine binding to $D_1$ and $D_2$, 179–182

Bovine cerebral cortex and aorta, $\alpha_2$-adrenergic receptors in, 67–68
Brain
 human, glycine receptors in, 233–237
 rat
  $\beta$-adrenergic receptor subtypes in, 73–80
  membrane fraction of, properties of benzodiazepine receptor binding to, 223–224
  morphological study on neurotransmitter receptors in, 245–257
Brain adenylate cyclase, labeling of GTP-binding regulatory protein of, 281–291
Butyrophenones ([$^3$H]BUTY) binding sites
 phenoxybenzamine-selective alkylation of, 130–131
 in striatum, DA receptors as, 127–129

Canine caudate nucleus, DA receptors and adenylate cyclase in, 175–182
Cardiac receptors, noradrenaline and, 83–89
Cardiac tissue, mechanisms of adrenergic-cholinergic interaction in, 22–24
Cat, spiperone inhibition of $^3$H-5-HT binding in, 105–108
Caudate, rat, regulation of $\beta_1$- or $\beta_2$-receptor density in, 76, 79–80
Caudate nucleus, canine, DA receptors and adenylate cyclase in, 175–182
Central nervous system, dopamine receptors in, 125–133
Central serotonin receptors, regulation mechanism of, 115–121
Cerebellum, rat, regulation of $\beta_1$- or $\beta_2$-receptor density in, 75–79
Cerebral benzodiazepine receptor, endogenous modulating mechanism of, 221–230
Cerebral cortex
 bovine, $\alpha_2$-adrenergic receptors in, 67–68
 rat, regulation of $\beta_1$- or $\beta_2$-receptor density in, 74–76
Chemical sympathectomy, with 6-OHDA, reciprocal alterations of splenic $\beta$-adrenergic and muscarinic receptors following, 45–47
Cholera toxin-catalyzed ADP-ribosylation, labeling of GTP-binding regulatory protein of rat brain adenylate cyclase by, 281–291
Cholinergic receptor protein, identification and isolation of, 10–11
Cholinergic receptors, presynaptic muscarinic, in splenic tissue, 43–50
Circling, measurement of, modification of DA transmission by TRH and, 190
Classes, two distinct, of DA receptor, mediating actions of antipsychotics, 163–171
Contractile response, decrease of, drugs and, 32–34
Contraction, regulation of, by muscarinic acetylcholine receptors, 31–35
Cryostat sections, receptor binding with, 246–249
Curare binding protein, identification and isolation of, 11–13
Cyclic AMP levels, in mouse striatum, modification of DA transmission by TRH and, 190–195

Cysteine sulfinic acid, specific binding of, to synaptic membrane fractions, 239–243

DA, see Dopamine
Desensitization, long-term, changes in muscarinic and α-adrenergic systems during, 32–35
Desmethylimipramine (DMI)
β-adrenergic receptors and, 84–86
muscarinic ACh receptors and, 85–87
Discrimination of multiple $^3$H-serotonin binding sites, by tryptamine analogues, 106,108–110
Dopamine (DA), inhibition of VIP-sensitive adenylate cyclase by, in rat anterior pituitary, 199–206
Dopamine binding, to $D_1$ and $D_2$
biochemical effects subsequent to, 179–182
inhibitory effects of 2-methoxy-benzamide derivatives on, 175–177
[$^3$H]dopamine-labeled $D_1$ and $D_2$, separation of, 177,179–180
Dopamine nerve terminals
mesolimbic, TRH and, 187–189
nigrostriatal, TRH and, 190
Dopamine receptor(s)
adenylate cyclase and, in canine caudate nucleus, 175–182
in central nervous system, 125–133
$D_1$
recognition binding subunit of, identification and localization of, 135–143
and $D_2$, biochemical events subsequent to dopamine binding to, 179–182
mediating actions of antipsychotics, two distinct classes of, 163–171
mediating inhibition of VIP-sensitive adenylate cyclase, pharmacological properties of, 201,203–205
pharmacological characterization of, 125
unitary, subunit composition of, 147–161
Dopaminergic agonists, regulation of antagonist binding by, 24–25
Dopaminergic transmission, modification of, by thyrotropin-releasing hormone, 185–196
Drugs, effects of, on decrease on mAChR and contractile response, 32–34

Endogenous modulating mechanism, of cerebral benzodiazepine receptor, 221–230
Ergopeptine molecule, structural modifications of, receptor binding sites and, 269–277

Feedback pathway-lateral habenula, SN and, 97–99
[$^3$H]flunitrazepam binding, induced by phospholipase C and phospholipase $A_2$, 228–229

Gamma-aminobutyric acid (GABA)
modulation of benzodiazepine receptor binding by, 214–217
in substantia nigra, 92–94
Glial receptors, for serotonin, 116–118
Glutamate, in substantia nigra, 94–96
Glycine receptors, in human brain, 233–237
GTP, see Guanosine triphosphate
Guanine nucleotide(s)
effects of, on inhibition of VIP-sensitive adenylate cyclase, 205–206

mAChR and, 35–40
regulation of muscarinic receptors
  by, 17–22
specific inactivation by trypsin of
  effect of, 39–40
Guanosine triphosphate (GTP), heat
  treatment-multiple effects
  mimicking, 131–132
Guanosine triphosphate-binding
  regulatory protein, of rat brain
  adenylate cyclase, labeling of,
  281–291

Heat treatment-multiple effects
  mimicking GTP, 131–132
Heterogeneous binding properties, of
  benzodiazepine receptor, 209–
  211
Heterogenity, of muscarinic receptor,
  15–27
Hormone, thyrotropin-releasing,
  modification of dopaminergic
  transmission by, 185–196
5-HT, see Serotonin entries
Human brain, glycine receptors in,
  233–237
6-hydroxydopa (6-OHDOPA)
  β-adrenergic receptor and, 84–86
  muscarinic ACh receptors and,
  85–87
6-hydroxydopamine (6-OHDA)
  chemical sympathectomy with,
    reciprocal alterations of
    splenic β-adrenergic and
    muscarinic receptors
    following, 45–47
  reduction of splenic NE
    concentration following, 46–
    47

Identification
  of acetylcholinesterase, 7–10
  of cholinergic receptor protein,
    10–11
  of curare binding protein, 11–13

of recognition binding subunit of
  $D_1$ DA receptor, 135–143
Inactivation
  radiation, of mAChR, 36–39
  specific, by trypsin, of effect of
    guanine nucleotide, 39–40
Inhibition
  spiperone, of $^3$H-5-HT binding, in
    cat, 105–108
  of VIP-sensitive adenylate cyclase,
    by DA, in rat anterior
    pituitary, 199–206
Inhibitory effects, of 2-methoxy-
  benzamide derivatives
  on apomorphine-induced
    stereotypy in rats, 177–179
  on [$^3$H]dopamine binding to $D_1$ and
    $D_2$, 175–177
Ionic effects, on muscarinic receptor
  binding, 25–26
Irreversible modification of DA
  receptors, 130–132
Isolation
  of acetylcholinesterase, 7–10
  of cholinergic receptor protein,
    10–11
  of curare binding protein, 11–13
Isoproterenol
  β-adrenergic receptors and, 84–
    86
  muscarinic ACh receptors and,
    85–87

Labeling, of GTP-binding regulatory
  protein, of rat brain adenylate
  cyclase, by cholera toxin-
  catalyzed ADP-ribosylation,
  281–291
Lateral habenula-feedback pathway,
  SN and, 97–99
Lesions, effects of, on stereospecific
  binding, 149–153, 157, 159
Localization
  neuroanatomical, of DA receptors
    in CNS, 132–133

Localization (contd.)
of recognition binding subunit of $D_1$ DA receptor, 135–143
Long-term desensitization, changes in muscarinic and α-adrenergic systems during, 32–35

mAChR, see Muscarinic acetylcholine receptors
Membrane fraction, of rat brain, properties of benzodiapine receptor binding to, 223–224
Mesolimbic dopamine nerve terminals, TRH and, 187–189
2-methoxy-benzamide derivatives, inhibitory effect of on apomorphine-induced stereotypy in rats, 177–179
on [$^3$H]dopamine binding to $D_1$ and $D_2$, 175–177
Modulating mechanism, endogenous, of cerebral benzodiazepine receptor, 221–230
Molecular nature, regulation of, by muscarinic acetylcholine receptors, 35–40
Morphological study on neurotransmitter receptors, in rat brain, 245–257
Multiple affinity states, of $α_2$-adrenergic receptor, 53–70
Multiple $^3$H-serotonin binding sites
discrimination of, by tryptamine analogues, 106,108–110
pharmacological and species differences of, 103–112
Muscarinic acetylcholine receptor(s) (mAChR), see also Muscarinic receptor(s)
decrease of, drugs and, 32–34
guanine nucleotide and, 35–40
6-OHDOPA, isoproterenol, DMI and, 85–87
radiation inactivation of, 36–39
in smooth muscles, 31–40
Muscarinic cholinergic receptors, presynaptic, in splenic tissue, 43–50
Muscarinic receptor(s), see also Muscarinic acetylcholine receptor(s)
heterogenity of, 15–27
regulation of, 15–27
guanine nucleotide, 17–22
in smooth muscle, 31–40
Muscarinic receptor binding, ionic effects on, 25–26
Muscarinic systems, changes in, during long-term desensitization, 32–35
Muscles, smooth, muscarinic acetylcholine receptors in, 31–40

NE, see Norepinephrine
Nerve terminals, DA
mesolimbic, TRH and, 187–189
nigrostriatal, TRH and, 190
Neuroanatomical localization, of DA receptors, in CNS, 132–133
Neuroblastoma × glioma (NG 108-15) cells
$α_2$-adrenergic receptors in, 63–67
opiate receptors of, sulfhydryl groups and, 259–267
Neuroleptics, comparison of, in antagonism of apomorphine-induced behaviors, 167–171
Neuronal receptors, for serotonin, 116–118
Neurotransmitter receptors, morphological study on, in rat brain, 245–257
Nigrostriatal dopamine nerve terminals, TRH and, 190
Noradrenaline, cardiac receptors and, 83–89

Norepinephrine (NE) concentration, splenic, reduction of, following 6-OHDA, 46–47

6-OHDA, see 6-hydroxydopamine
6-OHDOPA, see 6-hydroxydopa
Opiate receptors, of NG 108-15, sulfhydryl groups and, 259–267

Pharmacological characterization of dopamine receptors, 125
Pharmacological differences of $^3$H-serotonin binding sites, 103–112
Pharmacological properties of DA receptor mediating inhibition of VIP-sensitive adenylate cyclase, 201,203–205
Pharmacology, of D-2 and D-4 binding sites, 166–168
Phenoxybenzamine-selective alkylation, of [$^3$H]BUTY binding sites, 130–131
Phospholipase C and phospholipase A$_2$, [$^3$H]flunitrazepam binding induced by, 228–229
Phospholipids, modulation of benzodiazepine receptor binding by, 226–228
Pituitary
 anterior, rat, inhibition of VIP-sensitive adenylate cyclase by DA in, 199–206
 dopamine receptors in, radioligand binding to, 126–127
Platelets, $\alpha_2$-adrenergic receptors in, 55–64
Postsynaptic β-adrenergic receptors, in splenic tissue, 43–50
Postsynaptic serotonin receptor
 regulation mechanism of, 118–120
 tricyclic antidepressants and, 120–121

Presynaptic muscarinic cholinergic receptors, in splenic tissue, 43–50
[$^3$H]propyl β-carboline-3-carboxylate, binding of, with benzodiazepine receptors, 211–214
Protein
 cholinergic receptor, identification and isolation of, 10–11
 curare binding, identification and isolation of, 11–13
 GTP-binding regulatory, of rat brain adenylate cyclase, labeling of, 281–291
Proteolytic enzymes, effects of, on stereospecific binding, 153–161

Radiation inactivation, of mAChR, 36–39
Radioligand binding, to dopamine receptors in pituitary, 126–127
Rat brain
 β-adrenergic receptor subtypes in, 73–80
 membrane fraction of, properties of benzodiazepine receptor binding to, 223–224
 morphological study on neurotransmitter receptors in, 245–257
Rat brain adenylate cyclase, labeling of GTP-binding regulatory protein of, 281–291
Rats, apomorphine-induced stereotypy in, inhibitory effects of 2-methoxy-benzamide derivatives on, 177–179
Receptor(s)
 $\alpha_2$-adrenergic, multiple affinity states and regulation of, 53–70
 β-adrenergic
  6-OHDOPA, in isoproterenol, DMI and, 84–86

Receptor(s) (contd.)
   postsynaptic, in splenic tissue, 43–50
   subtypes of, in rat brain, 73–80
  benzodiazepine, 209–218
   cerebral, endogenous modulating mechanism of, 221–230
  dopamine, see Dopamine receptor(s)
  glial, for 5-HT, 116–118
  glycine, in human brain, 233–237
  inversely coupled to adenylate cyclase, $\alpha_2$-adrenergic receptor as, 53–70
  muscarinic, see Muscarinic receptor
  muscarinic acetylcholine, see Muscarinic acetylcholine receptor
  neuronal, for serotonin, 116–118
  neurotransmitter, in rat brain, morphological study on, 245–257
  opiate, of NG 108–15, sulfhydryl groups and, 259–267
  postsynaptic $\beta$-adrenergic, in splenic tissue, 43–50
  presynaptic muscarinic cholinergic, in splenic tissue, 43–50
  serotonin
   central, regulation mechanism of, 115–121
   neuronal, 116–118
   postsynaptic
    regulation mechanism of, 118–120
    tricyclic antidepressants and, 120–121
  splenic autonomic, 43–50
Receptor binding, with cryostat sections, 246–249
Receptor binding sites, see Binding sites
Receptor protein, cholinergic, identification and isolation of, 10–11
Reciprocal alterations, of splenic $\beta$-adrenergic and muscarinic cholinergic receptors, following chemical sympathectomy with 6-OHDA, 45–47
Recognition binding subunit, of $D_1$ DA receptor, identification and localization of, 135–143
Regulation
  of $\alpha_2$-adrenergic receptor, 53–70
  of antagonist binding, by dopaminergic agonists, 24–25
  of $\beta_1$- or $\beta_2$-receptor density
   in rat caudate, 76, 79–80
   in rat cerebellum, 75–79
   in rat cerebral cortex, 74–76
  of central serotonin receptors, 115–121
  by muscarinic acetylcholine receptors
   of contraction, 31–35
   of molecular nature, 35–40
  of muscarinic receptor, 15–27
   guanine nucleotide, 17–22
  of postsynaptic 5-HT receptor, 118–120
Regulatory protein, GTP-binding, of rat brain adenylate cyclase, labeling of, 281–291

$^3$H-Serotonin (5-HT) binding, in cat, spiperone inhibition of, 105–108
$^3$H-serotonin binding sites
  multiple discrimination of, by tryptamine analogues, 106, 108–110
  pharmacological and species differences of, 103–112

Serotonin receptors, central, regulation mechanism of, 115–121
Smooth muscles, muscarinic acetylcholine receptors in, 31–40
SN, see Substantia nigra
Solubilized fraction, properties of benzodiazepine receptor in, 224–226
Species differences, of $^3$H-serotonin binding sites, 103–112
Specific binding, of cysteine sulfinic acid, to synaptic membrane fractions, 239–243
Specific inactivation, by trypsin, of effect of guanine nucleotide, 39–40
Spiperone, inhibition of $^3$H-5-HT binding by, in cat, 105–108
Splenic autonomic receptors, 43–50
Splenic norepinephrine concentration, reduction of, following 6-OHDA, 46–47
Splenic tissue, presynaptic muscarinic cholinergic and postsynaptic β-adrenergic receptors in, 43–50
Stereospecific binding
 effects of lesions on, 149–153,157,159
 effects of proteolytic enzymes on, 153–161
Stereotypy, apomorphine-induced, in rats, inhibitory effects of 2-methoxy-benzamine derivatives on, 177–179
Striatum, dopamine receptors in, 127–130
Structure affinity analysis, 269–277
$^3$H-strychnine binding, characterization of, 233–237

Substance P, in substantia nigra, 96–97
Substantia nigra (SN), human, glycine receptors in, 233–237
Subunit, recognition binding, of $D_1$ DA receptor, identification and localization of, 135–143
Subunit composition, of unitary DA receptor, 147–161
Sulfhydryl groups, opiate receptors of NG 108–115 and, 259–267
Sympathectomy, chemical, with 6-OHDA, reciprocal alterations of splenic β-adrenergic and muscarinic receptors following, 45–47
Synaptic membrane fractions, specific binding of cysteine sulfinic acid to, 239–243

Terminals, DA nerve
 mesolimbic, TRH and, 187–189
 nigrostriatal, TRH and, 190
Thyrotropin-releasing hormone (TRH)
 mesolimbic DA nerve terminals and, 187–189
 modification of dopaminergic transmission by, 185–196
 nigrostriatal DA nerve terminals and, 190
Tricyclic antidepressants, postsynaptic 5-HT receptor and, 120–121
Trypsin, specific inactivation of effect of guanine nucleotide by, 39–40
Tryptamine analogues, discrimination of multiple $^3$H-5-HT binding sites by, 106,108–110
Two distinct classes of dopamine receptor, mediating actions of antipsychotics, 163–171

Unitary dopamine receptor, subunit composition of, 147–161

Vasoactive intestinal peptide (VIP)-sensitive adenylate cyclase, inhibition of, by DA, in rat anterior pituitary, 199–206